Fish Disease & Health Management

Fish Disease & Health Management

Editor

Neelima Watve

scitus
academics

Fish Disease & Health Management

Edited by **Neelima Watve**

ISBN: 978-1-68117-062-6

Library of Congress Control Number: 2015935460

SCITUS Academics LLC,
www.scitusacademics.com
Box No. 4766, 616 Corporate Way,
Suite 2, Valley Cottage,
NY 10989

Printed in United States of America on Acid Free Paper ♾

Contents

Preface

Like humans and other animals, fish suffer from diseases and parasites. Fish defenses against disease are specific and non-specific. Non-specific defenses include skin and scales, as well as the mucus layer secreted by the epidermis that traps microorganisms and inhibits their growth. If pathogens breach these defenses, fish can develop inflammatory responses that increase the flow of blood to infected areas and deliver white blood cells that attempt to destroy the pathogens. Specific defenses are specialized responses to particular pathogens recognized by the fish's body, that is adaptative immune responses. In recent years, vaccines have become widely used in aquaculture and ornamental fish, for example vaccines for furunculosis in farmed salmon and koi herpes virus in koi. Fish health management is a term used in aquaculture to describe management practices which are designed to prevent fish disease. Once fish get sick it can be difficult to salvage them. Successful fish health management begins with prevention of disease rather than treatment. Prevention of fish disease is accomplished through good water quality management, nutrition, and sanitation. Without this foundation it is impossible to prevent outbreaks of opportunistic diseases. The fish is constantly bathed in potential pathogens, including bacteria, fungi, and parasites. Daily observation of fish behavior and feeding activity allows early detection of problems when they do occur so that a diagnosis can be made before the majority of the population becomes sick. If treatment is indicated, it will be most successful if it is implemented early in the course of the disease while the fish are still in good shape.

Editor

Chapter 1

Comparative Pathogenomics of Bacteria Causing Infectious Diseases in Fish

Ponnerassery S. Sudheesh, Aliya Al-Ghabshi, Nashwa Al-Mazrooei, and Saoud Al-Habsi

Microbiology Laboratory, Fishery Quality Control Center, Ministry of Agriculture and Fisheries Wealth, 100 Muscat, Oman

ABSTRACT

Fish living in the wild as well as reared in the aquaculture facilities are susceptible to infectious diseases caused by a phylogenetically diverse collection of bacterial pathogens. Control and treatment options using vaccines and drugs are either inadequate, inefficient, or impracticable. The classical approach in studying fish bacterial pathogens has been looking at individual or few virulence factors. Recently, genome sequencing of a number of bacterial fish pathogens has tremendously increased our understanding of the biology, host adaptation, and virulence factors of these important pathogens. This paper attempts to compile the scattered literature on genome sequence information of fish pathogenic bacteria published and available to date. The genome sequencing has uncovered several complex adaptive evolutionary strategies mediated by horizontal gene transfer, insertion sequence elements, mutations and prophage sequences operating in fish pathogens, and how their genomes evolved from generalist environmental strains to highly virulent obligatory pathogens. In addition, the comparative genomics has allowed the identification of unique pathogen-specific gene clusters. The paper focuses on the comparative analysis of the virulogenomes of important fish bacterial pathogens, and the genes involved in their evolutionary adaptation to different ecological niches. The paper also proposes some new directions on finding novel vaccine and chemotherapeutic targets in the genomes of bacterial pathogens of fish.

INTRODUCTION

Genome sequencing has provided us with powerful insights into the genetic makeup of the microbial world. The microbial genomics today has progressed from the long drawnout individual genome sequencing projects in the past to a level of technological advancement, where sequencing and comparing the genomes of several strains of a single pathogen is accomplished in a very short period of time [1, 2]. We are currently passing through a period of explosive developments in the field and an overwhelming glut in the genome sequence data of microorganisms. To date, over 1800 microbial genomes have been published and the sequencing of more than 5200 microbial genome are in different stages of completion (http://www.ncbi.nlm.nih.gov/genomes/lproks.cgi).

The genomics information has categorically disproved the earlier thinking that microbial genomes are static and has demonstrated that genomic evolutionary processes are much more flexible and dynamic than previously thought. This has led to the emergence of new ideas such as "uprooting the tree of life" and the concept of "horizontal genomics" [3–8]. This new thinking about microbial genome evolution has emerged from the observations of lineage-specific genome reduction and horizontal gene transfer (HGT), frequently occurring in bacterial genomes. Increasingly, genome sequencing projects have identified an unexpected level of diversity among bacteria, which can often be linked to recombination and gene transfer between a variety of prokaryotic organisms.

There is large variation in size and content of bacterial genomes between different genera and species, and also among strains of the same species. Known genome sizes of bacteria range from under 0.6 to 10 megabases (Mb). The smallest bacterial genomes reported are for the mycoplasmas and related bacteria, with sizes as low as 530 kilobases [9]. It has been emphasized that the adaptive capability ("versatility") of bacteria directly correlates with genome size [10].

Genome sequencing of bacterial pathogens has produced exciting information on evolutionary relationships between pathogenic and nonpathogenic species and has demonstrated how each has developed special adaptations advantageous for each of their unique infectious lifestyles. In the longer term, an understanding of their genome and biology will enable scientists to design means of disrupting their infectious lifestyles.

The genomes of bacteria are made up of circular or linear chromosomes, extrachromosomal linear or circular plasmids as well as different combinations of these molecules. The functionally related genes are clustered together in very close proximity to each other, and those genes located on the "core" part of the chromosome present a relatively uniform G+C content and a specific codon usage. Closely related bacteria generally have very similar genomes [11].

The stability and integrity of the "core" sequences of the genome, however, is often interrupted by the presence of DNA fragments with a G+C content and a codon usage markedly different from those of the "core" genome. The "flexible" gene pool or the so-called "mobilome" [12], is created by the acquisition of strain-specific "assortments" of genetic information mainly represented by mobile genetic elements (MGE), such as plasmids, bacteriophages, genomic/pathogenicity islands (GEIs/PAIs), integrons, IS elements (ISEs), and transposons (see Figure 1). The flexible genes scattered in the genome provide the microbes with an additional repertoire of arsenal, for example, resistance to antibiotics, production of toxic compounds as well as other virulence factors [13].

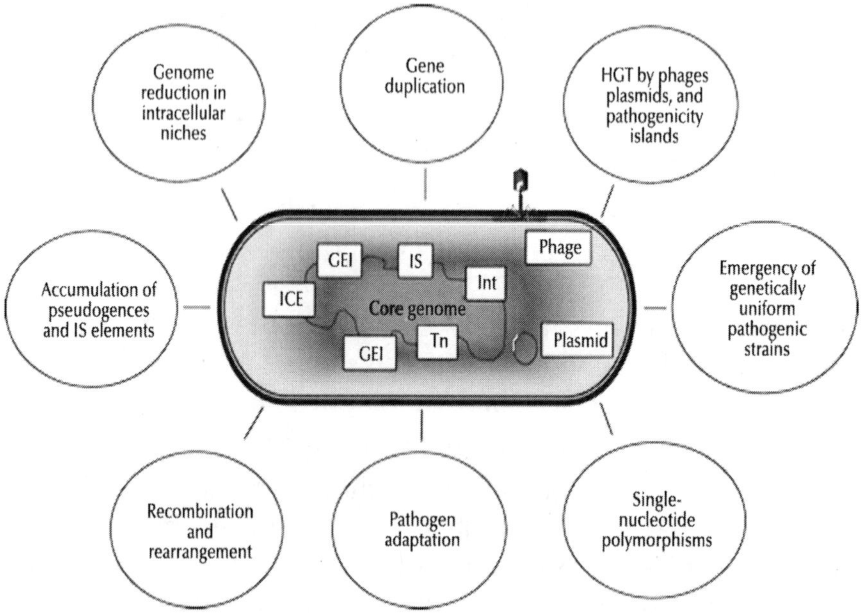

Figure 1: Major factors responsible for the pathogenomic evolution of bacteria (modified from [14, 15]; HGT: horizontal gene transfer, GEIs: genomic islands, ICEs: integrative conjugative elements, Int: integrons, Tn: conjugative transposons, IS: IS elements.

A fundamental question in biology is to define the minimum number of genes or functions to support cellular life. The size of bacterial genomes is primarily the result of two counteracting processes: the acquisition of new genes by gene duplication or by horizontal gene transfer; the deletion of nonessential genes. Genomic flux created by these gains and losses of genetic information can substantially alter gene content. This process drives divergence of bacterial species and eventually adaptation to new ecological niches [16].

Bacterial pathogens are a major cause of infectious diseases and mortality in wild fish stocks and fish reared in confined conditions. Disease problems constitute the largest single cause of economic losses in aquaculture [17]. Concurrent with the rapid growth and intensification of aquaculture, increased use of water bodies, pollution, globalization, and transboundary movement of aquatic fauna, the list of new pathogenic bacterial species isolated from fish has been steadily increasing [18]. In addition, the virulence and host range of existing pathogens has also been increasing, posing considerable challenge to fish health researchers, who are actively looking for more efficient vaccines and therapeutic drugs to combat bacterial fish diseases. The current treatment methods are ineffective and have many practical difficulties.

At the level of host-pathogen interaction, there is considerable pressure on pathogens to adapt to the harsh host environment as well as to adapt and evolve along with the ever changing external environment. The interplay between the host and the pathogen is a complex one, each driven by the need to secure the success of the species. Adaptations by one partner to exploit new environments will often stimulate the other to modify its characteristics to take advantage of the change. As a consequence of this cycle of interaction created by changing environments, new strains of pathogen will evolve. Over time, these strains may emerge as new species with characteristic disease symptoms.

The use of antibiotics to control fish diseases has met with limited success and has the potential danger of antibiotic resistance development in aquatic bacteria (World Health Organization antimicrobial resistance fact sheet 194, http://www.who.int/inf-fs/en/fact194.html) [19]. As aquaculture is one of the fastest growing food production industries in the world, demand for sustainable ways of combating fish diseases is gaining significance. There is tremendous scope for developing novel vaccines and therapeutic drugs against bacterial fish pathogens.

Genomic evolution and adaptive strategies of bacterial fish pathogens are poorly understood and lags far behind that of human and terrestrial animal pathogens. A detailed knowledge of the genome sequences of bacterial fish pathogens and how the genomes of the pathogenic species or strains evolved from nonpathogenic ancestors or counterparts will help us better understand their pathogenicity mechanisms and strategies of host adaptations. This information will help identifying novel vaccine and drug targets in the genomes of pathogens.

Recently, genome sequencing of a number of bacteria pathogenic to fish and other aquatic organisms have been completed. The genome sequence and genome characteristics of important bacterial fish pathogens completed and published to date are summarized in Table 1.

Table 1: Currently sequenced genomes of bacterial pathogens of fish

Organisms	Size (Mb)	CDS**	Unknown/ Hypothetical genes (%)	Pseudogenes prophages, ISE/GEI	% GC	Chromosomes	Plasmids
Vibrio anguillarum 775 serotype O1	4.117	3880	26	92	44.3	2	1
Vibrio anguillarum 96F serotype O1	4.065	3766	26	38	42	2	0
Vibrio anguillarum RV22 serotype O2β	4.022	3949	26	68	43.1	2	0
Vibrio ordalii ATCC 33509	3.415	3281	—	31	43.3	2	0
Vibrio harveyi ATCC BAA-1116*	6.054	—	—	—	45.4	2	1
Vibrio vulnificus YJ016 biotype 1	5.26	5028	34	—	46.1	2	1
Vibrio splendidus strain LGP32	4.974	4498	24.8	—	43.8	2	0
Aliivibrio salmonicida strain LFI1238	4.655	4286	—	1179	38.3	2	4
Flavobacterium psychrophilumJIP02/86	2.862	2432	45.3	94	32.5	1	1
Flavobacterium branchiophilumFL-15	3.56	2867	—	54	32.9	1	—
Flavobacterium columnareATCC 49512*	3.2	2896	—	—	32.0	1	—
Edwardsiella tarda EIB202	3.76	3486	28	97	59.7	1	1
Edwardsiella ictaluri 93–146*	3.812	3783	—	100	57.4	1	—
Aeromonas hydrophila ATCC 7966	4.744	5195	27.7	7	61.5	1	0
Aeromonas salmonicida A449	4.702	4437	—	258	58.5	1	5
Aeromonas veronii Strain B565	4.551	4057	—	—	58.7	1	—
A. caviae Ae398	4.43	—	—	6	61.4	1	1

Renibacterium salmoninarumATCC 33209	3.155	3507	25.3	151	56.3	1	0
Streptococcus parauberis	2.143	2641	21.3	—	35.6	1	0
Lactococcus garvieae UNIUD074	2.172	2101	21.8	224	38.7	1	0
Mycobacterium marinum M	6.636	5424	26	65	62.5	1	1

* Unpublished.

** Coding sequences.

The main aim of this paper is to put together and summarize the scattered genome sequencing information on important bacterial fish pathogens available in the literature to date. We sincerely believe that this paper will provide a genomic perspective on the adaptive evolutionary strategies of bacterial fish pathogens in different ecological niches and will help better understand the virulence mechanisms and pathogenesis of infections. It is hoped that this will lead to finding the most appropriate vaccine and therapeutic drug targets in the genomes and developing efficient control and treatment methods for fish diseases.

BACTERIAL PATHOGENS OF FISH

Although pathogenic species representing majority of existing bacterial taxa have been implicated in fish diseases, only a relatively small number of pathogens are responsible for important economic losses in cultured fish worldwide. Major bacterial pathogens responsible for infectious disease outbreaks in different species of fish are listed in Table 2. Major groups of bacteria causing infectious diseases in fish and the important genome characteristics of these bacteria are described in the following sections.

Table 2: Major bacterial pathogens of economically important fish

Causative agent/species	**Disease**	**Main host fish**
Gram-negatives		
Vibrio anguillarum	Vibriosis	Salmonids, turbot, sea bass, striped bass, eel, ayu, cod, and red sea bream
Aliivibrio salmonicida (formerly Vibrio salmonicida)	Vibriosis	Atlantic salmon, cod
Vibrio vulnificus	Vibriosis	Eels, tilapia
Vibrio ordalii	Vibriosis	Salmonids
Vibrio carchariae (syn.: Vibrio harveyi)	Vibriosis, infectious gastroenteritis	Shark, abalone, red drum, sea bream, sea bass, cobia, and flounder
Moritella viscosa (formerly Vibrio viscosus)	Winter ulcer	Atlantic salmon

Photobacterium damselae subsp. piscicida (formerly Pasteurella piscicida)	Photobacteriosis (pasteurellosis)	Sea bream, sea bass, sole, striped bass, and yellowtail
Pasteurella skyensis	Pasteurellosis	Salmonids and turbot
Tenacibaculum maritimum (formerly Flexibacter maritimus)	Flexibacteriosis	Turbot, salmonids, sole, sea bass, gilthead sea bream, red sea bream, and flounder
Flavobacterium psychrophilum	Coldwater disease	Salmonids, carp, eel, tench, perch, ayu
Flavobacterium branchiophila	Bacterial gill disease	A broad range of cultured cold water and warm water salmonid and nonsalmonid fishes
Flavobacterium columnare	Columnaris disease	cyprinids, salmonids, silurids, eel, and sturgeon
Pseudomonas anguilliseptica	Pseudomonadiasis, winter disease	Sea bream, eel, turbot, and ayu
Aeromonas salmonicida	Furunculosis	salmon, trout, goldfish, koi and a variety of other fish species
Aeromonas hydrophila Aeromonas veronii Biovar Sobria Aeromonas sobria Biovar Sobria (Motile aeromonads)	Motile aeromonas septicemia (MAS), hemorrhagic septicemia, ulcer disease or red-sore disease, and epizootic ulcerative syndrome (EUS)	A wide variety of salmonid and nonsalmonid fish, sturgeon, tilapia, catfish, striped bass, and eel
Edwardsiella ictaluri	Enteric septicemia	Catfish and tilapia
Edwardsiella tarda	Edwardsiellosis	Salmon, carps, tilapia, catfish, striped bass, flounder, and yellowtail
Yersinia ruckeri	Enteric redmouth	Salmonids, eel, minnows, sturgeon, and crustaceans
Piscirickettsia salmonis	Piscirickettsiosis	Salmonids
Gram-positives		
Lactococcus garvieae (formerly Enterococcus seriolicida)	Streptococcosis or lactococcosis	Yellowtail and eel
Streptococcus iniae	Streptococcosis	Yellowtail, flounder, sea bass, and barramundi
Streptococcus parauberis	Streptococcosis	Turbot
Streptococcus phocae	Streptococcosis	Atlantic salmon
Renibacterium salmoninarum	Bacterial kidney disease	Salmonids
Mycobacterium marinum	Mycobacteriosis	Sea bass, turbot, and Atlantic salmon

VIBRIOS

Bacteria in the genus Vibrio are mainly pathogenic to marine and brackish water fish. However, they are occasionally reported in freshwater species as well [20, 21]. The distribution of vibriosis is worldwide and causes great economic loss to the aquaculture industry [22]. Vibriosis, one of the major bacterial diseases affecting fish, bivalves, and crustaceans, is mainly caused by pathogenic species such as Vibrio anguillarum, V. harveyii (Syn. V. carchariae), V. ordalii, and Aliivibrio salmonicida (formerly Vibrio salmonicida) [23, 24].

Other species such as V. vulnificus [25, 26] and Moritella viscosa (formerly Vibrio viscosus) [27] have been implicated in fish diseases such as septicemia and winter ulcer, respectively; more pathogenic species have been isolated frequently and reported in the literature [28].

Genome sequences of four major fish pathogenic vibrios, V. anguillarum, V. ordalii, Aliivibrio salmonicida, and V.vulnificus have been completed and published [29–31]. Generally, they have two chromosomes, one larger and one smaller. The majority of genes that encode cell functions and pathogenic factors are located in the large one. The small chromosome usually contains genes for environmental adaptation.

Vibrio anguillarum is the most studied aetiological agent of vibriosis [32]. V. anguillarum typically causes a hemorrhagic septicemia. The O1 and O2 serotypes are the virulent strains frequently isolated from diseased fish [33, 34]. Many O1 serotype strains harbor 65 kb pJM1-type plasmids, which carry the siderophore anguibactin biosynthesis and transport genes, a main virulence factor of V. anguillarum, while one of the O1 serotype strains and other serotypes, such as all of the O2 strains, are plasmidless [28, 35, 36]. The O1 serotype strains cause disease in salmonid fish, whereas O2 β strains are usually isolated from cod and other nonsalmonids [28, 32].

Vibrio ordalii is a very close relative of V. anguillarum [37] and was previously recognized as V. anguillarumbiotype 2. Vibriosis caused by these two species are strikingly different based on histological evidences [38]. V. anguillarum has a special affinity for blood and loose connective tissue, whereas V. ordali is mostly present as aggregates in skeletal and cardiac muscles. V. ordalii has a lesser affinity for blood and develops bacteremia only at late stages of disease.

Genomic sequences of three different strains of V. anguillarum (the strain 775 containing plasmid pJM1, serotype O1 strain 96F, and plasmidless serotype O2 β strain RV22) and V. ordali have recently been published [31]. The pJM1 plasmid in the strain 775 contains 65 genes including the anguibactin biosynthesis and transport genes that are unique for the strain.

V. anguillarum 775 contains more transposase genes (about 53) than 96F (about 23), RV22 (about 42), and V. ordalii (about 18).

The genome comparison of V. anguillarum serotypes has revealed some interesting differences in the genomic composition, indicating horizontal acquisition of virulence genes and the evolution of different potential virulence mechanisms among the closely related serotypes [31]. The V. anguillarum 96F strain has a type III secretion system 2 (T3SS2) cluster, which is absent in the 775 strain. The T3SS2 genes are highly conserved with other T3SS2 genes reported in V. parahaemolyticus, V. cholera, and V. mimicus [39–41]. In the 775 strain, three transposase genes are present at the T3SS2 chromosomal location, one of which probably originated from the pJM1, indicating that the gene cluster is inactivated by a transposition, deletion, or inversion event [31]. The 775 strain also contains 10 genomic islands including integrase, transposase, and some novel sequences conferring genomic plasticity to adapt to specific ecological niches.

The strain RV22 genome contains the toxin-antitoxin systems, and genes encoding the accessory V. choleraeenterotoxin (Ace) and the Zonula occludens toxin (Zot), which is not present in the 775 strain. The yersiniabactin-like siderophore cluster, which is highly conserved in many Vibrio species and Photobacterium damselae subspecies piscicida [42], is present in strain RV22 and V. ordalii.

A striking feature of V. ordali genome is its significant reduction in size (3.4 Mb) compared to the V. anguillarum strains 775 (4.1 Mb), 96F (4.0 Mb), and RV22 (4.0 Mb). V. ordali lacks the ABC transporter genes, the type VI secretion systems, and the gene for microbial collagenase. The Syp biofilm formation cluster, which is conserved in many Vibrio species such as V. fischeri, V. vulnificus, and V. parahaemolyticus [43, 44], is present only in V. ordalii. Thus, it is probable that the transition of

V. anguillarum to V. ordalii is mediated by genome reductive evolution to become an endosymbiotic organism; V. ordali has the smallest genome of all vibrios.

Vibrio vulnificus includes three distinct biotypes. Biotype 1 strains cause human disease, while biotype 2 infects primarily eels, and biotype 3 infections has been associated with persons handling Tilapia, although the source and reservoir of biotype 3 have yet to be identified [45]. In another classification the terms clade 1 and clade 2 are used based on the multilocus sequence typing (MLST) [46]. Biotype 1 strains are present in both clades, whereas biotype 2 strains are present only in clade 1, and biotype 3 strains appear to be a hybrid between clades 1 and 2. Clade 1 strains are most often isolated from environmental samples, while clade 2 strains are mostly associated with human disease and are considered more virulent. Recent comparative genomic analysis of these biotypes or clades has clearly differentiated them based on the possession of an array of clade-specific unique genes including the presence of a virulence-associated genomic island XII in the highly virulent strains [30].

Aliivibrio salmonicida (formerly Vibrio salmonicida) causes coldwater vibriosis in marine fish such as farmed Atlantic salmon (Salmo salar), sea-farmed rainbow trout (Oncorhynchus mykiss), and captive Atlantic cod (Gadus morhua) [47]. The Gram-negative bacterium causes tissue degradation, hemolysis, and sepsis in vivo. Genome sequencing of Aliivibrio salmonicida has revealed a mosaic structure of the genome caused by large intrachromosomal rearrangements, gene acquisition, deletion, and duplication of DNA within the chromosomes and between the chromosomes and the plasmids [29].

The genome has many genes that appear to be recently acquired by HGT, and large sections of over 300 coding sequences (CDS) are disrupted by IS elements or contain point mutations causing frame shifts or premature stop codons [29]. The genomic islands (GIs) identified in the bacteria include major virulence-related genes encoding T6SS and Flp-type pilus and genes that appear to provide new functions to the bacteria. The Tad system has been proposed to represent a new subtype of T2SS and is essential for biofilm formation, colonization, and pathogenesis [48].

The genome analysis has unequivocally confirmed that Aliivibrio salmonicida has undergone extensive rearrangement of its genome by losing massive functional genes and acquiring new genes and become host-restricted, allowing the pathogen to adapt to new niches. IS expansion has been related to genome reduction in the evolution and emergence of pathogenicity [49], and accumulation of pseudogenes has been described for several other host restricted pathogens [50, 51].

AEROMONADS

Aeromonas hydrophila and other motile aeromonads are among the most common bacteria in a variety of aquatic environments worldwide, including bottled water, chlorinated water, well water, sewage, and heavily polluted waters, and are frequently associated with severe disease among cultured and feral fishes, amphibians, reptiles, and birds [52]. Aeromonads are also considered serious emerging pathogens of human beings [53]. Determination of the etiology of diseases involving aeromonad infections has been complicated by the genetic, biochemical, and antigenic heterogeneity of members of this group.

The genus Aeromonas has been conveniently divided into a group of nonmotile, psychrophilic species, prominently represented by Aeromonas salmonicida, which is an obligate fish pathogen and a second group of mostly human pathogenic, motile, and mesophilic species including A. hydrophila.

Genome sequencing of A. hydrophila ATCC 7966^T, A. salmonicida subsp. salmonicida A449, A. veronii strain B565, and A. caviae [54–57] has helped in resolving their taxonomic confusion and has brought new insights into the way these bacteria adapt to a myriad of ecological niches, their host adaptive evolution and virulence mechanisms.

Aeromonas salmonicida, the causative agent of furunculosis in salmonid and nonsalmonid fish, is a non-motile, Gram-negative bacterium; furunculosis is an important disease in wild and cultured stocks of fish inflicting heavy losses to aquaculture industry worldwide [58, 59]. A. hydrophila causes a septicemic disease in fish known variously as "motile aeromonas septicemia" (MAS), "hemorrhagic septicemia," "ulcer disease," or "red-sore disease" [60]. The disease caused by this bacterium primarily affects freshwater fish such as catfish, several species of bass, and many species of tropical or ornamental fish. A. veronii is the causative agent of bacterial hemorrhagic septicemia in fish and is becoming a major economic problem in the fish-farming industry [23].

Genome sequencing of the fish pathogen A. salmonicida A449 has confirmed the presence of fully functional genes for a type III secretion system (T3SS) that has been shown to be required for virulence in A. salmonicida[61], and genes for a typeVI secretion system (T6SS), which is disrupted by an IS element [55]. The ancestral state of the T3SS in A. salmonicida A449 is ambiguous because of the absence of the genes in A. hydrophilaATCC 7966^T, while other A. hydrophila strains carry T3SS operons on the chromosome [62]. The genome contains a multitude of virulence-related genes including several types of adhesins (e.g., surface layer, flagella, and pili), toxin genes (aerolysin, hemolysin, repeats in toxin (RTX) protein, and cytolytic delta-endotoxin), secreted enzymes (protease, phospholipase, nuclease, amylase, pullulanase, and chitinase), antibiotic resistance genes (tetA, β-lactamase gene, and efflux pumps), and genes involved in iron acquisition and quorum sensing.

Most of the above genes are present in A. hydrophila ATCC 7966^T genome and an expansion of gene families (paralogs) of ABC transporters, two-component signal transduction systems (TCSs), transcriptional regulators, FeS cluster-binding proteins involved in energy transduction at the membrane, and methyl-accepting chemotaxis proteins (MCPs). Interestingly, transposase, resolvase, or insertion sequence element sequences were not discovered in the A. hydrophila ATCC 7966^T genome, whereas these have been identified in A. salmonicida and A. caviae genomes. A. salmonicida possesses 88 copies of 10 different IS elements whereas A. caviae Ae398 has only five different IS elements, and A. hydrophila completely lacks IS elements.

Although A. hydrophila ATCC 7966^T has been demonstrated to be the second most virulent species amongAeromonas [63], a very important virulence determinant, T3SS, which is present in A. salmonicida A449 is strikingly absent in A. hydrophila ATCC 7966^T genome. A. caviae contains many putative virulence genes, including those encoding a type 2 secretion system, an RTX toxin, and polar flagella.

The genome of A. veronii strain B565 contains some putative virulence factors, such as chitinase, RTX protein, adhesion factor, flagella, and mannose-sensitive hemagglutinin (MSHA), all of which are shared with A. hydrophila ATCC 7966^{T} and A. salmonicida A449. On the other hand, 346 genes including some important putative virulence factors such as hemolysins and the type III secretion protein, which are shared by the latter two species are absent in A. veronii strain B565.

Many unique genes in A. hydrophila ATCC 7966^{T} and A. salmonicida A449 are virulence genes and often form large clusters, such as the rtx cluster in ATCC 7966^{T} and the flagellar gene cluster in A449, or are involved in mobile elements such as phages and transposons, highlighting their lateral transfer history [56].

The A. hydrophila ATCC 7966^{T} and A. salmonicida A449 genomes appear to be very closely related, encoding similar number of proteins with only 9% difference in gene content. However, there are many transposons, phage-related genes, and unique CDS in A. salmonicida A449 genome that are different from A. hydrophilaATCC 7966^{T} sequences, showing their distinct lineages and adaptive evolution that occurred while segregating into different species of the genus.

In sharp contrast to A. hydrophila ATCC 7966^{T} genome, the A. salmonicida A449 genome is characterized by the presence of large numbers of several different types of IS elements in multiple copies, with more than 20 genes being interrupted by IS elements. A. hydrophila ATCC 7966^{T} genome has no IS elements.

There is a higher tendency for genomic reduction in A. salmonicida A449 with the formation of many pseudogenes, and A. hydrophila ATCC 7966^{T} has only seven pseudogenes. The formation of pseudogenes has resulted in the loss of function of many genes including flagella and type IV pili, transcriptional regulators, genes encoding carbohydrate synthesis, and modification enzymes and genes for basic metabolic pathways, which are some characteristic features of pathogenomic evolution.

Thus, A. salmonicida A449 appears to have evolved much faster than A. hydrophila ATCC 7966^{T} through genetic rearrangements, genomic reduction, and HGT from common ancestral lineages by acquiring and forming multiple plasmids, prophages, a battery of IS elements, pseudogenes, and several individual genes and operons.

FLAVOBACTERIUM

The genus Flavobacterium includes over 30 species of which Flavobacterium psychrophilum, F. branchiophilum, and F. columnare are important disease agents for salmonids, catfish, and other cultured species [64, 65]. Flavobacteria are significant as they are ubiquitous in the soil, freshwater, and marine environments and are noted for their novel gliding motility and ability to degrade polymeric organic matter such as hydrocarbons [66].

F. psychrophilum is the etiological agent of bacterial coldwater disease (BCWD). It is a serious fish pathogen causing substantial economic losses and rearing difficulties to both commercial and conservation aquaculture.F. psychrophilum infections are found throughout the world. Juvenile rainbow trout and coho salmon are particularly susceptible to BCWD. However, F. psychrophilum infections have been reported in a wide range of hosts, Anguilla japonica, A. anguilla, Cyprinus carpio, Carassius carassius, Tinca tinca, Plecoglossus altivelis,Perca fluviatilis, and Rutilus rutilus [64, 67]. Fry and fingerlings with BCWD often have skin ulcerations on the peduncle, anterior to the dorsal fin, at the anus, or on the lower jaw and mortalities can go up to 70% [68].

F. branchiophilum is the causative organism of bacterial gill disease (BGD) in several parts of the world [69]. This disease is characterized by explosive morbidity and mortality rates attributable to massive bacterial colonization of gill lamellar surfaces and progressive branchial pathology stemming from high rates of lamellar epithelial necrosis [70].

F. columnare (formerly Cytophaga columnaris; Flexibacter columnaris) is the causative agent of columnaris disease of salmonids and other fishes in commercial aquaculture, the ornamental fish industry, and wild fish populations worldwide [71]. Classically, during outbreaks, its morbidity and mortality rates escalate more gradually than for BGD. Additionally, unlike the pattern of necrosis in BGD, fish with columnaris will have severe necrosis of all parts of the gill as the bacterium invades inwardly [72].

The taxonomy of the three species was initially based on phenotypic characteristics and has been revised several times during the years. The latest classification based on G+C content, DNA-ribosomal ribonucleic acid (rRNA) hybridisation, and fatty acid and protein profiles, has confirmed that all the three species now belong to the phylum/division Cytophaga-Flavobacterium-Bacteroides, family Flavobacteriaceae, and genusFlavobacterium [73].

The whole genome sequences of F. psychrophilum and F. branchiophilum have been published [74, 75]. The F. columnare genome sequence is yet to be completed and published [76].

Prominent features of F. psychrophilum infection include the strong adhesion to fish epithelial tissues followed by gliding motility, rapid and mass tissue destruction, and severe muscle tissue ulcerations. Hence, the identification of multiple genes encoding secreted proteases, adhesins, and gliding motility (gld) genes in F. psychrophilum genome indicates their possible involvement in the virulence of the pathogen. However, the gene sequence of a secreted collagenase was disrupted by an insertion sequence of the IS256 family in several strains isolated from rainbow trout [74] indicating the clonal dissemination of strains containing the disrupted gene. The F. psychrophilum seems to have horizontally acquired virulence associated genes from other unrelated bacteria. It has a hemolysin similar to the toxin VAH5, which is a virulence factor in Vibrio anguillarum [77]. It also has a gene encoding a protein that is similar to domains 1–3 of thiol-activated cytolysin family of pore-forming toxins (TACYs), which has been implicated in the pathogenicity of several Gram-positive bacteria [78]. Interestingly, F. psychrophilum lacks the type III and IV secretion systems usually present in Gram-negative pathogens; but, it has genes encoding PorT and PorR proteins, which are involved in transport and anchoring of virulence factors of the bacteria [79, 80]. In addition, the F. psychrophilum genome contains a large repertoire of genes involved in aerobic respiration, psychrotolerance, and stress response.

The sequencing of F. branchiophilum genome has revealed the existence of virulence mechanisms distinctly different from the closest species, F. psychrophilum. The F. branchiophilum genome has the first cholera-like toxin in a nonproteobacteria and an array of adhesins. A comparative analysis of its genome with genomes of other Flavobacterium species revealed a smaller genome size, large differences in chromosome organization, and fewer rRNA and tRNA genes, fitting with its more fastidious growth. In addition, identification of certain virulence factors, genomic islands, and CRISPR (clustered regularly interspaced short palindromic repeats) systems points to the adaptive evolution of F. branchiophilum by horizontal acquisition of genes.

EDWARDSIELLA

The genus Edwardsiella belongs to subgroup 3 of γ-proteobacteria, encompassing a group of Gram-negative enteric bacteria pathogenic to a variety of animals [81]. Two very closely related species, Edwardsiella tardaand E. ictaluri are important fish pathogens. Both are Gram-negative motile rods that are cytochrome oxidase negative and ferment glucose with production of acid and gas. The two species can be differentiated biochemically in that E. tarda produces both indol and hydrogen sulfide, whereas E. ictaluri produces neither. Moreover, the two species do not cross-react serologically. E. tarda has been isolated from many warm water fishes and some coldwater fishes, whereas E. ictaluri has been isolated only from a few species of warm water fishes (Table 2). Additionally, E. tarda causes disease in such other animals as marine mammals, pigs, turtles, alligators, ostriches, skunks, and snakes [81]. It has also occasionally infected humans [82, 83]. In contrast, E. ictaluri is limited to fish, and survivors of epizootics probably become carriers. The geographic range of E. tarda is worldwide, whereas that of E. ictaluri is still confined to the catfish growing areas in the United States [84].

E. tarda causes a disease condition in fish called systemic hemorrhagic septicemia with swelling skin lesions as well as ulcer and necrosis in internal organs such as liver, kidney, spleen, and musculature [85]. It has the ability of invading and multiplying in epithelial cells and macrophages in order to subvert the host immune system and to survive in the fish [86].

E. ictaluri is the causative agent of enteric septicemia of catfish (ESC), a major disease affecting the catfish industry. The disease can manifest as an acute form that is characterized by hemorrhagic enteritis and septicemia and a chronic disease that is characterized by meningoencephalitis [87]. Gross external symptoms include hemorrhages on the body, especially around the mouth and fins. Other signs include pale gills, exophthalmia, and small ulcerations on the body [84].

The whole genome sequencing of the two species has recently been completed and published allowing comparative genomic analysis of these very important fish pathogens [88, 89]. The genome sequencing of the two closely related species E. tarda and E. ictaluri has revealed a high level of genomic plasticity with a high content of mobile genetic elements, IS elements, genomic islands, phage-like products, integrases, or recombinases. E. ictaluri displays high biochemical homogeneity with only one serotype, but possess many IS elements in the genome. In addition, highly variable G+C content and a large quantity of variable number of tandem repeats (VNTRs) or direct repeat sequences were identified in the E. tarda genome indicating the rapid genomic evolution undergoing in the species [88]. An interesting feature is the identification of insertion sequence IS Saen1 of Salmonella enterica serovar Enteritidis [90] in both E. tarda EIB202 and E. ictaluri 93–146 genomes. Conversely, the difference in genomic islands among the three species may partially explain their rapid evolutionary changes and diverging lineage from a common ancestor.

The E. tarda genome has a gene cluster sharing high similarities to the pvsABCDE-psuA-pvuA operon, which encodes the proteins for the synthesis and utilization of vibrioferrin, an unusual type of siderophore requiring nonribosomal peptide synthetase (NRPS) independent synthetases (NIS) and usually mediating the iron uptake systems in V. parahaemolyticus and V. alginolyticus [91, 92]. But E. ictaluri genome lacks siderophore biosynthesis genes, even though it possesses heme binding/transport genes.

E. tarda genome is smaller than that of E. ictaluri and other sequenced genomes of Enterobacteriaceae, justifying the hypothesis that E. tarda may not be present as a free living microorganism in natural waters but multiply intracellularly in protozoans and transmitted to fish, reptile, and other animals or humans [81].

The E. tarda and E. ictaluri genomes have a multitude of virulence factors including P pilus, type 1 fimbriae, nonfimbrial adhesins, invasins and hemagglutinins and various secretion pathways including sec-dependent transport system, the components of the main terminal branch of the general secretory pathway (GSP), the signal recognition particle (SRP), and the sec-independent twin arginine transport (Tat), T1SS, TTSS, and T6SS indicating their evolutionary fitness and ability to adapt to a variety of demanding ecological niches and harsh host intracellular environments.

YERSINIA RUCKERI

Yersinia ruckeri, the causal agent of enteric redmouth (ERM) disease, which is a systemic bacterial infection of fishes, but is principally known for its occurrence in rainbow trout, Salmo gairdneri [93]. Y. ruckeri was initially isolated from rainbow trout in the Hagerman Valley, Idaho, USA, in the 1950s [94] and is now widely found in fish populations throughout North America, Australia, South Africa, and Europe [95]. Outbreaks of ERM usually begin with low mortalities which slowly escalate and may result in high losses. The problem may become large-scaled if chronically infected fish are exposed to stressful conditions such as high stocking densities and poor water quality [96]. Y. ruckeri is a nonspore-forming bacterium which does not possess a capsule, but often has a flagellum [97].

Historically, Y. ruckeri is fairly homogenous in biochemical reactions. However, Y. ruckeri strains have recently been grouped into clonal types on the basis of biotype, serotype, and outer membrane protein (OMP) profiles [98]. Strains of serovars I and II [99], equivalent to serotypes O1a and O2b, respectively [100], cause most epizootic outbreaks in cultured salmonids, serovar I being predominant in rainbow trout [101]. Within serovar I, six clonal OMP types have been recognized, but only two are associated with major disease outbreaks: clonal group 5, which includes the so-called Hagerman strain and clonal group 2 [98, 102]. Clonal group 5 comprises the majority of isolates, all of them motile and with a widespread distribution (Europe, North America, and South Africa). Clonal group 2 includes only nonmotile strains isolated in the UK.

More recently, multilocus sequence typing has revealed distinct phylogenetic divergence of Y. ruckeri from the rest of the Yersinia genus raising doubts about its taxonomic position [103]. This view has gained credibility after the genome sequencing of Y. ruckeri, which has a substantially reduced total genome size (3.58 to 3.89 Mb), compared with the 4.6 to 4.8 Mb seen in the genus generally [104]. In addition, Y. ruckeri was found to be the most evolutionarily distant member of the genus with a number of features distinct from other members of the genus.

Several common Yersinia genes were missing in Y. ruckeri. These included genes involved in xylose utilization, urease activity, B12-

related metabolism, and the mtnKADCBEU gene cluster that comprises the majority of the methionine salvage pathway [104]. The genomic reduction achieved by losing these and other genes is suggestive of its means of adaptation to an obligatory life style in fish hosts.

RENIBACTERIUM SALMONINARUM

Renibacterium salmoninarum is a small Gram-positive diplobacillus, and the causative agent of bacterial kidney disease (BKD), which is a slowly progressive, systemic infection in salmonid fishes with a protracted course and an insidious nature [105]. The pathogen can be transmitted from fish to fish [106] or from adults to their progeny via eggs [107]. Infected fish may take months to show signs of disease. bacterial kidney disease is one of the most difficult bacterial diseases of fish to treat [108], mainly due to its ability to evade phagocytosis and invade and survive in host cells [109, 110]. R. salmoninarum is very slow growing, and it is extremely difficult to apply genetic manipulation techniques to study its gene functions.

R. salmoninarum, despite being an obligate intracellular pathogen of fish, is phylogenetically closest to the non-pathogenic environmental Arthrobacter species [51]. Based on 16S rRNA phylogenetic analysis, R. salmoninarum has been included in the actinomycetes subdivision and was found related to a subgroup harboring morphologically and chemotaxonomically rather heterogeneous taxa, including Arthrobacter, Micrococcus, Cellulomonas, Jonesia, Promicromonospora, Stomatococcus, and Brevibacterium [111]. In fact,Arthrobacter davidanieli is commercially used as a vaccine (commercially known as Renogen) and can provide significant cross-protection in Atlantic salmon, though not in Pacific salmon [112]. The genome sequencing ofR. salmoninarum ATCC 33209 strain and two Arthrobacter strains, the TC1 and FB24, has revealed many interesting aspects of how this obligates fish pathogen evolved, via genomic reduction and horizontal gene acquisition, from members of the nonpathogenic genus Arthrobacter [51, 113]. A total of 1562 ORF clusters were similar in R. salmoninarum and Arthrobacter spp. demonstrating the genetic basis for the efficiency and cross-protection of the A. davidanieli vaccine.

There is significant genome reduction in R. salmoninarum genome, which is 1.44 Mb smaller than the chromosome of TC1 and 1.55 Mb smaller than the chromosome of FB24. The two Arthrobacter strains have several large plasmids that are not present in the ATCC 33209 strain. In addition, these plasmids do not have high levels of similarity to sequences in the R. salmoninarum chromosome [51].

The presence of many IS elements, pseudogenes, and genomic islands in R. salmoninarum genome coupled with a lack of restriction-modification systems contribute to the extensive disruption of ORFs as a strategy to reduce many pathways in the bacteria. Moreover, the highly homogeneous nature of R. salmoninarum with respect to the overall genomic structure, biochemical properties, and surface antigens [114, 115] points to the evolution of this pathogen towards a strictly intracellular life style.

Several virulence factors including capsular synthesis genes, heme acquisition operons, genes encoding possible hemolysins, and the poorly characterized msa genes identified in the R. salmoninarum genome seems to be horizontally acquired. Arthrobacter spp. lacks most of these gene sequences, thus underlining the differential evolution and adaptation of these two very closely related species to contrasting ecological niches.

STREPTOCOCCUS AND LACTOCOCCUS

Gram-positive cocci belonging to the genera Streptococcus and Lactococcus are increasingly being recognized as important fish pathogens all over the world [116]. There are several different species of Gram-positive cocci, including Streptococcus parauberis, S. iniae, S. agalactiae (syn. Streptococcus difficilis), S. phocae [117, 118],Lactococcus garvieae (syn. Enterococcus seriolicida) [119], L. piscium [120–123], Vagococcus salmoninarum, and Carnobacterium piscicola [124], implicated in infectious diseases of warm water as well as cold water fishes.

Streptococcosis appears to have very few limitations in regard to geographic boundaries or host range, with outbreaks occurring in aquaculture facilities worldwide and in many different cultured species. S. iniae, S.parauberis, S. agalactiae, and L. garvieae are known as the major pathogens of streptococcosis and lactococcosis in

Oncorhynchus mykiss, Seriola quinqueradiata, Siganus canaliculatus, and Tilapia spp. [125].Recently, S. iniae and L. garvieae are also recognized as emerging zoonotic pathogens, causing diseases in both fish and human beings [23, 126].

S. iniae is a β-haemolytic, Gram-positive coccus that causes generalized septicaemia and meningoencephalitis in a variety of warm water fishes [127], whereas S. parauberis is an α-hemolytic, Gram-positive coccus, mainly pathogenic in cultured turbot (Scophthalmus maximus) and olive flounder, Paralichthys olivaceus. L. garvieaecauses a hyperacute and haemorrhagic septicemia in fishes particularly during the summer time. General pathological symptoms of streptococcosis and lactococcosis in fishes are hemorrhage, congestion, lethargy, dark pigmentation, erratic swimming, and exophthalmos with clouding of the cornea [117, 128].

Complete genome sequences of different strains of S. parauberis and L. garvieae, important pathogenic species isolated from both fish and human, have been published [129–132].

S. parauberis is recognized as the dominant etiological agent of streptococcosis in fish [117], whereas both S. parauberis and S. uberis are involved the causation of bovine mastitis in dairy cow [133, 134].

S. parauberis is closer to S. uberis than with other Streptococcus spp. and is biochemically and serologically indistinguishable from S. uberis [135]. Both species were earlier considered as type I and II of S. uberis, but later shown to be phylogenetically distinct and renamed the type I as S. uberis and type II as S. parauberis[134].

The S. parauberis strain KCTC11537BP genome size falls in the middle of the 1.8 to 2.3 Mb range of streptococcal genomes sequenced to date and the average G+C content of 35.6% is significantly lower than those of S. pyogenes [132]. About 78% of genes are shared between the genomes of S. parauberis strain KCTC11537BP and S. uberis NC_012004, but they differ significantly at two regions of the genome, demonstrating the genomic basis for their separation into two species.

S. parauberis genome encodes an M-like protein of S. iniae (SiM), which is an important virulence factor in S. iniae [136]. It also encodes hasA and hasB genes that may be involved in capsule production for resistance against phagocytosis. The genome analysis indicates that S. parauberis could possibly possess the ability to regulate the metabolism of more carbohydrates than other Streptococcus species and to synthesize all the aminoacids and regulatory factors required to adapt and survive in a highly hostile host environment.

Complete genome sequences of L. garvieae strain UNIUD074, isolated from diseased rainbow trout in Italy, a virulent strain Lg2 (serotype KG2) and a nonvirulent strain ATCC 49156 (serotype KG+), both isolated from diseased yellowtail in Japan have recently been published [130, 131]. In addition, genome sequence of L. garvieae strain 21881, isolated from a man suffering from septicemia has been published [129].

The strains Lg2 and ATCC 49156 have 99% sequence identity and share 1944 orthologous genes, but are different in 24 Lg2-specific genes that were absent in the ATCC 49156 genome. One of the Lg2-specific genes is a 16.5 kb capsule gene cluster, which confirms the earlier transmission electron microscopic finding that Lg2 is encapsulated, and ATCC 49156 is nonencapsulated [137]. In fact, the capsule gene cluster has the features of a horizontally acquired genomic island conferring virulence to the Lg2 strain but might have been lost from the ATCC 49156 strain while subculturing in the laboratory [131]. Both genomes carried three types of IS elements, prophage sequences, and integrase genes and were found smaller than those of at least five sequenced L. lactis genomes. The Lg2 genome lacks several aminoacid biosynthesis genes, which is a characteristic feature of pathogenic bacteria with reduced genomes. The Lg2 strain contains hemolysins, NADH oxidase and superoxide dismutase (SOD), adhesins and sortase, which are known virulence factors [137–139]. It also encodes a gene for phosphoglucomutase, a virulence factor conferring the resistance to peptide antimicrobials in S. iniae [140].

Although L. garvieae and L. lactis genomes share 75% CDS, about 25% genes are Lg2-specific hypothetical proteins and proteins of unknown functions, which may be involved in the virulence of the Lg2 strain. These findings indicate that L. garvieae and L. lactis have significantly diverged from the common ancestor, and theL. garvieae is evolving into a pathogenic species equipped with virulence features suitable for living in the host environment.

MYCOBACTERIA

Chronic infections in fish caused by different species of mycobacteria have been well recognized [23, 141, 142]. Several slow growing as well as fast growing species of mycobacteria such as Mycobacterium marinum, M. fortuitum, M. chelonae, and M. avium have been isolated from wild and cultured fish suffering from mycobacteriosis in different parts of the world [143–145]. Among them, M. marinum is the most important fish pathogen, frequently isolated from a variety of fish species with granulomas [146]. It is also a known zoonotic pathogen, transmitted to man though fish handling in aquariums and aquaculture tanks, producing superficial and self-limiting lesions called "fish tank or aquarium tank granuloma" involving the cooler parts of the body such as hands, forearms, elbows, and knees [147, 148]. Although strain variation has been reported [149], there is significant intraspecies sequence homogeneity among different M. mrinum strains [150]. However, it is hypothesized that only certain strains of M. marinum have zoonotic potential [151]. Phylogenetic studies have shown that M. marinum is most closely related to M. ulcerans followed by M. tuberculosis [150]. Owing to this, M. marinum and M. tuberculosis share many virulence factors and significant pathological features and respond to similar antibiotics [152, 153]. Hence, M. marinum is also an important model organism to study the pathogenesis of tuberculosis [152, 153].

Interestingly, the genome of M. marinum is 50% bigger than that of M. tuberculosis and seems to have acquired a number of genes encoding NRPSs and the huge repertoire of PE, PPE, and ESX systems probably by HGT [154]. Both species might have evolved differently from a common environmental mycobacteria. M. tuberculosis might have adapted to its host intracellular life by extensive genome reduction and M. marinum, by and large retained or obtained genes required for its dual lifestyle and broad-host range.

11. Genome Sequencing to Find Novel Vaccine and Drug Targets in Fish Pathogens

Our understanding of the molecular basis of virulence of certain well-studied fish bacterial pathogens has increased dramatically during the past decade. This has resulted from the application of recombinant DNA technology and cell biology to investigate bacterial infections, and the development of genetic techniques for identifying virulence genes.

More recently, genome sequence information of several bacterial fish pathogens has become available from genome sequencing projects. There is strong reason to believe that this understanding will be exploited to develop new interventions against fish bacterial infections.

The relevance of sequencing projects for drug and vaccine discovery is obvious. During the "pregenomic" era, the vaccine candidate genes were individually identified by tedious gene knockout studies and virulence attenuation. But now, the complete genome sequencing provides information on every virulence gene and all potential vaccine candidates, and the sequence databases will become indispensable for research in fish vaccinology and drug development.

After sequencing, the open reading frames (ORFs) are searched against available databases for sequence similarity with genes of known functions in other organisms. There are several strategies for gene annotation employing the tools of predictive bioinformatics programs combined with analyses of the published literature.

Multiple target vaccine candidate genes can be chosen and deleted simultaneously by various strategies including global transposon mutagenesis and gene replacement techniques [155, 156] to study their effect on virulence and essentiality. A number of important virulence determinants identified in the sequenced genome can be targeted. For example, the sortase enzyme in Gram-positive fish pathogens would be a very attractive universal vaccine and therapeutic drug target, as it mediates covalent anchoring of many surface displayed antigenic and/or virulence related proteins in Gram-positive bacteria [139]. The inactivation or inhibition of the sortase enzyme can simultaneously prevent the surface display of a number of virulence factors, thus effectively attenuating the virulence of the pathogen [110, 157].

The availability of sequences of the complete surface antigenic repertoire of pathogens, including protein and noprotein antigens would facilitate strategies for rational design of vaccines and drugs. In addition, the recent availability of large collections of the "virulogenome" of fish bacterial pathogens will provide enormous virulence sequence information for DNA vaccination studies. The whole complement of IS elements, prophages, and pathogenicity islands that can harbor virulence, and antimicrobial resistance gene clusters can be easily identified in the genomes. The comparison of genomes of different strains of the same bacteria or closely related species can reveal how these strains or species behave differently while infecting fish hosts, thus opening exciting opportunities for functional genomic analysis of infection processes and pathogenesis. However, experimental validation of predicted functions of genes identified from sequencing projects has lagged far behind the speed of annotation, and the major challenge of researchers in the field today is to understand the functional framework of the sequenced genomes.

CONCLUSIONS

There has been a steady increase in the number of species of bacteria implicated in fish diseases. The common fish pathogenic bacterial species belong to the genera Vibrio, Aeromonas, Flavobacterium, Yersinia, Edwardsiella, Streptococcus, lactococcus, Renibacterium, and Mycobacterium [23]. However, there is growing indications that the pathogenic species spectrum as well as the geographic and host range is widening among fish pathogens [158–161], leading to the emergence of new pathogens. Unlike the situation in human and animal medicine, fish diseases pose unique and daunting challenges. Fish are always bathed in a continuous medium of water, and fish disease treatment is essentially a population medicine. In addition, the current treatment methods are largely ineffective, and the biology and genetics of most fish bacterial pathogens are poorly understood, limiting the application of modern science-based pathogen intervention strategies.

Rapid growth and expansion of genome sequencing of human and animal pathogens enabled better understanding of their biology, evolution, and host adaptation strategies, and helped in combating many major diseases. Unfortunately, such developments and progress in the genomics and functional genomics of fish pathogenic bacteria have been very slow. However, recent availability of cost-effective high-throughput sequencing technologies has set the pace of sequencing of more fish pathogenic bacteria. Genome sequencing of a number of important bacterial pathogens of fish has helped us to better understand their biology and genetics. The sequencing projects have unearthed exciting new information on the adaptive evolution of fish pathogens, for example, how the nonpathogenic and ubiquitous soil bacteria such as Arthrobacter sp. has evolved into a strictly obligate fish pathogen, R. salmoninarum, by shedding functional genes through genomic reduction to lead to a very cosy intracellular life style.

On the other hand, phenotypically similar strains of the same species differ in certain set of virulence gene clusters, acquired through HGT and become highly virulent. The capsule gene cluster in the L. garvieae Lg2 strain confers virulence compared to noncapsulated ATCC 49156, which lacks the gene cluster. Nonpathogenic strains acquire genomic islands from distantly related pathogenic species and emerge as new pathogens of fish.

Comparative pathogenomics of closely related bacteria has increased our knowledge of how they vary in their virulence and their ability to adapt to different ecological niches. This is clearly evident in the difference in virulence of various strains of V. anguillarum and V. vulnificus, and among the closely related species of the genus Flavobacterium. As more strain-specific sequence information on bacterial pathogens of fish becomes available, we will have a better understanding of the subtle genomic differences among strains with varying virulence characteristics.

The typical pathogen evolutionary strategy of acquiring, shuffling and shedding genes mediated by IS elements, pseudogenes, prophage sequences, and HGT is also observed in most bacterial pathogens of fish. It is certain that the new genomic information will bring paradigm changes in bacterial pathogenesis and should provide new perspectives to our current thinking on the evolutionary and adaptive strategies of aquatic bacteria and how they colonize and establish in wider ecological niches and new host species. Moreover, the identification of key virulence factors in pathogenic strains should help us design efficient drugs and vaccines to combat major bacterial pathogens of fish.

However, it should be stressed that the genomic information will provide only a snapshot of the microorganism. Highly virulent clones armed with one or more acquired virulence factors can suddenly develop from the existing harmless microorganisms in the face of environmental, antibiotic, and host-induced selective pressures.

More intriguingly, about 40% of the genes in sequenced bacterial genomes constitute new putative genes and hypothetical proteins with mysterious functions and are conserved among several different species of bacteria. Even in Escherichia coli, the most studied of all bacteria, only 54% genes have currently been functionally characterized based on experimental evidence [162]. A close scrutiny of the sequenced genomes of fish pathogens reveals that the above situation is essentially true for these pathogens as well. Although current advances in functional genomics, structural genomics and bioinformatics have contributed immensely to deciphering and extracting useful biological information from the vast genomic data, understanding and assigning functionality to the unique and new gene sequences discovered in the genomes will be the major task of genome biologists in the coming years.

ACKNOWLEDGMENTS

This work was financially supported by various research fundings from the Ministry of Agriculture and Fisheries Wealth, Oman.

REFERENCES

1. J. M. Rothberg and J. H. Leamon, "The development and impact of 454 sequencing," Nature Biotechnology, vol. 26, no. 10, pp. 1117–1124, 2008.
2. J. Zhang, R. Chiodini, A. Badr, and G. Zhang, "The impact of next-generation sequencing on genomics,"Journal of Genetics and Genomics, vol. 38, no. 3, pp. 95–109, 2011.
3. E. Pennisi, "Genome data shake tree of life," Science, vol. 280, no. 5364, pp. 672–674, 1998.
4. W. F. Doolittle, "Phylogenetic classification and the universal tree," Science, vol. 284, no. 5423, pp. 2124–2128, 1999.
5. W. F. Doolittle, "Lateral genomics," Trends in Cell Biology, vol. 9, no. 12, pp. M5–M8, 1999.
6. E. Pennisi, "Is it time to uproot the tree of life?" Science, vol. 284, no. 5418, pp. 1305–1307, 1999.
7. W. F. Doolittle, "Uprooting the tree of life," Scientific American, vol. 282, no. 2, pp. 90–95, 2000.

8. E. V. Koonin, K. S. Makarova, and L. Aravind, "Horizontal gene transfer in prokaryotes: quantification and classification," Annual Review of Microbiology, vol. 55, pp. 709–742, 2001.
9. N. A. Moran, "Microbial minimalism: genome reduction in bacterial pathogens," Cell, vol. 108, no. 5, pp. 583–586, 2002.
10. A. Mira, L. Klasson, and S. G. E. Andersson, "Microbial genome evolution: sources of variability,"Current Opinion in Microbiology, vol. 5, no. 5, pp. 506–512, 2002.
11. L. Holm, "Codon usage and gene expression," Nucleic Acids Research, vol. 14, no. 7, pp. 3075–3087, 1986.
12. L. S. Frost, R. Leplae, A. O. Summers, and A. Toussaint, "Mobile genetic elements: the agents of open source evolution," Nature Reviews Microbiology, vol. 3, no. 9, pp. 722–732, 2005.
13. U. Dobrindt, B. Hochhut, U. Hentschel, and J. Hacker, "Genomic islands in pathogenic and environmental microorganisms," Nature Reviews Microbiology, vol. 2, no. 5, pp. 414–424, 2004.
14. U. Dobrindt and J. Hacker, "How bacterial pathogens were constructed," in Bacterial Virulence: Basic Principles, Models and Global Approaches, P. Sansonetti, Ed., pp. 3–15, Wiley-VCH, GmbH & Co. KGaA, Weinheim, Germany, 2010.
15. M. J. Pallen and B. W. Wren, "Bacterial pathogenomics," Nature, vol. 449, no. 7164, pp. 835–842, 2007.
16. J. G. Lawrence and J. R. Roth, "Genomic flux: genome evolution by gene loss and acquisition," inOrganization of the Prokaryotic Genome, R. L. Charlebois, Ed., pp. 263–289, American Society for Microbiology, Washington, DC, USA, 1999.
17. F. P. Meyer, "Aquaculture disease and health management.," Journal of Animal Science, vol. 69, no. 10, pp. 4201–4208, 1991.
18. C. D. Harvell, K. Kim, J. M. Burkholder et al., "Emerging marine diseases—climate links and anthropogenic factors," Science, vol. 285, no. 5433, pp. 1505–1510, 1999.
19. R. Subasinghe, "Fish health and quarantine; review of the state of the World aquaculture," in FAO Fisheries Circular, no. 886, pp. 45–49, Rome, Italy, Food and Agriculture Organization of the United Nations, 1997.

20. B. Hjeltnes and R. J. Roberts, "Vibriosis," in Bacterial Diseases of Fish, R. J. Roberts, N. R. Bromag, andV. Inglis, Eds., pp. 109–121, Blackwell Scientific, Oxford, UK, 1993.
21. D. V. Lightner and R. M. Redman, "Shrimp diseases and current diagnostic methods," Aquaculture, vol. 164, no. 1–4, pp. 201–220, 1998.
22. O. Bergh, F. Nilsen, and O. B. Samuelsen, "Diseases, prophylaxis and treatment of the Atlantic halibutHippoglossus hippoglossus: a review," Diseases of Aquatic Organisms, vol. 48, no. 1, pp. 57–74, 2001.
23. B. Austin and D. A. Austin, Bacterial Fish Pathogens: Disease in Farmed and Wild Fish, Springer, New York, NY, USA, 3rd edition, 1999.
24. B. Austin and X. H. Zhang, "Vibrio harveyi: a significant pathogen of marine vertebrates and invertebrates," Letters in Applied Microbiology, vol. 43, no. 2, pp. 119–124, 2006.
25. C. Amaro, E. G. Biosca, C. Esteve, et al., "Comparative study of phenotypic and virulence properties inVibrio vulnificus biotypes 1 and 2 obtained from a European eel farm experiencing mortalities," Diseases of Aquatic Organisms, vol. 13, pp. 29–35, 1992.
26. E. G. Biosca, H. Llorens, E. Garay, and C. Amaro, "Presence of a capsule in Vibrio vulnificus biotype 2 and its relationship to virulence for eels," Infection and Immunity, vol. 61, no. 5, pp. 1611–1618, 1993.
27. E. Benediktsdóttir, L. Verdonck, C. Spröer, S. Helgason, and J. Swings, "Characterization of Vibrio viscosus and Vibrio wodanis isolated at different geographical locations: a proposal for reclassification ofVibrio viscosus as Moritella viscosa comb. nov.," International Journal of Systematic and Evolutionary Microbiology, vol. 50, no. 2, pp. 479–488, 2000.
28. L. A. Actis, M. E. Tolmasky, and J. H. Crosa, "Vibriosis," in Fish Diseases and Disorders, Viral, Bacterial, and Fungal Infections, P. T. K. Woo and D. W. Bruno, Eds., vol. 3, pp. 570–605, CABI International, Oxfordshire, UK, 2nd edition, 2011.
29. E. Hjerde, M. Lorentzen, M. T. G. Holden et al., "The genome sequence of the fish pathogen Aliivibrio salmonicida strain

LFI1238 shows extensive evidence of gene decay," BMC Genomics, vol. 9, article 616, 2008.

30. P. A. Gulig, V. D. Crécy-Lagard, A. C. Wright, B. Walts, M. Telonis-Scott, and L. M. McIntyre, "SOLiD sequencing of four Vibrio vulnificus genomes enables comparative genomic analysis and identification of candidate clade-specific virulence genes," BMC Genomics, vol. 11, no. 1, article 512, 2010.
31. H. Naka, G. M. Dias, C. C. Thompson, C. Dubay, F. L. Thompson, and J. H. Crosa, "Complete genome sequence of the marine fish pathogen Vibrio anguillarum harboring the pJM1 virulence plasmid and genomic comparison with other virulent strains of V. anguillarum and V. ordalii," Infection and Immunity, vol. 79, no. 7, pp. 2889–2900, 2011.
32. J. L. Larsen, K. Pedersen, and I. Dalsgaard, "Vibrio anguillarum serovars associated with vibriosis in fish," Journal of Fish Diseases, vol. 17, no. 3, pp. 259–267, 1994.
33. U. B. S. Sorensen and J. L. Larsen, "Serotyping of Vibrio anguillarum," Applied and Environmental Microbiology, vol. 51, no. 3, pp. 593–597, 1986.
34. A. E. Toranzo and J. L. Barja, "A review of the taxonomy and seroepizootiology of Vibrio anguillarum, with special reference to aquaculture in the NorthWest Spain," Diseases of Aquatic Organisms, vol. 9, pp. 73–82, 1990.
35. J. H. Crosa, "A plasmid associated with virulence in the marine fish pathogen Vibrio anguillarumspecifies an iron-sequestering system," Nature, vol. 284, no. 5756, pp. 566–568, 1980.
36. A. E. Toranzo, J. L. Barja, S. A. Potter, et al., "Molecular factors associated with virulence of marine vibrios isolated from striped bass in Chesapeake Bay," Infection and Immunity, vol. 39, no. 3, pp. 1220–1227, 1983.
37. M. H. Schiewe, T. J. Trust, and J. H. Crosa, "Vibrio ordalii sp. nov.: a causative agent of vibriosis in fish,"Current Microbiology, vol. 6, no. 6, pp. 343–348, 1981.
38. D. P. Ransom, C. N. Lannan, J. S. Rohovec, and J. L. Fryer, "Comparison of histopathology caused byVibrio anguillarum and Vibrio ordalii in three species of Pacific salmon," Journal of Fish Diseases, vol. 7, pp. 107–115, 1984.

39. K. Makino, K. Oshima, K. Kurokawa et al., "Genome sequence of Vibrio parahaemolyticus: a pathogenic mechanism distinct from that of V. cholerae," The Lancet, vol. 361, no. 9359, pp. 743–749, 2003.
40. N. Okada, S. Matsuda, J. Matsuyama et al., "Presence of genes for type III secretion system 2 in Vibrio mimicus strains," BMC Microbiology, vol. 10, article 302, 2010.
41. A. Alam, K. A. Miller, M. Chaand, J. S. Butler, and M. Dziejman, "Identification of Vibrio cholerae type III secretion system effector proteins," Infection and Immunity, vol. 79, no. 4, pp. 1728–1740, 2011.
42. C. R. Osorio, S. Juiz-Rio, and M. L. Lemos, "A siderophore biosynthesis gene cluster from the fish pathogen Photobacterium damselae subsp. piscicida is structurally and functionally related to the Yersinia high-pathogenicity island," Microbiology, vol. 152, no. 11, pp. 3327–3341, 2006.
43. E. S. Yip, B. T. Grublesky, E. A. Hussa, and K. L. Visick, "A novel, conserved cluster of genes promotes symbiotic colonization and σ-dependent biofilm formation by Vibrio fischeri," Molecular Microbiology, vol. 57, no. 5, pp. 1485–1498, 2005.
44. H. S. Kim, S. J. Park, and K. H. Lee, "Role of NtrC-regulated exopolysaccharides in the biofilm formation and pathogenic interaction of Vibrio vulnificus," Molecular Microbiology, vol. 74, no. 2, pp. 436–453, 2009.
45. E. Sanjuan, B. Fouz, J. D. Oliver, and C. Amaro, "Evaluation of genotypic and phenotypic methods to distinguish clinical from environmental Vibrio vulnificus strains," Applied and Environmental Microbiology, vol. 75, no. 6, pp. 1604–1613, 2009.
46. N. Bisharat, D. I. Cohen, M. C. Maiden, D. W. Crook, T. Peto, and R. M. Harding, "The evolution of genetic structure in the marine pathogen, Vibrio vulnificus," Infection, Genetics and Evolution, vol. 7, no. 6, pp. 685–693, 2007.
47. M. B. Schrøder, S. Espelid, and T. Ø. Jørgensen, "Two serotypes of Vibrio salmonicida isolated from diseased cod (Gadus morhua L.); virulence, immunological studies and vaccination experiments," Fish and Shellfish Immunology, vol. 2, no. 3, pp. 211–221, 1992.

48. M. Tomich, P. J. Planet, and D. H. Figurski, "The tad locus: postcards from the widespread colonization island," Nature Reviews Microbiology, vol. 5, no. 5, pp. 363–375, 2007.
49. P. Siguier, J. Filee, and M. Chandler, "Insertion sequences in prokaryotic genomes," Current Opinion in Microbiology, vol. 9, no. 5, pp. 526–531, 2006.
50. J. Parkhill, G. Dougan, K. D. James et al., "Complete genome sequence of a multiple drug resistantSalmonella enterica serovar Typhi CT18," Nature, vol. 413, no. 6858, pp. 848–852, 2001.
51. G. D. Wiens, D. D. Rockey, Z. Wu et al., "Genome sequence of the fish pathogen Renibacterium salmoninarum suggests reductive evolution away from an environmental Arthrobacter ancestor,"Journal of Bacteriology, vol. 190, no. 21, pp. 6970–6982, 2008.
52. A. Martin-Carnahan and S. W. Joseph, "Aeromonadaceae," in Bergey›s Manual of Systematic Bacteriology, G. M. Garrity, Ed., vol. 2, pp. 556–580, Springer, New York, NY, USA, 2nd edition, 2005.
53. M. J. Figueras, "Clinical relevance of Aeromonas sM503," Reviews in Medical Microbiology, vol. 16, no. 4, pp. 145–153, 2005.
54. R. Seshadri, S. W. Joseph, A. K. Chopra et al., "Genome sequence of Aeromonas hydrophila ATCC 7966T: jack of all trades," Journal of Bacteriology, vol. 188, no. 23, pp. 8272–8282, 2006.
55. M. E. Reith, R. K. Singh, B. Curtis et al., "The genome of Aeromonas salmonicida subsp. salmonicidaA449: Insights into the evolution of a fish pathogen," BMC Genomics, vol. 9, article 427, 2008.
56. Y. Li, Y. Liu, Z. Zhou et al., "Complete genome sequence of Aeromonas veronii strain B565," Journal of Bacteriology, vol. 193, no. 13, pp. 3389–3390, 2011.
57. S. A. Beatson, M. D. G. de Luna, N. L. Bachmann et al., "Genome sequence of the emerging pathogenAeromonas caviae," Journal of Bacteriology, vol. 193, no. 5, pp. 1286–1287, 2011.
58. E. M. Bernoth, "Furunculosis: the history of the diseases and of disease research," in Furunculosis, Multidisciplinary Fish Disease Research, E. M. Bernoth, A. E. Ellis, P. J. Midtlyng, G. Olivier, and P. Smith, Eds., pp. 1–20, Academic Press, London, UK, 1997.

59. M. Hiney and G. Olivier, "Furunculosis (Aeromonas salmonicida)," in Fish Diseases and Disorders III: Viral, Bacterial and Fungal Infections, P. T. K. Woo and D. W. Bruno, Eds., pp. 341–425, CAB Publishing, Oxford, UK, 1999.
60. C. Paniagua, O. Rivero, J. Anguita, and G. Naharro, "Pathogenicity factors and virulence for rainbow trout (Salmo gairdneri) of motile Aeromonas spp. isolated from a river," Journal of Clinical Microbiology, vol. 28, no. 2, pp. 350–355, 1990.
61. S. E. Burr, D. Pugovkin, T. Wahli, H. Segner, and J. Frey, "Attenuated virulence of an Aeromonas salmonicida subsp. salmonicida type III secretion mutant in a rainbow trout model," Microbiology, vol. 151, no. 6, pp. 2111–2118, 2005.
62. J. Sha, L. Pillai, A. A. Fadl, C. L. Galindo, T. E. Erova, and A. K. Chopra, "The type III secretion system and cytotoxic enterotoxin alter the virulence of Aeromonas hydrophila," Infection and Immunity, vol. 73, no. 10, pp. 6446–6457, 2005.
63. J. M. Janda and R. P. Kokka, "The pathogenicity of Aeromonas strains relative to genospecies and phenospecies identification," FEMS Microbiology Letters, vol. 90, no. 1, pp. 29–33, 1991.
64. J. Madetoja, I. Dalsgaard, and T. Wiklund, "Occurrence of Flavobacterium psychrophilum in fish-farming environments," Diseases of Aquatic Organisms, vol. 52, no. 2, pp. 109–118, 2002. A. Nematollahi, A. Decostere, F. Pasmans, and F. Haesebrouck, "Flavobacterium psychrophiluminfections in salmonid fish," Journal of Fish Diseases, vol. 26, no. 10, pp. 563–574, 2003.
65. J. G. Leahy and R. R. Colwell, "Microbial degradation of hydrocarbons in the environment,"Microbiological Reviews, vol. 54, no. 3, pp. 305–315, 1990.
66. J. Lehmann, D. Mock, F. J. Stuerenberg, and J. F. Bernardet, "First isolation of Cytophaga psychrophilafrom a systemic disease in eel and cyprinids," Diseases of Aquatic Organisms, vol. 10, pp. 217–220, 1991.
67. R. A. Holt, Cytophaga psychrophila, the causative agent of bacterial cold-water disease in salmonid fish, Ph.D. thesis, Oregon State University, Corvallis, Ore, USA, 1987.
68. G. J. Heo, K. Kasai, and H. Wakabayashi, "Occurrence of Flavobacterium branchiophila associated with bacterial gill

disease at a trout hatchery," Fish Pathology, vol. 25, pp. 99–105, 1990.

69. V. E. Ostland, J. S. Lumsden, D. D. MacPhee, and H. W. Ferguson, "Characteristics of Flavobacterium branchiophilum, the cause of salmonid bacterial gill disease in Ontario," Journal of Aquatic Animal Health, vol. 6, no. 1, pp. 13–26, 1994.
70. J. F. Bernardet, "Flexibacter columnaris: first description in France and comparison with bacterial strains from other origins," Diseases of Aquatic Organisms, vol. 6, pp. 37–44, 1989.
71. D. J. Speare and H. W. Ferguson, "Clinical and pathological features of common gill diseases of cultured salmonids in Ontario," Canadian Veterinary Journal, vol. 30, pp. 882–887, 1989.
72. J. F. Bernardet, P. Segers, M. Vancanneyt, F. Berthe, K. Kersters, and P. Vandamme, "Cutting a gordian knot: emended classification and description of the genus Flavobacterium, emended description of the family Flavobacteriaceae, and proposal of Flavobacterium hydatis nom. nov. (basonym, Cytophaga aquatilis Strohl and Tait 1978)," International Journal of Systematic Bacteriology, vol. 46, no. 1, pp. 128–148, 1996.
73. E. Duchaud, M. Boussaha, V. Loux et al., "Complete genome sequence of the fish pathogenFlavobacterium psychrophilum," Nature Biotechnology, vol. 25, no. 7, pp. 763–769, 2007.
74. M. Touchon, P. Barbier, J. F. Bernardet, et al., "Complete genome sequence of the fish pathogenFlavobacterium branchiophilum," Applied and Environmentl Microbiology, vol. 77, no. 21, pp. 7656–7662, 2011.
75. M. L. Lawrence, A. Karsi, H. C. Tekedar, et al., "Comparative genomics of Flavobacterium columnareisolates from two genetic divisions and with different pathogenic potential for channel catfish (Ictalurus punctatus)," in Proceedings of the Conference on FLAVOBACTERIUM, Paris, France, September 2009.
76. C. Rodkhum, I. Hirono, J. H. Crosa, and T. Aoki, "Four novel hemolysin genes of Vibrio anguillarumand their virulence to rainbow trout," Microbial Pathogenesis, vol. 39, no. 4, pp. 109–119, 2005.
77. M. Palmer, "The family of thiol-activated, cholesterol-binding cytolysins," Toxicon, vol. 39, no. 11, pp. 1681–1689, 2001.

78. M. Shoji, D. B. Ratnayake, Y. Shi et al., "Construction and characterization of a nonpigmented mutant ofPorphyromonas gingivalis: Cell surface polysaccharide as an anchorage for gingipanis," Microbiology, vol. 148, no. 4, pp. 1183–1191, 2002.
79. K. Sato, E. Sakai, P. D. Veith et al., "Identification of a new membrane-associated protein that influences transport/ maturation of gingipains and adhesins of Porphyromonas gingivalis," The Journal of Biological Chemistry, vol. 280, no. 10, pp. 8668–8677, 2005.
80. S. L. Abbott and J. M. Janda, "The genus Edwardsiella," Prokaryotes, vol. 6, pp. 72–89, 2006.
81. J. E. Clarridge, D. M. Musher, V. Fanstein, and R. J. Wallace Jr., "Extra-intestinal human infection caused by Edwardsiella tarda," Journal of Clinical Microbiology, vol. 11, no. 5, pp. 511–514, 1980.
82. P. Nagel, A. Serritella, and T. J. Layden, "Edwardsiella tarda gastroenteritis associated with a pet turtle,"Gastroenterology, vol. 82, no. 6, pp. 1436–1437, 1982.
83. W. A. Rogers, "Edwardsiellosis in fishes," in Antigens of Fish Pathogens. Les Antigenes des Microorganisms Pathogenes des Poissons, D. P. Anderson, M. Dorson, and Ph. Dubourget, Eds., pp. 153–159, Fondation Marcel Merieux, Lyon, France, 1983.
84. F. P. Meyer and G. L. Bullock, "Edwardsiella tarda, a new pathogen of channel catfish (Ictalurus punctatus)," Applied Microbiology, vol. 25, no. 1, pp. 155–156, 1973.
85. S. H. M. Ling, X. H. Wang, L. Xie, T. M. Lim, and K. Y. Leung, "Use of green fluorescent protein (GFP) to study the invasion pathways of Edwardsiella tarda in in vivo and in vitro fish models," Microbiology, vol. 146, no. 1, pp. 7–19, 2000.
86. J. C. Newton, L. G. Wolfe, J. M. Grizzle, and J. A. Plumb, "Pathology of experimental enteric septicaemia in channel catfish, Ictalurus punctatus (Rafinesque), following immersion-exposure to Edwardsiella ictaluri," Journal of Fish Diseases, vol. 12, no. 4, pp. 335–347, 1989.
87. Q. Wang, M. Yang, J. Xiao et al., "Genome sequence of the versatile fish pathogen Edwardsiella tardaprovides insights into its adaptation to broad host ranges and intracellular niches," PLoS One, vol. 4, no. 10, Article ID e7646, 2009.

88. M. L. Williams, A. F. Gillaspy, D. W. Dyer, et al., "Genome sequence of Edwardsiella ictaluri 93–146, a strain associated with a natural channel catfish outbreak of enteric septicemia of catfish," Journal of Bacteriology, vol. 194, no. 3, pp. 740–741, 2012.
89. S. R. Partridge and R. M. Hall, "The IS1111 family members IS4321 and IS5075 have sub-terminal inverted repeats and target the terminal inverted repeats of Tn21 family transposons," Journal of Bacteriology, vol. 185, no. 21, pp. 6371–6384, 2003.
90. T. Tanabe, T. Funahashi, H. Nakao, S. I. Miyoshi, S. Shinoda, and S. Yamamoto, "Identification and characterization of genes required for biosynthesis and transport of the siderophore vibrioferrin inVibrio parahaemolyticus," Journal of Bacteriology, vol. 185, no. 23, pp. 6938–6949, 2003.
91. Q. Wang, Q. Liu, Y. Ma, L. Zhou, and Y. Zhang, "Isolation, sequencing and characterization of cluster genes involved in the biosynthesis and utilization of the siderophore of marine fish pathogen Vibrio alginolyticus," Archives of Microbiology, vol. 188, no. 4, pp. 433–439, 2007.
92. M. D. Furones, C. J. Rodgers, and C. B. Munn, "Yersinia ruckeri, the causal agent of enteric redmouth disease (ERM) in fish," Annual Review of Fish Diseases, vol. 3, no. C, pp. 105–125, 1993.
93. R. R. Rucker, "Redmouth disease of rainbow trout (Salmo gairdneri)," Bulletin de l›Office International des Epizooties, vol. 65, no. 5, pp. 825–830, 1966.
94. E. Tobback, A. Decostere, K. Hermans, F. Haesebrouck, and K. Chiers, "Yersinia ruckeri infections in salmonid fish," Journal of Fish Diseases, vol. 30, no. 5, pp. 257–268, 2007.
95. M. T. Horne and A. C. Barnes, "Enteric redmouth disease (Y. ruckeri)," in Fish Diseases and Disorders: Viral, Bacterial and Fungal Infections, P. T. K. Woo and D. W. Bruno, Eds., vol. 3, pp. 455–477, CABI Publishing, Oxfordshire, UK, 1999.
96. A. J. Ross, R. R. Rucker, and W. H. Ewing, "Description of a bacterium associated with redmouth disease of rainbow trout (Salmo gairdneri)," Canadian Journal of Microbiology, vol. 12, no. 4, pp. 763–770, 1966.

97. R. L. Davies, "Virulence and serum-resistance in different clonal groups and serotypes ofYersinia ruckeri,"Veterinary Microbiology, vol. 29, no. 3-4, pp. 289–297, 1991.
98. R. M. V. Stevenson and D. W. Airdrie, "Serological variation among Yersinia ruckeri strains," Journal of Fish Diseases, vol. 7, pp. 247–254, 1984.
99. J. L. Romalde, B. Magarinos, J. L. Barja, and A. E. Toranzo, "Antigenic and molecular characterization ofYersinia ruckeri proposal for a new intraspecies classification," Systematic and Applied Microbiology, vol. 16, no. 3, pp. 411–419, 1993.
100. R. M. Stevenson, "Immunization with bacterial antigens: yersiniosis," Developments in Biological Standardization, vol. 90, pp. 117–124, 1997.
101. R. L. Davies, "Yersinia ruckeri produces four iron-regulated proteins but does not produce detectable siderophores," Journal of Fish Diseases, vol. 14, pp. 563–570, 1991.
102. M. Kotetishvili, A. Kreger, G. Wauters, J. G. Morris, A. Sulakvelidze, and O. C. Stine, "Multilocus sequence typing for studying genetic relationships among Yersinia species," Journal of Clinical Microbiology, vol. 43, no. 6, pp. 2674–2684, 2005.
103. P. E. Chen, C. Cook, A. C. Stewart et al., "Genomic characterization of the Yersinia genus," Genome Biology, vol. 11, no. 1, article R1, 2010.
104. J. E. Sanders and J. L. Fryer, "Renibacterium salmoninarum gen. nov., sp. nov., the causative agent of bacterial kidney disease in salmonid fishes," International Journal of Systematic Bacteriology, vol. 30, no. 2, pp. 496–502, 1980.
105. D. L. Mitchum and L. E. Sherman, "Transmission of bacterial kidney disease from wild to stocked hatchery trout," Canadian Journal of Fisheries and Aquatic Sciences, vol. 38, pp. 547–551, 1981.
106. G. L. Bullock, Bacterial Kidney Disease of Salmonid Fishes Caused by Renibacterium salmoninarum, no. 60, U.S. Fish and Wildlife Service, Fish Disease Leaflet, Washington, DC, USA, 1980.
107. K. E. Wolf and C. E. Dunbar, "Test of 34 therapeutic agents for control of kidney disease in trout,"Transactions of American Fisheries Society, vol. 88, pp. 117–124, 1959.

108. S. K. Gutenberger, J. R. Duimstra, J. S. Rohovec, and J. L. Fryer, "Intracellular survival of Renibacterium salmoninarum in trout mononuclear phagocytes," Disease of Aquatic Organisms, vol. 28, no. 2, pp. 93–106, 1997.
109. P. S. Sudheesh, S. Crane, K. D. Cain, and M. S. Strom, "Sortase inhibitor phenyl vinyl sulfone inhibitsRenibacterium salmoninarum adherence and invasion of host cells," Diseases of Aquatic Organisms, vol. 78, no. 2, pp. 115–127, 2007.
110. E. Stackebrandt, U. Wehmeyer, H. Nader, and F. Fiedler, "Phylogenetic relationship of the fish pathogenic Renibacterium salmoninarum to Arthrobacter, Micrococcus and related taxa," FEMS Microbiology Letters, vol. 50, no. 2-3, pp. 117–120, 1988.
111. K. Salonius, C. Siderakis, A. M. MacKinnon, and S. G. Griffiths, "Use of Arthrobacter davidanieli as a live vaccine against Renibacterium salmoninarum and Piscirickettsia salmonis in salmonids,"Developments in Biologicals, vol. 121, pp. 189–197, 2005.
112. E. F. Mongodin, N. Shapir, S. C. Daugherty et al., "Secrets of soil survival revealed by the genome sequence of Arthrobacter aurescens TC1," PLoS Genetics, vol. 2, no. 12, article e214, 2006.
113. R. G. Getchell, J. S. Rohovec, and J. L. Fryer, "Comparison of Renibacterium salmoninarum isolates by antigenic analysis," Fish Pathology, vol. 20, pp. 149–159, 1985.
114. F. Fiedler and R. Draxl, "Biochemical and immunochemical properties of the cell surface ofRenibacterium salmoninarum," Journal of Bacteriology, vol. 168, no. 2, pp. 799–804, 1986.
115. T. Kitao, "Streptococcal infections," in Bacterial Disease of Fish, V. Inglis, R. J. Roberts, and N. R. Bromage, Eds., pp. 196–210, Blackwell Scientific, Oxford, UK, 1993.
116. A. Domenech, J. F. Fernandez-Garayzabal, C. Pasqual, et al., "Streptococcosis in cultured turbot,Scophthalmus maximus (L.), associated with Streptococcus parauberis," Journal of Fish Diseases, vol. 19, pp. 33–38, 1996.
117. J. L. Romalde, C. Ravelo, I. Valdés et al., "Streptococcus phocae, an emerging pathogen for salmonid culture," Veterinary Microbiology, vol. 130, no. 1-2, pp. 198–207, 2008.
118. D. Vendrell, J. L. Balcázar, I. Ruiz-Zarzuela, I. de Blas, O. Gironés, and J. L. Múzquiz, "Lactococcus garvieae in fish: a

review," Comparative Immunology, Microbiology and Infectious Diseases, vol. 29, no. 4, pp. 177–198, 2006.

119. M. D. Collins, J. A. E. Farrow, B. A. Phillips, and O. Kandler, "Streptococcus garvieae sp. nov. andStreptococcus plantarum sp. nov.," Journal of General Microbiology, vol. 129, no. 11, pp. 3427–3431, 1983.
120. A. M. Williams, J. L. Fryer, and M. D. Collins, "Lactococcus piscium sp. nov. a new Lactococcus species from salmonid fish," FEMS Microbiology Letters, vol. 68, no. 1-2, pp. 109–113, 1990.
121. A. Domenech, J. Prieta, J. F. Fernandez-Garayzabal, et al., "Phenotypic and phylogenetic evidence for a close relationship between Lactococcus garvieae and Enterococcus seriolicida," Microbiologia SEM, vol. 9, no. 1, pp. 63–68, 1993.
122. A. Eldar, C. Ghittino, L. Asanta et al., "Enterococcus seriolicida is a junior synonym of Lactococcus garvieae, a causative agent of septicemia and meningoencephalitis in fish," Current Microbiology, vol. 32, no. 2, pp. 85–88, 1996.
123. S. Wallbanks, A. J. Martinez-Murcia, J. L. Fryer, B. A. Phillips, and M. D. Collins, "16S rRNA sequence determination for members of the genus Carnobacterium and related lactic acid bacteria and description of Vagococcus salmoninarum sp. nov.," International Journal of Systematic Bacteriology, vol. 40, no. 3, pp. 224–230, 1990.
124. E. S. Bromage and L. Owens, "Infection of barramundi Lates calcarifer with Streptococcus iniae: effects of different routes of exposure," Diseases of Aquatic Organisms, vol. 52, no. 3, pp. 199–205, 2002.
125. J. A. Elliott, M. D. Collins, N. E. Pigott, and R. R. Facklam, "Differentiation of Lactococcus lactis andLactococcus garvieae from humans by comparison of whole-cell protein patterns," Journal of Clinical Microbiology, vol. 29, no. 12, pp. 2731–2734, 1991.
126. R. P. Perera, S. K. Johnson, M. D. Collins, and D. H. Lewis, "Streptococcus iniae associated with mortality of Tilapia nilotica X T.aurea hybrids," Journal of Aquatic Animal Health, vol. 6, no. 4, pp. 335–340, 1994.
127. R. Kusuda, K. Kawai, F. Salati, C. R. Banner, and J. L. Fryer, "Enterococcus seriolicida sp. nov., a fish pathogen," International

Journal of Systematic Bacteriology, vol. 41, no. 3, pp. 406–409, 1991.

128. M. Aguado-Urda, G. H. López-Campos, M. M. Blanco et al., "Genome sequence of Lactococcus garvieae21881, isolated in a case of human septicemia," Journal of Bacteriology, vol. 193, no. 15, pp. 4033–4034, 2011.
129. P. Reimundo, M. Pignatelli, L. D. Alcaraz, G. D›Auria, A. Moya, and J. A. Guijarro, "Genome sequence of Lactococcus garvieae UNIUD074, isolated in Italy from a lactococcosis outbreak," Journal of Bacteriology, vol. 193, no. 14, pp. 3684–3685, 2011.
130. H. Morita, H. Toh, K. Oshima et al., "Complete genome sequence and comparative analysis of the fish pathogen Lactococcus garvieae," PLoS One, vol. 6, no. 8, Article ID e23184, 2011.
131. S. W. Nho, J. I. Hikima, I. S. Cha et al., "Complete genome sequence and immunoproteomic analyses of the bacterial fish pathogen Streptococcus parauberis," Journal of Bacteriology, vol. 193, no. 13, pp. 3356–3366, 2011.
132. J. L. Watts, "Etiological agents of bovine mastitis," Veterinary Microbiology, vol. 16, no. 1, pp. 41–66, 1988.
133. A. M. Williams and M. D. Collins, "Molecular taxonomic studies on Streptococcus uberis types I and II. Description of Streptococcus parauberis sp. nov.," Journal of Applied Bacteriology, vol. 68, no. 5, pp. 485–490, 1990.
134. R. W. Bentley, J. A. Leigh, and M. D. Collins, "Intrageneric structure of Streptococcus based on comparative analysis of small-subunit rRNA sequences," International Journal of Systematic Bacteriology, vol. 41, no. 4, pp. 487–494, 1991.
135. J. B. Locke, R. K. Aziz, M. R. Vicknair, V. Nizet, and J. T. Buchanan, "Streptococcus iniae M-like protein contributes to virulence in fish and is a target for live attenuated vaccine development," PLoS One, vol. 3, no. 7, Article ID e2824, 2008.
136. M. Kawanishi, T. Yoshida, M. Kijima et al., "Characterization of Lactococcus garvieae isolated from radish and broccoli sprouts that exhibited a KG+ phenotype, lack of virulence and absence of a capsule,"Letters in Applied Microbiology, vol. 44, no. 5, pp. 481–487, 2007.

137. T. J. Mitchell, "The pathogenesis of streptococcal infections: from tooth decay to meningitis," Nature Reviews. Microbiology, vol. 1, no. 3, pp. 219–230, 2003.
138. L. A. Marraffini, A. C. Dedent, and O. Schneewind, "Sortases and the art of anchoring proteins to the envelopes of gram-positive bacteria," Microbiology and Molecular Biology Reviews, vol. 70, no. 1, pp. 192–221, 2006.
139. J. T. Buchanan, J. A. Stannard, X. Lauth et al., "Streptococcus iniaephosphoglucomutase is a virulence factor and a target for vaccine development," Infection and Immunity, vol. 73, no. 10, pp. 6935–6944, 2005.
140. G. N. Frerichs, "Acid-fast fish pathogens," in Bacterial Diseases of Fish, V. Inglis, R. J. Roberts, and N. R. Bromage, Eds., pp. 217–233, Blackwell Scientific, Oxford, UK, 1993.
141. E. J. Noga, Fish disease diagnosis and treatment, Mosby, St. Louis, Mo, USA, 1996.
142. L. G. Wayne, G. P. Kubica, et al., "Genus Mycobacterium Lehmann and Neumann 1896, 363AL," inBergey›s Manual of Systematic Bacteriology, P. H. A. Sneath, N. S. Mair, M. E. Sharpe, and J. G. Holt, Eds., vol. 2, pp. 1436–1457, Williams & Wilkins, Baltimore, Md, USA, 1986.
143. C. O. Thoen and T. A. Schliesser, "Mycobacterial infections in cold-blooded animals," in The Mycobacteria, G. P. Kubica and L. G. Wayne, Eds., part B, p. 1471, 1st edition, 1984.
144. G. E. Sanders and L. E. Swaim, "Atypical piscine Mycobacteriosis in Japanese medaka (Oryzias latipes),"Comparative Medicine, vol. 51, no. 2, pp. 171–175, 2001.
145. M. K. Stoskopf, Fish Medicine, WB Saunders, Philadelphia, Pa, USA, 1993.
146. D. T. Smith and H. P. Willett, "Other Mycobacterium species," in Zinsser Microbiology, K. Joklik, H. P. Willet, and D. B. Amos, Eds., pp. 674–698, Appleton-Century-Crofts, New York, NY, USA, 17th edition, 1980.
147. D. Huminer, S. D. Pitlik, C. Block, et al., "Aquarium-borne Mycobacterium marinum skin infection. Report of a case and review of the literature," Archives of Dermatology, vol. 122, no. 6, pp. 698–703, 1986.

148. M. Ucko, A. Colorni, H. Kvitt, A. Diamant, A. Zlotkin, and W. R. Knibb, "Strain variation inMycobacterium marinum fish isolates," Applied and Environmental Microbiology, vol. 68, no. 11, pp. 5281–5287, 2002.

149. M. J. Yip, J. L. Porter, J. A. M. Fyfe et al., "Evolution of Mycobacterium ulcerans and other mycolactone-producing mycobacteria from a common Mycobacterium marinum progenitor," Journal of Bacteriology, vol. 189, no. 5, pp. 2021–2029, 2007.

150. M. Ucko and A. Colorni, "Mycobacterium marinum infections in fish and humans in Israel," Journal of Clinical Microbiology, vol. 43, no. 2, pp. 892–895, 2005.

151. H. E. Volkman, H. Clay, D. Beery, J. C. W. Chang, D. R. Sherman, and L. Ramakrishnan, "Tuberculous granuloma formation is enhanced by a Mycobacterium virulence determinant," PLoS Biology, vol. 2, no. 11, article e367, 2004.

152. L. E. Swaim, L. E. Connolly, H. E. Volkman, O. Humbert, D. E. Born, and L. Ramakrishnan, "Mycobacterium marinum infection of adult zebrafish causes caseating granulomatous tuberculosis and is moderated by adaptive immunity," Infection and Immunity, vol. 74, no. 11, pp. 6108–6117, 2006.

153. T. P. Stinear, T. Seemann, P. F. Harrison et al., "Insights from the complete genome sequence ofMycobacterium marinum on the evolution of Mycobacterium tuberculosis," Genome Research, vol. 18, no. 5, pp. 729–741, 2008.

154. J. McFadden, "Recombination in mycobacteria," Molecular Microbiology, vol. 21, no. 2, pp. 205–211, 1996.

155. N. R. Salama, B. Shepherd, and S. Falkow, "Global transposon mutagenesis and essential gene analysis ofHelicobacter pylori," Journal of Bacteriology, vol. 186, no. 23, pp. 7926–7935, 2004.

156. P. Cossart and R. Jonquières, "Sortase, a universal target for therapeutic agents against Gram-positive bacteria?" Proceedings of the National Academy of Sciences of the United States of America, vol. 97, no. 10, pp. 5013–5015, 2000.

157. M. Maher, R. Palmer, F. Gannon, and T. Smith, "Relationship of a novel bacterial fish pathogen toStreptobacillus monilifomris and the fusobacteria group, based on 16S ribosomal RNA analysis,"Systematic and Applied Microbiology, vol. 18, no. 1, pp. 79–84, 1995.

158. J. L. Fryer and M. J. Mauel, "The rickettsia: an emerging group of pathogens in fish," Emerging Infectious Diseases, vol. 3, no. 2, pp. 137–144, 1997.
159. T. H. Birkbeck, L. A. Laidler, A. N. Grant, and D. I. Cox, "Pasteurella skyensis sp. nov., isolated from Atlantic salmon (Salmo salar L.)," International Journal of Systematic and Evolutionary Microbiology, vol. 52, no. 3, pp. 699–704, 2002.
160. C. Michel, J. F. Bernardet, P. Daniel, S. Chilmonczyk, M. Urdaci, and P. de Kinkelin, "Clinical and aetiological aspects of a summer enteritic syndrome associated with the sporulating segmented filamentous bacterium "Candidatus Arthromitus" in farmed rainbow trout, Oncorhynchus mykiss(Walbaum)," Journal of Fish Diseases, vol. 25, no. 9, pp. 533–543, 2002.
161. M. Riley, T. Abe, M. B. Arnaud et al., "Escherichia coli K-12: a cooperatively developed annotation snapshot—2005," Nucleic Acids Research, vol. 34, no. 1, pp. 1–9, 2006.

Chapter 2

Mercury Toxicity and Treatment: A Review of the Literature

Robin A. Bernhoft[1],

[1]Bernhoft Center for Advanced Medicine, Suite 208, 11677 San Vicente Boulevard, Los Angeles, CA 90049, USA

[2]Los Angeles Center for Advanced Medicine, Brentwood Gardens Suite 208, 11677 San Vicente Boulevard, Los Angeles, CA 90049, USA

ABSTRACT

Mercury is a toxic heavy metal which is widely dispersed in nature. Most human exposure results from fish consumption or dental amalgam. Mercury occurs in several chemical forms, with complex pharmacokinetics. Mercury is capable of inducing a wide range of clinical presentations. Diagnosis of mercury toxicity can be challenging but can be obtained with reasonable reliability. Effective therapies for clinical toxicity have been described.

INTRODUCTION

Mercury is a heavy metal of known toxicity, noted for inducing public health disasters in Minamata Bay, Japan [1] and in Iraq [2–4]. The clinical impact of smaller mercury exposures remains controversial. It exists in several forms: inorganic mercury, which includes metallic mercury and mercury vapor (Hg^0) and mercurous (Hg_2^{++}) or mercuric (Hg^{++}) salts; and organic mercury, which includes compounds in which mercury is bonded to a structure containing carbon atoms (methyl, ethyl, phenyl, or similar groups). The biological behavior, pharmacokinetics, and clinical significance of the various forms of mercury vary with chemical structure. There is some interconversion in vivo between the various forms of mercury. Inhaled elemental mercury vapor, for example, is easily absorbed through mucus membranes and the lung and rapidly oxidized to other forms (but not so quickly as to prevent considerable deposition of elemental mercury in the brain). Methyl mercury is easily absorbed through the gut and deposits in many tissues, but does not cross the blood-brain barrier as efficiently as elemental mercury; however, on entering the brain it is progressively demethylated to elemental mercury [5]. Mercury salts, in contrast, tend to be insoluble, relatively stable, and poorly absorbed.

Human toxicity varies with the form of mercury, the dose and the rate of exposure. The target organ for inhaled mercury vapor is primarily the brain [5]. Mercurous and mercuric salts chiefly damage the gut lining and kidney [5], while methyl mercury is widely distributed throughout the body [5]. Toxicity varies with dosage: large acute exposures to elemental mercury vapor induce severe pneumonitis, which in extreme cases can be fatal [5]. Low-grade chronic exposure to elemental or other forms of mercury induces subtler symptoms and clinical findings, as discussed hereinafter.

There is considerable controversy about the clinical significance of exposure to the various forms of mercury and some disagreement regarding techniques for clinical assessment of mercury burden. This paper is intended to review published data on these issues and to assess published clinical experience using DMPS to remove mercury from the human body. Most of the authors cited hereinafter consider DMPS to be a stronger chelator than DMSA, with one exception citing evidence that DMSA is more effective at removing organic mercury

[6]. This is a complicated issue. The absorption of DMPS and DMSA by ingestion is highly variable from one patient to the next; DMPS can be given intravenously, while DMSA cannot. DMPS is considerably safer than penicillamine or British anti-Lewisite, as discussed hereinafter. It is available for compounding in the United States and is available over the counter in Germany.

SOURCES OF MERCURY EXPOSURE

Most human exposure to mercury is caused by outgassing of mercury from dental amalgam, ingestion of contaminated fish, or occupational exposure, according to the World Health Organization [7, 8].

Mercury exists in nature primarily as elemental mercury or as a sulfide and is found in the earth's crust at approximately 0.5 parts per million. Atmospheric exposures occur from outgassing from rock or through volcanic activity. Human sources of atmospheric mercury include coal burning [9] and mining (mercury and gold in particular). Atmospheric elemental mercury settles in water, where it is converted by microorganisms into organic (methyl or ethyl) mercury, which is ingested by smaller creatures which are eventually consumed by larger fish. Fish at the top of the food chain (e.g., tuna, swordfish, or shark) may concentrate considerable mercury in their tissues.

Human mercury exposures occur chiefly [7, 8] through inhalation of elemental mercury vapor via occupational or dental amalgam exposure or through ingestion of mercury bonded to organic moieties (methyl, dimethyl, or ethyl mercury), primarily from seafood. Most human metallic mercury exposure comes from mercury vapor outgassing from amalgam fillings, at a rate of 2 to 28 micrograms per facet surface per day, of which about 80% is absorbed, according to the World Health Organization [7, 8] and Berglund et al. [10]. A less common source of mercury vapor is spilled mercury [11], and there is a report in the literature of Idiopathic Thrombocytopenic Purpura [12] caused by vacuuming spilled mercury (thereby producing a major acute exposure to mercury vapor).

Methyl and dimethyl mercury (organic mercury) usually originate from biological sources, chiefly fresh or salt water fish. Over three thousand lakes in the United States have been closed to fishing due to mercury contamination [5] and many species of ocean fish are also tainted with considerable concentrations of mercury [13].

PHARMACOKINETICS OF MERCURY EXPOSURE

Inorganic Mercury

Elemental or Metallic (Hg^0) Mercury

Approximately 80% of metallic mercury vapor outgassed from amalgams is absorbed through inhalation [10,14, 15], compared with about 7 to 10% absorption of ingested metallic mercury [5], and about 1% absorption of metallic mercury through skin contact [5]. On entry to the body, mercury vapor has great affinity for sulfhydryl groups and bonds to sulfur-containing amino acids throughout the body. Mercury vapor is transported to the brain [16], either dissolved in serum or adherent to red cell membranes. Metallic mercury passes easily through the blood brain barrier [17] and through the placenta, where it lodges in the fetal brain [18]. Metallic mercury is, however, rapidly oxidized to mercuric mercury on entry to the blood stream [5], although not so quickly as to prevent considerable uptake by the central nervous system while still in the metallic form.

In addition to the brain [16, 19–26], metallic mercury is also deposited in the thyroid [5, 19, 21], breast [27], myocardium [28, 29], muscles [5, 21], adrenals [5], liver [5, 30–32], kidneys [5, 7, 8, 19, 20, 23, 30–32], skin [5,7, 8], sweat glands [5], pancreas [5], enterocytes [5, 30], lungs [5, 23, 30], salivary glands [5], testes, and prostate [5] and may be associated with dysfunction of those organs. Mercury also has affinity for binding sites on the surface of T cells and for sulfhydryl groups influencing T cell function [33, 34]. Mercury deposits readily in placenta and fetal tissues and is found in breast milk. [5, 18, 31, 35]

Metallic mercury is largely excreted as mercuric mercury [5]. The excretory half lives of metallic and mercuric mercury vary widely, depending on the organ of deposition and redox state, with values ranging from a few days to several months [5], with some pools (e.g., CNS) having a half life exceeding several years [5]. Hair mercury does not correlate with brain content of metallic mercury [5]. These complexities make accurate assessment of body burden challenging (see Section 9 hereinafter).

Mercurous (Hg_2^{++}) Mercury

Mercurous mercury salt in the form of Hg_2Cl_2 (calomel) is poorly soluble in water and poorly absorbed by the intestine, although some portion is thought to undergo oxidation to more readily absorbable forms [36]. It is doubtful that mercurous mercury survives in the body, other than as a transitional form between metallic and mercuric mercury [5].

Some absorption evidently occurs, however, as calomel is occasionally associated with pink disease, or acrodynia.

Mercuric (Hg^{++}) Mercury

Historically, mercuric chloride ($HgCl_2$) was used as a preservative and for development of photographic film and was ingested accidentally or as a suicide measure. It is a component of some skin-lightening creams. Only about 2% of ingested mercuric chloride is absorbed initially [37], although it is believed that its corrosive effect on the intestine may increase permeability and, hence, absorption, with prolonged exposure [38]. Available data on skin penetration of mercuric mercury are insufficient to make quantitative comparison with ingestion or with metallic mercury.

Like metallic mercury, mercuric mercury in the bloodstream adheres to sulfhydryl groups on erythrocytes, metallothionein, or glutathione or is suspended in plasma [26]. Mercuric mercury does not cross the blood-brain barrier efficiently, but it does accumulate in quantity in the placenta, fetal tissues, and amniotic fluid [35]. Evidence exists showing transport of mercuric mercury via one or more amino acid transporters [39], particularly that for cysteine, which may account for accumulation in the brain [5]. Much of the body burden of mercuric mercury resides in the proximal convoluted renal tubule [40] bonded to metallothionein [41]. Significant deposition also occurs periportally in the liver [42] and lesser amounts in epithelial tissues, choroidal plexus, and testes.

Excretion of mercuric mercury is largely through urine and stool, although significant amounts are shed through sweat, tears, breast milk, and saliva [5, 43]. Half lives appear to be multiphasic, as with metallic mercury, with human studies suggesting an effective half life of 42 days for 80% of an oral tracer dose; the other 20% did not appear to have a measureable rate of excretion [44]. This may reflect demethylation to metallic mercury in the brain and other organs or mechanisms yet to be determined.

Organic Mercury Compounds

Most available data on organic mercury compounds refer to methyl mercury, which is a major source of human mercury exposure, is found naturally in fish, and is relatively stable. Ethyl mercury behaves in a similar fashion to methyl mercury at the cellular level, but with an excretory half life about one third as long [5].

Methyl mercury vapor is absorbed with similar (80%) efficiency as metallic mercury vapor [5]. Intestinal absorption of methyl mercury from fish is also fairly efficient, as is absorption through the skin [5]. On entry to the bloodstream, methyl mercury adheres to sulfhydryl groups, particularly to those in cysteine. Methyl mercury is deposited throughout the body, with equilibrium between blood and body occurring approximately four days after exposure [45]. Distribution to peripheral tissues seems to occur through one or more transporters, especially the cysteine transporter, probably adherent to the sulfhydryl group in cysteine [5].

Concentration of methyl mercury occurs in the brain, liver, kidneys, placenta, and fetus, especially in the fetal brain, as well as in peripheral nerves and bone marrow [5]. Deposited methyl mercury slowly undergoes demethylation to inorganic mercury [46].

The excretory half life of methyl mercury in man is about 70 days, with approximately 90% being excreted in stool. Some degree of enterohepatic circulation apparently occurs. Perhaps 20% of methyl mercury is excreted in breast milk, with the actual amount varying with severity of exposure [5]. Hair mercury reflects blood methyl mercury at the time of incorporation, but not elemental mercury [47], and hence is not a good index of total body burden [5], given the short half life of methyl mercury in blood.

Dimethyl mercury is also efficiently absorbed through the skin, and there is a reported death of a scientist caused by minimal skin contact [48].

TOXICITY

Inorganic Mercury

Metallic Mercury Vapor

Mercury in all forms poisons cellular function by altering the tertiary and quaternary structure of proteins and by binding with sulfhydryl and selenohydryl groups. Consequently, mercury can potentially impair function of any organ, or any subcellular structure. The chief target organ of mercury vapor is the brain, but peripheral nerve function, renal function, immune function, endocrine and muscle function, and several types of dermatitis have been described [49].

With massive acute exposure to mercury vapor, erosive bronchitis and bronchiolitis potentially leading to respiratory failure may be accompanied by CNS symptoms such as tremor or erethism [50].

Chronic exposure to clinically significant doses of mercury vapor usually produces neurological dysfunction. At low-level exposures, nonspecific symptoms like weakness, fatigue, anorexia, weight loss, and gastrointestinal disturbance have been described [51]. Higher exposure levels are associated with mercurial tremor: fine muscle fasciculations punctuated every few minutes by coarse shaking. Erethism may also be observed: severe behavior and personality changes, emotional excitability, loss of memory, insomnia, depression, fatigue, and in severe cases delirium and hallucination [10]. Gingivitis and copious salivation have been described [5].

These symptoms may regress with cessation of exposure, but in many cases do not. Persistent neurological symptoms are common [52].

Mercurous Mercury

Calomel (Hg_2Cl_2) is still used in some regions of the world as a laxative. Although poorly absorbed, some is converted to mercuric mercury, which is absorbed, and induces toxicity as expected with mercuric mercury.

Mercuric Mercury

Acute poisoning with mercuric salts (typically $HgCl_2$) generally targets the gastrointestinal tract and the kidneys. Extensive precipitation of enterocyte proteins occurs, with abdominal pain, vomiting, and bloody diarrhea with potential necrosis of the gut mucosa. This may produce death either from peritonitis or from septic or hypovolemic shock. Surviving patients commonly develop renal tubular necrosis with anuria [53].

Chronic poisoning with mercury salts is rare, usually also involving concomitant occupational exposure to mercury vapor. Kidney toxicity involves either renal tubular necrosis or autoimmune glomerulonephritis, or both [53]. Immune dysfunctions include hypersensitivity reactions to mercury exposure, including asthma and dermatitis, various types of autoimmunity [54], and suppression of natural killer cells [55] and disruption of various other lymphocyte subpopulations [5].

Brain dysfunction is less evident than with other forms of mercury. Thyroid dysfunction seems associated with inhibition of the 5′ deiodonases, with decreased free T3 and increased reverse T3 [56]. Accumulation in the testicles appears to inhibit spermatogenesis [57]. Atrophy and capillary damage have been described in thigh muscle [58].

Organic Mercury

Methyl mercury reacts with sulfhydryl groups throughout the body, therefore potentially interfering with the function of any cellular or subcellular structure. Mercury is believed to interfere with DNA transcription and protein synthesis [59], including protein synthesis in the developing brain, with destruction of endoplasmic reticulum and disappearance of ribosomes [60]. Evidence suggests disruption of numerous subcellular elements in the central nervous system and other organs and in mitochondria; adverse effects have also been described on heme synthesis [61], cell membrane integrity in many locations [5], free radical generation [27,62, 63], neurotransmitter disruption, and stimulation of neural excitoxins [5], resulting in damage to many parts of the brain and peripheral nervous system [5].

Methyl mercury has been associated with reduction in Natural Killer cell activity [64–67], as well as an imbalance in Th2 : Th1 ratios favoring autoimmunity [34, 68, 69]. Mercury is also possibly associated with disruption of DNA repair [5, 27]. The affinity of mercury for sulfhydryl groups of the mitochondrial oxidative phosphorylation complex [70] associated with destruction of mitochondrial membranes may contribute to chronic fatigue syndrome.

CLINICAL PRESENTATION

Inorganic

Elemental (Metallic) Mercury

Acute exposure to a large quantity of mercury vapor induces pneumonitis, as discussed previously. Symptoms of low-grade chronic exposure are more subtle and nonspecific: weakness, fatigue, anorexia, weight loss, and gastrointestinal distress [5], sometimes referred to as micromercurialism [71]. At higher exposures, the mercurial fine tremor punctuated by coarse shaking occurs; erethism, gingivitis, and excessive salivation have also been described [5], as has immune dysfunction [34].

Objective findings include altered evoked potentials and decreased peripheral nerve conduction velocity [72]. Objective measures of short-term memory may be inversely correlated with urinary mercury in chloralkali workers [73]. Reduced color vision and visual acuity have also been observed [74]. Changes in coordination, tremor, mental concentration capacity, facial expression, and emotional state are also described [75], as are polyarthritis, various forms of dermatitis, and a syndrome mimicking pheochromocytoma [76].

Subtler clinical findings among dentists have been documented, including delayed reaction time, poor fine motor control, and deficits in mental concentration, vocabulary, task switching, and the One Hole test, as well as mood lability, all correlating with urinary mercury excretion [75]. Evidence also links elemental mercury to depression, excessive anger, and anxiety [77], as well as acute myocardial infarction, lipid peroxidation, and carotid atherosclerosis, in Finland [78]; the Finnish experience may possibly be explained by dietary selenium deficiency, since selenium antagonizes mercury toxicity. Other investigators, however, have described associations between mercury and hypertension, lipid peroxidation, ischemic heart disease, and stroke [79].

Mercuric Salts

Ingestion of mercuric chloride produces extensive precipitation of intestinal mucosal proteins, mucosal necrosis, generalized abdominal pain, bloody diarrhea, and shock. If the patient survives, acute renal failure may follow [5].

Organic Mercury

Methyl mercury and ethyl mercury produce similar signs and symptoms. Most published data refer to methyl mercury. Symptoms relate more to magnitude of methyl mercury retention than to the rate of deposition. Acute exposures tend to have a latency period of one or more weeks; once acquired, toxic doses are cleared slowly, if at all [5].

Massive prenatal poisoning may induce a form of cerebral palsy [5]. Lesser prenatal doses have been associated with neurodevelopmental delays and cognitive deficits [80–82].

Postnatal exposures generate a range of symptoms ranging from paresthesias, with lesser exposures, to ataxia, visual, auditory, and extrapyramidal impairments with moderate exposures and clonic seizures in more severe exposures, as in Minamata [1] and Iraq [2–4].

Objective physical findings are similar to those seen with elemental mercury exposure.

LABORATORY ASSESSMENT OF MERCURY EXPOSURE

Given the wide range of excretory half lives of the various mercury pools, discussion of laboratory assessment will combine the various forms into one discussion. It is important to recall that blood, hair, and urine mercury levels reflect recent exposure and do not correlate with total body burden [83–86]. Blood and urine levels correlate fairly well to each other, but not to total body burden [87]. With half life of all mercury pools in the blood estimated to be in the range of three to five days [88], during which either excretion or deposition in solid organs occurs, more accurate means of estimating body burden have been required.

That being said, the US federal biological exposure index (BEI) is currently set at 50 mcg/L urine. Aside from the obvious problems associated with basing a monitoring index on a measurement which only reflects current or recent exposure, and not overall body burden, several clinical studies show objective symptoms well below 50 mcg/L, with many proband values extending down into the low end of the reference range for urinary mercury excretion [75, 89–94], effectively rendering the US federal BEI useless for clinical or investigational purposes. Similar criticisms have been made of the EPA Reference Dose for methylmercury [95]. As summarized by Kazantzis, "it has not been possible to set a level for mercury in blood or urine below which mercury related symptoms will not occur" [96].

Because of these difficulties, provocation with a chelator has been proposed as providing a more reliable estimate of body burden, and DMPS (2,3 Dimercapto-1-Propanesulfonate) has been found by a number of investigators to provide a reliable estimate of body burden, safer than British Anti-Lewisite and more potent than DMSA [75, 97–101].

DMPS: SAFETY

DMPS is an analog of British Anti-Lewisite (BAL) with high affinity for mercury. Due to its superior safety, it has been widely used in Germany for the past fifty years and is available over the counter in that country.

Protocols determining the pharmacokinetics of DMPS and evaluating its use for diagnostic purposes have been published in Germany [101], Sweden [102, 103], New Zealand [100], and Mexico [104] and in the United States [105–109].

Maiorino et al. [106] gave his volunteers DMPS 300 mg orally; over 90% of the absorbed DMPS was converted rapidly to disulfide forms. Published absorption of ingested DMPS varies from 39% [107] to 60% [110]. The excretory half life of unaltered DMPS was 4 . 4 ± 1 . 1 hours. The excretory half life of the disulfide forms of DMPS was9 . 9 ± 1 . 6hours.

Hurlbut et al.'s [107] volunteers were given an unusually large dose of DMPS (3 mg/kg intravenously over 5 minutes). Two subjects had a transient 20 mmHg drop in systolic blood pressure during infusion, without other changes in vital signs. Excretory half life of unaltered DMPS ranged from 1.3 to 4.0 hours. Half life of the altered DMPS was from 19.8 to 37.5 hours.

In each of the cited studies, mercury output following provocation with DMPS correlated significantly with amalgam number and/or occupational or dietary exposure. There were no significant complications in any of the trials. Consequently, all the investigators but one [111] concluded that urine output provoked by DMPS represented a fair estimate of body burden.

DMPS: EFFICACY

Each of the test trials cited in the previous section and others [112] showed statistically significant increases in urinary mercury output with administration of DMPS. With prolonged treatment, evidence of decreased body burden has been inferred [113].

Several controlled clinical trials support this conclusion. The largest was undertaken in the Phillippines in a gold mining area [114]. Workers in gold mining who sustained ongoing exposure to elemental mercury were compared to people living downstream who ate fish, which contained considerable methyl mercury, and to controls without significant known mercury exposure. Probands from the two exposed areas were chosen with elevated blood, urine and hair mercury levels, and appropriate symptoms (tremor, sleeplessness, memory loss, etc.) [115]; controls had normal levels and were asymptomatic.

One hundred six probands completed the fourteen-day trial with oral DMPS 400 mg per day. The only complication was an allergic rash in one patient, who was excluded from the trial. Blood mercury did not decrease during the trial, despite increases in urine mercury up to 85-fold.

Despite the short (fourteen-day) duration of the trial, significant improvements were observed in objective measures like hypomimia, Romberg test, tests for tremor and ataxia, pencil tapping, and Frostig visual perception. Most of the patients reported subjective improvement in memory, sleeplessness, metallic taste, fatigue, anxiety, and paresthesias. Treatment efficacy was similar in the metallic mercury group (miners) and in the methyl mercury group (downstream fish eaters). Similar results were presented in a parallel study by Drasch et al. [115].

A university case report from the United States of treatment of occupational exposures to mercury vapor [116] showed relief of muscle twitching, arthralgias, paresthesias, night sweats, weight loss, and excessive salivation following two weeks of oral DMPS 100 mg TID followed by DMPS 100 mg QID for an additional six weeks. Reduction of symptoms closely paralleled urine mercury output, which tapered over time.

DISCUSSION

Mercury toxicity is not often included in the differential diagnosis of common subjective complaints such as fatigue, anxiety, depression, odd paresthesias, weight loss, memory loss, and difficulty concentrating, but these are the symptoms of low-grade chronic mercury exposure described by the investigators cited previously. Given the ability of the various forms of mercury to deposit in most parts of the human body, the range of symptoms potentially caused by mercury is quite large.

Animal studies linking mercury toxicity to neurodegenerative diseases [117, 118] raise clinical concern, as do a series of associations between mercury and neurodegenerative diseases in humans [119–123].

Mercury exposure is not insignificant according to WHO, as cited previously, and the NHANES reports suggest widespread exposure in the United States, especially among women [124, 125].

Diagnosis of mercury overload is difficult. The commonly used modalities (blood, urine, and/or hair levels) do not correlate with total body burden and offer little diagnostically useful information. Provocation with DMPS appears to offer a more accurate assessment of body burden.

Since provocation is safe and inexpensive, indications for provocation must rest on clinical grounds: does the patient have multiple, vague symptoms similar to those described in the mercury literature, without other plausible, and potentially reversible, explanation? Is there a significant history of mercury exposure: multiple amalgam fillings, high seafood intake, and history of multiple thimerosal-containing vaccinations or significant occupational exposures? Is there a family history of Alzheimer's, Parkinson's, or other diseases with postulated links to mercury exposure? Is there a history of known glutathione transferase (GST) polymorphisms, which decrease the body's ability to clear heavy metals like mercury?

If so, then provocation with a chelator may be indicated. Published protocols [126–130] exist which call for provocation with DMPS with or without EDTA, in sequence. These are designed for safety, and for diagnostic breadth. DMPS has far better affinity for mercury than EDTA, but EDTA is more effective in removing lead, cadmium, nickel, and other toxic metals. Provocation with both gives a fuller picture of overall metal burden. Patients with GST enzyme abnormalities may also receive glutathione to expedite excretion of chelated metal. For unknown reasons, patients with GST polymorphisms tend to excrete mercury later in their course of treatment than other heavy metals [131]; this can sometimes produce early false negatives for mercury, due to preferential excretion of lead and other metals. All effective chelation protocols call for replacement of beneficial minerals, which are also removed by EDTA and DMPS.

There are currently no consensus criteria for the diagnosis of mercury overload, nor for overload of other toxic metals. Clinicians who specialize in this area generally consider a provoked urine metal output more than 2 standard deviations above the NHANES reference range a positive result.

Further research is required to clarify the relation between provoked urine results and clinical disease and to document clinical outcomes.

REFERENCES

1. Environmental Health Department, Ministry of the Environment, Minimata Disease: The History and Measures, Ministry of the Environment, Government of Japan, Tokyo, Japan, 2002.
2. F. Bakir, S. F. Damluji, and I. Amin Zaki, "Methylmercury poisoning in Iraq: an interuniversity report,"Science, vol. 181, no. 4096, pp. 230–241, 1973.
3. S. B. Skerfving and J. F. Copplestone, "Poisoning caused by the consumption of organomercury dressed seed in Iraq," Bulletin of the World Health Organization, vol. 54, no. 1, pp. 101–112, 1976.
4. T. W. Clarkson, L. Magos, and C. Cox, "Tests of efficacy of antidotes for removal of methylmercury in human poisoning during the Iraq outbreak," Journal of Pharmacology and Experimental Therapeutics, vol. 218, no. 1, pp. 74–83, 1981.
5. M. Berlin, R. K. Zalups, and B. A. Fowler, "Mercury," in Handbook on the Toxicology of Metals, G. F. Nordberg, B. A. Fowler, M. Nordberg, and L. T. Friberg, Eds., chapter 33, Elsevier, New York, NY, USA, 3rd edition, 2007.
6. H. V. Aposhian, "DMSA and DMPS—water soluble antidotes for heavy metal poisoning," Annual Review of Pharmacology and Toxicology, vol. 23, pp. 193–215, 1983.
7. World Health Organization, "Inorganic mercury: environmental health criteria 118," in International Programme on Chemical Safety, World Health Organization, Geneva, Switzerland, 1991.
8. M. Richardson, The Safety of Dental Amalgam, ISBN 0-662-24873-2, Minister of Health, Canada, 1996.
9. H. M. Boylan, R. D. Cain, and H. M. Kingston, "A new method to assess mercury emissions: a study of three coal-fired electric-generating power station configurations," Journal of the Air and Waste Management Association, vol. 53, no. 11, pp. 1318–1325, 2003.
10. A. Berglund, L. Pohl, S. Olsson, and M. Bergman, "Determination of the rate of release of intra-oral mercury vapor from amalgam," Journal of Dental Research, vol. 67, no. 9, pp. 1235–1242, 1988.

11. P. Zeitz, M. F. Orr, and W. E. Kaye, "Public health consequences to mercury spills: hazardous substances emergency events surveillance system, 1993–1998," Environmental Health Perspectives, vol. 110, no. 2, pp. 129–132, 2002.
12. J. G. Schwartz, T. E. Snider, and M. M. Montiel, "Toxicity of a family from vacuumed mercury,"American Journal of Emergency Medicine, vol. 10, no. 3, pp. 258–261, 1992.
13. J. Burger, C. Jeitner, and M. Gochfeld, "Locational differences in mercury and selenium levels in 19 species of saltwater fish from New Jersey," Journal of Toxicology and Environmental Health, vol. 74, no. 13, pp. 863–874, 2011.
14. F. N. Kudsk, "The influence of ethyl alcohol on the absorption of mercury vapour from the lungs in man," Acta Pharmacologica et Toxicologica, vol. 23, no. 2, pp. 263–274, 1965.
15. J. B. Hursh, T. W. Clarkson, and M. G. Cherian, "Clearance of mercury (Hg-197, Hg-203) vapor inhaled by human subjects," Archives of Environmental Health, vol. 31, no. 6, pp. 302–309, 1976.
16. D. W. Eggleston and M. Nylander, "Correlation of dental amalgam with mercury in brain tissue," The Journal of Prosthetic Dentistry, vol. 58, no. 6, pp. 704–707, 1987.
17. G. F. Nordberg and F. Serenius, "Distribution of inorganic mercury in the guinea pig brain," Acta Pharmacologica et Toxicologica, vol. 27, no. 4, pp. 269–283, 1969.
18. T. W. Clarkson, L. Magos, and M. R. Greenwood, "The transport of elemental mercury into fetal tissues," Biology of the Neonate, vol. 21, no. 3, pp. 239–244, 1972.
19. G. Guzzi, M. Grandi, C. Cattaneo et al., "Dental amalgam and mercury levels in autopsy tissues: food for thought," American Journal of Forensic Medicine and Pathology, vol. 27, no. 1, pp. 42–45, 2006.
20. J. W. Reinhardt, "Side-effects: mercury contribution to body burden from dental amalgam," Advances in Dental Research, vol. 6, pp. 110–113, 1992.
21. L. Björkman, B. F. Lundekvam, T. Lægreid et al., "Mercury in human brain, blood, muscle and toenails in relation to exposure: an autopsy study," Environmental Health, vol. 6, article 30, 2007.

22. D. Wenstrup, W. D. Ehmann, and W. R. Markesbery, "Trace element imbalances in isolated subcellular fractions of Alzheimer's disease brains," Brain Research, vol. 533, no. 1, pp. 125–131, 1990.
23. M. Nylander, L. Friberg, and B. Lind, "Mercury concentrations in the human brain and kidneys in relation to exposure from dental amalgam fillings," Swedish Dental Journal, vol. 11, no. 5, pp. 179–187, 1987.
24. J. Mutter, A. Curth, J. Naumann, R. Deth, and H. Walach, "Does inorganic mercury play a role in Alzheimer's disease? A systematic review and an integrated molecular mechanism," Journal of Alzheimer's Disease, vol. 22, no. 2, pp. 357–374, 2010.
25. R. L. Siblerud, "The relationship between mercury from dental amalgam and mental health," American Journal of Psychotherapy, vol. 43, no. 4, pp. 575–587, 1989.
26. T. W. Clarkson, J. Gatzy, and E. Dalton, UR-582, Division of Radiation Chemistry and Toxicology, University of Rochester Atomic Energy Project, Rochester, NY, USA, 1961.
27. M. E. Crespo-López, G. L. Macêdo, S. I. D. Pereira et al., "Mercury and human genotoxicity: critical considerations and possible molecular mechanisms," Pharmacological Research, vol. 60, no. 4, pp. 212–220, 2009.
28. A. Frustaci, N. Magnavita, C. Chimenti et al., "Marked elevation of myocardial trace elements in idiopathic dilated cardiomyopathy compared with secondary cardiac dysfunction," Journal of the American College of Cardiology, vol. 33, no. 6, pp. 1578–1583, 1999.
29. N. Matsuo, T. Suzuki, and H. Akagi, "Mercury concentration in organs of contemporary Japanese,"Archives of Environmental Health, vol. 44, no. 5, pp. 298–303, 1989.
30. L. J. Hahn, R. Kloiber, M. J. Vimy, Y. Takahashi, and F. L. Lorscheider, "Dental 'silver' tooth fillings: a source of mercury exposure revealed by whole-body image scan and tissue analysis," FASEB Journal, vol. 3, no. 14, pp. 2641–2646, 1989.
31. M. J. Vimy, Y. Takahashi, and F. L. Lorscheider, "Maternal-fetal distribution of mercury released from dental amalgam fillings," American Journal of Physiology, vol. 258, no. 4, pp. R939–R945, 1990.

32. G. Danscher, P. Horsted-Bindslev, and J. Rungby, "Traces of mercury in organs from primates with amalgam fillings," Experimental and Molecular Pathology, vol. 52, no. 3, pp. 291–299, 1990.

33. P. Hultman, "Immunotoxicology of metals," in Handbook on the Toxicology of Metals, G. F. Nordberg, B. A. Fowler, M. Nordberg, and L. T. Friberg, Eds., pp. 205–206, Elsevier, Amsterdam, The Netherlands, 3rd edition, 2007.

34. S. H. Park, S. Araki, A. Nakata et al., "Effects of occupational metallic mercury vapour exposure on suppressor-inducer (CD4+CD45RA+) T lymphocytes and CD57+CD16+ natural killer cells," International Archives of Occupational and Environmental Health, vol. 73, no. 8, pp. 537–542, 2000.

35. T. Suzuki, T. I. Takemoto, S. Shishido, and K. Kani, "Mercury in human amniotic fluid," Scandinavian Journal of Work, Environment and Health, vol. 3, no. 1, pp. 32–35, 1977.

36. Goodman and Gilman, The Pharmacological Basis of Therapeutics, 8th edition, 1990.

37. T. Norseth and T. W. Clarkson, "Intestinal transport of ^{203}Hg-labeled methyl mercury chloride. Role of biotransformation in rats," Archives of Environmental Health, vol. 22, no. 5, pp. 568–577, 1971.

38. K. Kostial, D. Kello, and S. Jugo, "Influence of age on metal metabolism and toxicity," Environmental Health Perspectives, vol. 25, pp. 81–86, 1978.

39. T. Jansson, "Amino acid transporters in the human placenta," Pediatric Research, vol. 49, no. 2, pp. 141–147, 2001.

40. R. Taugner, K. zum Winkel, and J. Iravani, "The localization of mercuric chloride concentration in the rat kidney," Virchows Archiv, vol. 340, no. 4, pp. 369–383, 1966.

41. M. G. Cherian and T. W. Clarkson, "Radioactive mercury distribution in biological fluids and excretion in human subjects after inhalation of mercury vapor," Archives of Environmental Health, vol. 33, no. 3, pp. 109–114, 1978.

42. M. Berlin and S. Ullberg, "Accumulation and retention of mercury in the mouse. I. An autoradiographic study after a single intravenous injection of mercuric chloride," Archives of Environmental Health, vol. 6, pp. 589–601, 1963.

43. K. A. Björnberg, M. Vahter, B. Berglund, B. Niklasson, M. Blennow, and G. Sandborgh-Englund, "Transport of methylmercury and inorganic mercury to the fetus and breast-fed infant," Environmental Health Perspectives, vol. 113, no. 10, pp. 1381–1385, 2005.
44. T. Rahola, T. Hattula, and A. Lorolainen, "The Elimination of ^{203}Hg-methylmercury in man,"Scandinavian Journal of Clinical and Laboratory Investigation, vol. 27, supplement 116, p. 77, 1971.
45. T. G. Kershaw, T. W. Clarkson, and P. H. Dhahir, "The relationship between blood levels and dose of methylmercury in man," Archives of Environmental Health, vol. 35, no. 1, pp. 28–36, 1980.
46. I. Suda and H. Takahashi, "Degradation of methyl and ethyl mercury into inorganic mercury by other reactive oxygen species besides hydroxyl radical," Archives of Toxicology, vol. 66, no. 1, pp. 34–39, 1992.
47. M. Berglund, B. Lind, K. A. Björnberg, B. Palm, O. Einarsson, and M. Vahter, "Inter-individual variations of human mercury exposure biomarkers: a cross-sectional assessment," Environmental Health, vol. 4, article 20, 2005.
48. D. W. Nierenberg, R. E. Nordgren, M. B. Chang et al., "Delayed cerebellar disease and death after accidental exposure to dimethylmercury," New England Journal of Medicine, vol. 338, no. 23, pp. 1672–1676, 1998.
49. M. Berlin, Dental Materials and Health, Statens Offentliga Utredningar, Stockholm, 2003.
50. R. Garnier, J. M. Fuster, and F. Conso, "Acute mercury vapour poisoning," Toxicological European Research, vol. 3, no. 2, pp. 77–86, 1981.
51. L. Friberg and G. F. Nordberg, Eds., Mercury in the Environment, CRC Press, Boca Raton, Fla, USA, 1972.
52. G. Baldi, E. C. Vigliani, and N. Zurlo, "Mercury poisoning in hat industry," La Medicina del Lavoro, vol. 44, no. 4, pp. 160–199, 1953.
53. J. L. Barnes, E. M. McDowell, and J. S. McNeil, "Studies on the pathophysiology of acute renal failure. V. Effect of chronic saline loading on the progression of proximal tubular injury

and functional impairment following administration of mercuric chloride in the rat," Virchows Archiv Abteilung B Cell Pathology, vol. 32, no. 3, pp. 233–260, 1980.

54. G. de Vos, S. Abotaga, Z. Liao, E. Jerschow, and D. Rosenstreich, "Selective effect of mercury on Th2-type cytokine production in humans," Immunopharmacology and Immunotoxicology, vol. 29, no. 3-4, pp. 537–548, 2007.
55. N. G. Ilback, J. Sundberg, and A. Oskarsson, "Methyl mercury exposure via placenta and milk impairs natural killer (NK) cell function in newborn rats," Toxicology Letters, vol. 58, no. 2, pp. 149–158, 1991.
56. D. G. Ellingsen, J. Efskind, E. Haug, Y. Thomassen, I. Martinsen, and P. I. Gaarder, "Effects of low mercury vapour exposure on the thyroid function in chloralkali workers," Journal of Applied Toxicology, vol. 20, no. 6, pp. 483–489, 2000.
57. M. V. Rao and P. S. N. Sharma, "Protective effect of vitamin E against mercuric chloride reproductive toxicity in male mice," Reproductive Toxicology, vol. 15, no. 6, pp. 705–712, 2001.
58. E. Nadorfy-Lopez, S. H. Torres, H. Finol, M. Mendez, and B. Bello, "Skeletal muscle abnormalities associated with occupational exposure to mercury vapours," Histology and Histopathology, vol. 15, no. 3, pp. 673–682, 2000.
59. D. W. Gruenwedel and D. S. Lu, "Changes in the sedimentation characteristics of DNA due to methylmercuration," Biochemical and Biophysical Research Communications, vol. 40, no. 3, pp. 542–548, 1970.
60. S. P. Herman, R. Klein, F. A. Talley, and M. R. Krigman, "An ultrastructural study of methylmercury-induced primary sensory neuropathy in the rat," Laboratory Investigation, vol. 28, no. 1, pp. 104–118, 1973.
61. B. A. Fowler and J. S. Woods, "Ultrastructural and biochemical changes in renal mitochondria during chronic oral methyl mercury exposure. The relationship to renal function," Experimental and Molecular Pathology, vol. 27, no. 3, pp. 403–412, 1977.
62. G. Olivieri, C. Brack, F. Müller-Spahn et al., "Mercury induces cell cytotoxicity and oxidative stress and increases β- amyloid secretion and tau phosphorylation in SHSY5Y neuroblastoma

cells," Journal of Neurochemistry, vol. 74, no. 1, pp. 231–236, 2000.

63. S. Yee and B. H. Choi, "Oxidative stress in neurotoxic effects of methylmercury poisoning,"NeuroToxicology, vol. 17, no. 1, pp. 17–26, 1996.
64. N. G. Ilback, J. Sundberg, and A. Oskarsson, "Methyl mercury exposure via placenta and milk impairs natural killer (NK) cell function in newborn rats," Toxicology Letters, vol. 58, no. 2, pp. 149–158, 1991.
65. S. H. Park, S. Araki, A. Nakata et al., "Effects of occupational metallic mercury vapour exposure on suppressor-inducer (CD4+CD45RA+)T lymphocytes and CD57+CD16+ natural killer cells,"International Archives of Occupational and Environmental Health, vol. 73, no. 8, pp. 537–542, 2000.
66. L. Santarelli, M. Bracci, and E. Mocchegiani, "In vitro and in vivo effects of mercuric chloride on thymic endocrine activity, NK and NKT cell cytotoxicity, cytokine profiles (IL-2, IFN-γ, IL-6): role of the nitric oxide-l-arginine pathway," International Immunopharmacology, vol. 6, no. 3, pp. 376–389, 2006.
67. L.Vimercati, L. Santarelli, G. Pesola et al., "Monocyte-macrophage system and polymorphonuclear leukocytes in workers exposed to low levels of metallic mercury," Science of the Total Environment, vol. 270, no. 1–3, pp. 157–163, 2001.
68. G. de Vos, S. Abotaga, Z. Liao, E. Jerschow, and D. Rosenstreich, "Selective effect of mercury on Th2-type cytokine production in humans," Immunopharmacology and Immunotoxicology, vol. 29, no. 3-4, pp. 537–548, 2007.
69. T. Tanigawa, H. Takehashi, and A. Nakata, "Naïve (CD4+CD45RA+) T cell subpopulation is susceptible to various types of hazardous substances in the workplace," International journal of immunopathology and pharmacology, vol. 17, supplement 2, pp. 109–114, 2004.
70. D. W. Gruenwedel and M. K. Cruickshank, "Effect of methylmercury(II) on the synthesis of deoxyribonucleic acid, ribonucleic acid and protein in HeLa S3 cells," Biochemical Pharmacology, vol. 28, no. 5, pp. 651–655, 1979.
71. L. Friberg and G. F. Nordberg, Eds., Mercury in the Environment, CRC Press, Boca Raton, Fla, USA, 1972.

72. A. Andersen, D. G. Ellingsen, T. Morland, and H. Kjuus, "A neurological and neurophysiological study of chloralkali workers previously exposed to mercury vapour," Acta Neurologica Scandinavica, vol. 88, no. 6, pp. 427–433, 1993.
73. P. J. Smith, G. D. Langolf, and J. Goldberg, "Effects of occupational exposure to elemental mercury on short term memory," British Journal of Industrial Medicine, vol. 40, no. 4, pp. 413–419, 1983.
74. A. Cavalleri, L. Belotti, F. Gobba, G. Luzzana, P. Rosa, and P. Seghizzi, "Colour vision loss in workers exposed to elemental mercury vapour," Toxicology Letters, vol. 77, no. 1–3, pp. 351–356, 1995.
75. D. Echeverria, N. J. Heyer, M. D. Martin, C. A. Naleway, J. S. Woods, and A. C. Bittner Jr., "Behavioral effects of low-level exposure to Hg° among dentists," Neurotoxicology and Teratology, vol. 17, no. 2, pp. 161–168, 1995.
76. C. Kosan, A. K. Topaloglu, and B. Ozkan, "Chronic mercury intoxication simulating pheochromocytoma: effect of captopril on urinary mercury excretion," Pediatrics International, vol. 43, no. 4, pp. 429–430, 2001.
77. R. L. Siblerud, J. Motl, and E. Kienholz, "Psychometric evidence that mercury from silver dental fillings may be an etiological factor in depression, excessive anger, and anxiety," Psychological Reports, vol. 74, no. 1, pp. 67–80, 1994.
78. J. T. Salonen, K. Seppanen, K. Nyyssonen et al., "Intake of mercury from fish, lipid peroxidation, and the risk of myocardial infarction and coronary, cardiovascular, and any death in Eastern Finnish men,"Circulation, vol. 91, no. 3, pp. 645–655, 1995.
79. H. M. Chan and G. M. Egeland, "Fish consumption, mercury exposure, and heart diseases," Nutrition Reviews, vol. 62, no. 2, pp. 68–72, 2004.
80. S. Booth and D. Zeller, "Mercury, food webs, and marine mammals: implications of diet and climate change for human health," Environmental Health Perspectives, vol. 113, no. 5, pp. 521–526, 2005.
81. P. Grandjean, P. Weihe, R. F. White et al., "Cognitive deficit in 7-year-old children with prenatal exposure to methylmercury," Neurotoxicology and Teratology, vol. 19, no. 6, pp. 417–428, 1997.

82. G. B. Ramirez, O. Pagulayan, H. Akagi et al., "Tagum study II: follow-up study at two years of age after prenatal exposure to mercury," Pediatrics, vol. 111, no. 3, pp. 289–295, 2003.
83. A. Aitio, S. Valkonen, H. Kivisto, and E. Yrjanheikki, "Effect of occupational mercury exposure on plasma lysosomal hydrolases," International Archives of Occupational and Environmental Health, vol. 53, no. 2, pp. 139–147, 1983.
84. M. Berlin, J. Fazackerley, and G. Nordberg, "The uptake of mercury in the brains of mammals exposed to mercury vapor and to mercuric salts," Archives of Environmental Health, vol. 18, no. 5, pp. 719–729, 1969.
85. M. Berlin and S. Gibson, "Renal uptake, excretion, and retention of mercury. I. A study in the rabbit during infusion of mercuric chloride," Archives of Environmental Health, vol. 6, pp. 617–625, 1963.
86. G. Drasch, E. Wanghofer, and G. Roider, "Are blood, urine, hair, and muscle valid biomonitors for the internal burden of men with the heavy metals mercury, lead and cadmium? An investigation on 150 deceased," Trace Elements in Medicine, vol. 14, no. 3, pp. 116–123, 1997.
87. R. G. Smith, A. J. Vorwald, L. S. Patil, and T. F. Mooney, "Effects of exposure to mercury in the manufacture of chlorine," American Industrial Hygiene Association journal, vol. 31, no. 6, pp. 687–700, 1970.
88. "3rd National report on human exposure to environmental chemicals," Tech. Rep., Centers for Disease Control and Prevention, 2005.
89. M. W. Haut, L. A. Morrow, D. Pool, T. S. Callahan, J. S. Haut, and M. D. Franzen, "Neurobehavioral effects of acute exposure to inorganic mercury vapor," Applied Neuropsychology, vol. 6, no. 4, pp. 193–200, 1999.
90. D. B. Chaffin, D. B. Dinman, J. M. Miller, et al., "Final report NIOSH," Tech. Rep. contract no HSM-099-71-62, University of Michigan, Ann Arbor, Mich, USA, 1973.
91. M. Meyer-Baron, M. Schaeper, and A. Seeber, "A meta-analysis for neurobehavioural results due to occupational mercury exposure," Archives of Toxicology, vol. 76, no. 3, pp. 127–136, 2002.

92. R. Lucchini, I. Cortesi, P. Facco et al., "Neurotoxic effect of exposure to low doses of mercury," Medicina del Lavoro, vol. 93, no. 3, pp. 202–214, 2002.
93. D. Echeverria, H. Vasken Aposhian, J. S. Woods et al., "Neurobehavioral effects from exposure to dental amalgam Hg^0: new distinctions between recent exposure and Hg body burden," FASEB Journal, vol. 12, no. 11, pp. 971–980, 1998.
94. H. A. Roels, P. Hoet, and D. Lison, "Usefulness of biomarkers of exposure to inorganic mercury, lead, or cadmium in controlling occupational and environmental risks of nephrotoxicity," Renal Failure, vol. 21, no. 3-4, pp. 251–262, 1999.
95. D. C. Rice, "The US EPA reference dose for methylmercury: sources of uncertainty," Environmental Research, vol. 95, no. 3, pp. 406–413, 2004.
96. G. Kazantzis, "Mercury exposure and early effects: an overview," Medicina del Lavoro, vol. 93, no. 3, pp. 139–147, 2002.
97. H. V. Aposhian, A. Arroyo, M. E. Cebrian et al., "DMPS-arsenic challenge test. I: increased urinary excretion of monomethylarsonic acid in humans given dimercaptopropane sulfonate," Journal of Pharmacology and Experimental Therapeutics, vol. 282, no. 1, pp. 192–200, 1997.
98. G. Kazantzis, "Diagnosis and treatment of metal poisoning—general aspects," in Handbook on The Toxicology of Metals, G. F. Nordberg, Ed., chapter 15, pp. 313–314, Elsevier, New York, NY, USA, 3rd edition, 2007.
99. V. R. Schiele, K. H. Schaller, and D. Weltle, "Aus dem Institut fur Arbeits-und Sozialmedizin und der Poliklinik fur Berufskrankheiten de Universitat Erlangen-Nurnberg," pp. 249–251, 1989.
100. M. Godfrey and N. Campbell, "Confirmation of mercury retention and toxicity using 2,3 dimercapto-1-propane sulphonic acid sodium salt (DMPS)," Journal of Advancement in Medicine, vol. 7, no. 1, pp. 19–30, 1994.
101. M. Daunderer, "Mobilization test for environmental metal poisonings," Forum des Praktischen und Allgemein-Arztes, vol. 28, no. 3, pp. 88–94, 1989.
102. M. Molin, A. Schutz, S. Skerfving, and G. Sallsten, "Mobilized mercury in subjects with varying exposure to elemental

mercury vapour," International Archives of Occupational and Environmental Health, vol. 63, no. 3, pp. 187–192, 1991.

103. J. Aaseth, D. Jacobsen, O. Andersen, and E. Wickstrom, "Treatment of mercury and lead poisonings with dimercaptosuccinic acid and sodium dimercaptopropanesulfonate. A review," Analyst, vol. 120, no. 3, pp. 853–854, 1995.

104. O. Torres-Alanis, L. Garza-Ocanas, and A. Pineyro-Lopez, "Evaluation of urinary mercury excretion after administration of 2,3-dimercaptol-propane sulfonic acid to occupationally exposed men," Journal of Toxicology—Clinical Toxicology, vol. 33, no. 6, pp. 717–720, 1995.

105. H. V. Aposhian, R. M. Maiorino, M. Rivera et al., "Human studies with the chelating agents, DMPS and DMSA," Journal of Toxicology—Clinical Toxicology, vol. 30, no. 4, pp. 505–528, 1992.

106. R. M. Maiorino, R. C. Dart, D. E. Carter, and H. V. Aposhian, "Determination and metabolism of dithiol chelating agents. XII. Metabolism and pharmacokinetics of sodium 2,3-dimercaptopropane-1-sulfonate in humans," Journal of Pharmacology and Experimental Therapeutics, vol. 259, no. 2, pp. 808–814, 1991.

107. K. M. Hurlbut, R. M. Maiorino, M. Mayersohn, R. C. Dart, D. C. Bruce, and H. V. Aposhian, "Determination and metabolism of dithiol chelating agents XVI: pharmacokinetics of 2,3-dimercapto-1-propanesulfonate after intravenous administration to human volunteers," Journal of Pharmacology and Experimental Therapeutics, vol. 268, no. 2, pp. 662–668, 1994.

108. H. V. Aposhian, "Mobilization of mercury and arsenic in humans by sodium 2,3-dimercapto-1-propane sulfonate (DMPS)," Environmental Health Perspectives, vol. 106, no. 4, pp. 1017–1025, 1998.

109. H. V. Aposhian, R. M. Maiorino, D. Gonzalez-Ramirez et al., "Mobilization of heavy metals by newer, therapeutically useful chelating agents," Toxicology, vol. 97, no. 1–3, pp. 23–38, 1995.

110. "2,3 Dimercapto-1-propane sulfonic acid (DMPS) in the treatment of heavy metal poisoning," FDA Docket 98-n-0182 entry for DMPS and Nguyen H. T., 1999,http://www.fda.gov/ohrms/dockets/DOCKETS/98n0182/nom005b.pdf.

111. G. Sallsten, L. Barregard, and A. Schutz, "Clearance half life of mercury in urine after the cessation of long term occupational exposure: influence of a chelating agent (DMPS) on excretion of mercury in urine," Occupational and Environmental Medicine, vol. 51, no. 5, pp. 337–342, 1994.

112. O. Torres-Alanis, L. Garza-Ocanas, and A. Pineyro-Lopez, "Evaluation of urinary mercury excretion after administration of 2,3-dimercaptol-propane sulfonic acid to occupationally exposed men," Journal of Toxicology—Clinical Toxicology, vol. 33, no. 6, pp. 717–720, 1995.

113. D. Gonzalez-Ramirez, M. Zuniga-Charles, A. Narro-Juarez et al., "DMPS (2,3-dimercaptopropane-1-sulfonate, dimaval) decreases the body burden of mercury in humans exposed to mercurous chloride,"Journal of Pharmacology and Experimental Therapeutics, vol. 287, no. 1, pp. 8–12, 1998.

114. S. Böse-O'Reilly, G. Drasch, C. Beinhoff et al., "The Mt. Diwata study on the Philippines 2000—Treatment of mercury intoxicated inhabitants of a gold mining area with DMPS (2,3-Dimercapto-1-propane-sulfonic acid, Dimaval®)," Science of the Total Environment, vol. 307, no. 1–3, pp. 71–82, 2003.

115. G. Drasch, S. Böse-O›Reilly, C. Beinhoff, G. Roider, and S. Maydl, "The Mt. Diwata study on the Philippines 1999—Assessing mercury intoxication of the population by small scale gold mining," Science of the Total Environment, vol. 267, no. 1–3, pp. 151–168, 2001.

116. J. R. Campbell, T. W. Clarkson, and M. D. Omar, "The therapeutic use of 2,3-dimercaptopropane-1-sulfonate in two cases of inorganic mercury poisoning," Journal of the American Medical Association, vol. 256, no. 22, pp. 3127–3130, 1986.

117. J. C. Pendergrass, B. E. Haley, M. J. Vimy, S. A. Winfield, and F. L. Lorscheider, "Mercury vapor inhalation inhibits binding of GTP to tubulin in rat brain: similarity to a molecular lesion in Alzheimer diseased brain," NeuroToxicology, vol. 18, no. 2, pp. 315–324, 1997.

118. M. Fujimura, F. Usuki, M. Sawada, and A. Takashima, "Methylmercury induces neuropathological changes with tau hyperphosphorylation mainly through the activation of the c-jun-N-terminal kinase pathway in the cerebral cortex, but not in the

hippocampus of the mouse brain," NeuroToxicology, vol. 30, no. 6, pp. 1000–1007, 2009.

119. F. Monnet-Tschudi, M. G. Zurich, C. Boschat, A. Corbaz, and P. Honegger, "Involvement of environmental mercury and lead in the etiology of neurodegenerative diseases," Reviews on Environmental Health, vol. 21, no. 2, pp. 105–117, 2006.

120. M. Aschner, N. Onishchenko, and S. Ceccatelli, "Toxicology of alkylmercury compounds," Metal Ions in Life Sciences, vol. 7, pp. 403–423, 2010.

121. J. Mutter, A. Curth, J. Naumann, R. Deth, and H. Walach, "Does inorganic mercury play a role in Alzheimer›s disease? A systematic review and an integrated molecular mechanism," Journal of Alzheimer›s Disease, vol. 22, no. 2, pp. 357–374, 2010.

122. F. O. Johnson and W. D. Atchison, "The role of environmental mercury, lead and pesticide exposure in development of amyotrophic lateral sclerosis," NeuroToxicology, vol. 30, no. 5, pp. 761–765, 2009.

123. D. J. Yang, S. Shi, L. F. Zheng, T. M. Yao, and L. N. Ji, "Mercury(II) promotes the in vitro aggregation of tau fragment corresponding to the second repeat of microtubule-binding domain: coordination and conformational transition," Biopolymers, vol. 93, no. 12, pp. 1100–1107, 2010.

124. "(NHANES III) 3rd National report on human exposure to environmental chemicals," Tech. Rep., Centers for Disease Control and Prevention, 2005.

125. "(NHANES IV) 4th National Report on Human Exposure to Environmental Chemicals," Tech. Rep., Centers for Disease Control and Prevention, 2009.

126. "Toxicological profile for mercury," U.S. Department of Health and Human Services, Public Health Service, 1999, http://www.atsdr.cdc.gov/toxprofiles/tp46.pdf.

127. "Diagnostic and Treatment Protocols for safer, effective mercury human biohazard management," Consensus Development Working Group of the International College of Integrative Medicine, 2003.

128. Chelation Module, American College for Advancement in Medicine, Irvine, Calif, USA, 2010.

129. Advanced Medical Education and Services Physician Association, Introduction to Clinical Metal Toxicology, Advanced Medical Education and Services Physician Association, San Antonio, Tex, USA, 2007.

130. Clinician Seminar Level 1, Autism Research Institute, San Diego, Calif, USA, 2010.

131. R. A. Bernhoft and R. A. Buttar, "Autism: a multi-system oxidative and inflammatory disorder,"Townsend Letter, pp. 86–90, 2008.

Chapter 3

Use of Probiotics in Aquaculture

Patricia Martínez Cruz[1,2], Ana L. Ibáñez[3], Oscar A. Monroy Hermosillo[4], and Hugo C. Ramírez Saad

[1]Departamento de Sistemas Biológicos, Universidad Autónoma Metropo-litana-Xochimilco, Calzada del Hueso 1100, 04960 Mexico City, Mexico

[2]Universidad Autónoma Metropolitana-Xochimilco, Calzada del Hueso 1100, 04960 Mexico City, Mexico

[3]Departamento de Hidrobiología, Universidad Autónoma Metropolitana-Iztapalapa, Av. San Rafael Atlixco 186, 09340 Mexico City, Mexico

[4]Departamento de Biotecnología, Universidad Autónoma Metropolitana-Iztapalapa, Av. San Rafael Atlixco 186, 09340 Mexico City, Mexico

ABSTRACT

The growth of aquaculture as an industry has accelerated over the past decades; this has resulted in environmental damages and low productivity of various crops. The need for increased disease resistance, growth of aquatic organisms, and feed efficiency has brought about the use of probiotics in aquaculture practices. The first application of probiotics occurred in 1986, to test their ability to increase growth of hydrobionts (organisms that live in water). Later, probiotics were used to improve water quality and control of bacterial infections. Nowadays, there is documented evidence that probiotics can improve the digestibility of nutrients, increase tolerance to stress, and encourage reproduction. Currently, there are commercial probiotic products prepared from various bacterial species such as Bacillus sp., Lactobacillus sp., Enterococcussp., Carnobacterium sp., and the yeast Saccharomyces cerevisiae among others, and their use is regulated by careful management recommendations. The present paper shows the current knowledge of the use of probiotics in aquaculture, its antecedents, and safety measures to be carried out and discusses the prospects for study in this field.

INTRODUCTION

Aquaculture is the farming of aquatic organisms by intervention in the rearing process to enhance production and private ownership of the stock being cultivated. Compared to fishing, this activity allows a selective increase in the production of species used for human consumption, industry or sport fishing. Due to overfishing of wild populations, aquaculture has become an economic activity of great importance around the world. Aquaculture's contribution to world food production, raw materials for industrial and pharmaceutical use, and aquatic organisms for stocking or ornamental trade has increased dramatically in recent decades. The report World Aquaculture 2012 found that global production of fish from aquaculture grew more than 30 percent between 2006 and 2011, from 47.3 million tons to 63.6 million tons. It also forecasts that by 2012 more than 50 percent of the world's food fish consumption will come from aquaculture, so it is expected to overtaking capture fisheries as a source of edible fish. This growth rate is due to several factors: (1) many fisheries have reached their maximum sustainable exploitation, (2) consumer concerns about security and safety of their food, (3) the market demand for high-quality, healthy, low-calorie, and high-protein aquatic products, and (4) aquatic breeding makes only a minimum contribution to carbon dioxide emission [1, 2].

Aquaculture has a long history, originating at least in the year 475 B.C. in China [3], but became important in the late nineteen-forties, since the methods of aquaculture could be used to restock the waters as a complement to natural spawning. Nowadays, aquaculture is a lucrative industry [2, 4]. However, the intensification of aquaculture practices requires cultivation at high densities, which has caused significant damage to the environment due to discharges of concentrated organic wastes, that deplete dissolved oxygen in ponds, giving rise to toxic metabolites (such as hydrogen sulfide, methane, ammonia, and nitrites), that often are responsible for mortality. Additionally, aquaculture has appropriated of water bodies used for recreational purpose, and sometimes makes a water's waste because this natural resource is not reused in extensive aquaculture systems [5, 6]. Moreover, under these conditions of intensive production, aquatic species are subjected to high-stress conditions, increasing the incidence of diseases and causing a decrease in productivity [7].

Outbreaks of viral, bacterial, and fungal infections have caused devastating economic losses worldwide, that is, China reported disease-associated losses of $750 million in 1993, while India reported $210 million losses from 1995 to 1996. Added to this, significant stock mortality has been reported due to poor environmental conditions on farms, unbalanced nutrition, generation of toxins, and genetic factors [8]. In recent decades, prevention and control of animal diseases has focused on the use of chemical additives and veterinary medicines, especially antibiotics, which generate significant risks to public health by promoting the selection, propagation, and persistence of bacterial-resistant strains [9–11].

Resistance to antibiotics is acquired in two ways: chromosomal mutation or acquisition of plasmids. Chromosomal mutations are not transferred laterally to other bacteria but resistance plasmids can be transferred very rapidly, producing a high percentage of pathogenic bacteria that develop mediated plasmid-resistance in a short period of time [12]. This can be an important public health issue as well. For example, transfer of multidrug resistance occurred in Ecuador during the cholera epizootic happened between 1991 and 1994, which originated from shrimp farm workers. Although the original epidemic strain Vibrio cholera 01 was susceptible to 12 antimicrobial agents tested, on the coast of Ecuador it acquired multidrug resistance due to transfer of resistance genes from other Vibrio species that were pathogenic to shrimp [13]. Probiotic is a relatively new term which is used to name microorganisms that are associated with the beneficial effects for the host. Kozasa made the first empirical application of probiotics in aquaculture [14], considering the benefits exerted by the use of probiotics on humans and poultry. He used spores of Bacillus toyoi as feed additive to increase the growth rate of yellow tail, Seriola quinqueradiata. In 1991, Porubcan [15,16] documented the use of Bacillus spp, to test its ability to increase productivity of Penaeus monodonfarming and to improve water quality by decreasing the concentrations of ammonia and nitrite. In order to avoid or reduce the use of certain antimicrobials, biological control was tested, described as the use of natural enemies to reduce the damage caused by harmful organisms. Strictly speaking, a probiotic should not be classified as a biological control agent because it is not necessarily a natural enemy of the pathogen [17]. However, certain probiotics have the ability to inhibit the growth of pathogenic bacteria. Moriarty determined the ability of Bacillus spp. to decrease the proportion of Vibrio spp. in shrimp ponds, especially in sediments [18]. Further studies have stressed probiotics ability to stimulate appetite, improve absorption of nutrients, and strengthen the host immune system [19, 20]. The aim of this paper is to present an updated concept of probiotics, current uses in aquaculture, commercial presentations, and a final approach to prospect applications in this area.

DEFINITION OF PROBIOTIC

The term "probiotic" comes from Greek pro and bios meaning "prolife" [56], having different meanings over the years. In 1905, Dr. Elie Metchnikoff was the first to describe the positive role played by some bacteria among farmers who consumed pathogen-containing milk and that "reliance on gut microbes for food makes it possible to take steps to change the flora of our bodies and to replace harmful microbes by beneficial microbes" [57]. However, the term probiotic was introduced until 1965 by Lilly and Stillwell [58] as a modification of the original word "probiotika." It was used to describe substances produced by a microorganism that prolong the logarithmic growth phase in other species. It was described as an agent which has the opposite function of antibiotics. Later, Sperti [59] modified the concept of "tissue extracts that stimulate microbial growth."

The first use of the term to describe a microbial feed/food supplement was by Parker in 1974 [60]. He defined it as "organisms and substances that contribute to intestinal microbial balance." Fuller [61] expanded the definition to "live microbial food supplement that benefits the host (human or animal) by improving the microbial balance of the body" and said that it would be effective in a range of extreme temperatures and salinity variations. Afterwards, it was suggested that probiotics were "monocultures or mixed cultures of microorganisms applied to animals or humans, that benefit the host by improving properties of indigenous microflora" [62]. In 1998, Guarner and Schaafsma assumed that probiotics are live microorganisms which, when consumed in adequate amounts, confer health benefits to the host [63]. Gatesoupe in 1999, defined them as "microbial cells administered in a certain way, which reaches the gastrointestinal tract and remain alive with the aim of improving health" [25]. In the same year, studies were carried out on the inhibition of pathogens using probiotics, this expanded the definition to "... live microbial supplement which benefits the host by improving its microbial balance" [34].

Knowledge of probiotics has increased, currently it is known that these microorganisms have an antimicrobial effect through modifying the intestinal microbiota, secreting antibacterial substances (bacteriocins and organic acids), competing with pathogens to prevent their adhesion to the intestine, competing for nutrients necessary for pathogen survival, and producing an antitoxin effect. Probiotics are also capable of modulating the immune system, regulating allergic response of the body, and reducing proliferation of cancer in mammals. Because of this, when provided at certain concentration and viability, probiotics favorably affect host health [64]. In fact, terms such as "friendly bacteria," "friendly," or "healthy" are commonly used to describe probiotics [19].

For many years, studies focused on microorganisms characteristic from intestinal microbiota, and the term "probiotic" was mainly restricted to gram-positive lactic acid bacteria [65], particularly representative of the genera Bifidobacterium, Lactobacillus, and Streptococcus [66]. In contrast to terrestrial animals, gastrointestinal microbiota of aquatic species is particularly dependent on the external environment due to the flow of water passing through the digestive tract. Thus, the majority of bacteria are transient in the intestine, due to constant intake of water and food, together with microorganisms present in them. Although in the gastrointestinal tract (GIT) of aquatic animals have been reported potentially pathogenic bacteria such as Salmonella, Listeria, and Escherichia coli, probiotic bacteria and other microorganisms have also been identified. These include gram-positive bacteria such as Bacillus, Carnobacterium, Enterococcus, and several species of Lactobacillus; gram-negative, facultative anaerobic such as Vibrio and Pseudomonas, as well as certain fungi, yeasts, and algae of the genera Debaryomyces, Saccharomyces, and Tetraselmis, respectively [20,67, 68]. Due to the increasing interest of probiotics in aquaculture, Moriarty [18] proposed extending the definition of these to "living microbial additives that benefit the health of hydrobionts and therefore increase productivity."

A more general and common concept of probiotic is "one or more microorganisms with beneficial effects for the host, able to persist in the digestive tract because of its tolerance to acid and bile salts" [20]. Although the use of probiotics in aquaculture is relatively recent, interest in them has increased due to their potential in disease control [19]; however, gradually other applications have been proposed (summarized in Table 1), that will be addressed in detail later.

Table 1: Different applications of probiotics in aquaculture

Application	Identity of the probiotic	Applied to aquatic species	Reference
Growth promoter	Bacillus sp. S11	Penaeus monodon	[21]
	Bacillus sp.	Catfish	[22]
	Carnobacterium divergens	Gadus morhua	[23]
	Alteromonas CA2	Crassostrea gigas	[24]
	Lactobacillus helveticus	Scophthalmus maximus	[25]
	Lactobacillus lactis AR21	Brachionus plicatilis	[26]
	Streptococcus thermophilus	Scophthalmus maximus	[25]
	Streptomyces	Xiphophorus helleri	[27]
	L. casei	Poeciliopsis gracilis	[28]
	Bacillus NL 110, Vibrio NE 17	Macrobrachium rosenbergii	[29]
	Bacillus coagulans	Cyprinus carpio koi	[30]

Pathogen inhibition	Bacillus sp.	Penaeids	[18]
	Enterococcus faecium SF 68	Anguilla anguilla	[31]
	L. rhamnosus ATCC53103	Oncorhynchus mykiss	[32]
	Micrococcus luteus A1-6	Oncorhynchus mykiss	[33]
	Pseudomonas fluorescens	Oncorhynchus mykiss	[34]
	P. fluorescens AH2	Oncorhynchus mykiss	[35]
	Pseudomonassp.	Oncorhynchus mykiss	[36]
	Roseobacter sp. BS. 107	Scallop larvae	[37]
	Saccharomyces cerevisiae, S. exiguous, Phaffia rhodozyma	Litopenaeus vannamei	[38]
	Vibrio alginolyticus	Salmonids	[39]
	V. fluvialis	Oncorhynchus mykiss	[33]
	Tetraselmis suecica	Salmo salar	[40]
	Carnobacterium sp. Hg4-03	Hepialus gonggaensis larvae	[41]
	Lactobacillus acidophilus	Clarias gariepinus	[42]
	Bacillus spp., Enterococcussp.	Farfantepenaeus brasiliensis	[43]
	Lactococcus lactis	Epinephelus coioides	[44]
Nutrient digestibility	L. helveticus	Scophthalmus maximus	[25]
	Bacillus NL 110, Vibrio NE 17	Macrobrachium rosenbergii	[29]
	Carnobacterium sp. Hg4-03	Hepialus gonggaensis larvae	[41]
	Lactobacillus acidophilus	Clarias gariepinus	[45]
	Shewanella putrefaciens Pdp11	Solea senegalensis	[46]
	Bacillus sp. 48	Penaeus monodon	[19]
	Bacillus NL 110, Vibrio sp. NE 17	Macrobrachium rosenbergii	[29]
Water quality	Lactobacillus acidophilus	Clarias gariepinus	[45]
	B. coagulans SC8168	Pennaeus vannamei	[47]
	Bacillus sp., Saccharomyces sp.	Penaeus monodon	[48]
	Lactobacillus delbrueckii	Dicentrarchus labrax	[49]
	Alteromonas sp.	Sparus auratus	[50]
Stress tolerance	B. subtilis, L. acidophilus, S. cerevisiae	Paralichthys olivaceus	[51]
	L. casei	Poecilopsis gracilis	[28]
	Pediococcus acidilactici	Litopenaeus stylirostris	[52]
	Shewanella putrefaciens Pdp11	Makimaki	[46]
Reproduction improvement	Bacillus subtilis	Poecilia reticulata, Xiphophorus maculatus	[53]
	L. rhamnosus	Danio rerio	[54]
	L. acidophilus, L. casei, Enterococcus faecium, Bifidobacterium thermophilum	Xiphophorus helleri	[55]

COMMERCIAL PREPARATIONS

The interest in probiotics as an environmentally friendly alternative is increasing and its application is both empirical and scientific. According to Soccol et al. [69], the global market for probiotic ingredients, supplements and foods, reached US $15,900 million in 2008 and is projected to increase to US $19,600 million in 2013, representing an annual growth rate of 4.3%. At present, there are several commercial preparations of probiotics that contain one or more live microorganisms, which have been introduced to improve the cultivation of aquatic organisms. Probiotics can be used as a food additive added directly to the culture tank or mixed with food.

Apart from laboratory preparation of bacteria, some commercially available products are now available. One of the first evaluations of commercial products focussed on a bacterial preparation called Biostart that is derived from Bacillus isolates. It was used during the production of cultured catfish studying the effect of inoculum concentration [22]. In 1998, Moriarty reported that the use of commercial probiotic strains ofBacillus spp. increased the quality and viability of pond-raised shrimp [18]. Meanwhile, Chang and Liu [31] evaluated the effect of Enterococcus faecium SF68 and Bacillus toyoi isolates present in Cernivet LBC and Toyocerin, respectively, to decrease the mortality of the European eel because of the edwardsielosis, ensuring greater efficiency with E. faecium SF68. It is relevant to note that E. faecium has long been known as a probiotic for humans, whereas B. toyoi has been used with terrestrial animals. Moreover, a B. subtilis strain combined with hydrolytic enzymes to produce Biogen, was used to supplement the feed of Oreochromis niloticus, obtaining significant increases in productivity [70].

The lactic acid-producing bacteria have been the focus of much interest. The human probiotic, Lactobacillus rhamnosus ATCC (American Type Culture Collection, Rockville, MD, USA), was used in rainbow trout for 51 days to reduce mortality by Aeromonas salmonicida, the causative agent of the fish disease "furunculosis" (one of the major fish diseases in many parts of world). Mortality was reduced from 52.6 to 18.9% when 10^9cells g^{-1} were administered with feed, when probiotic dose was increased to 10^{12} cells g^{-1} of feed the mortality reached 46.3% [32]. Apparently, increasing dosage does not necessarily improve protection. Abasali and Mohamad [55] increased the gonadosomatic index and the production of fingerlings in females of reproductive age, using mixed cultures consisting of L. acidophilus, L. casei, E. faecium, and B. thermophilum(Primalac).

Studies with Penaeus vannamei showed that using mixed cultures of probiotics increases survival, feed conversion, and the final production of farmed shrimp [71]. Meanwhile, Taoka et al. [72] used Alchem Poseidon and Alchem Korea CO and Wonju Korea CO, which have mixed cultures of bacteria (Bacillus subtilis, Lactobacillus acidophilus, and Clostridium butyricum) and yeast (Saccharomyces cerevisiae), enhanced nonspecific immune parameters of tilapia Oreochromis niloticus such as lysozyme activity, migration onf neutrophils, and plasma bactericidal activity, resulting in improvement of resistance to Edwardsiella tardainfection. Previous studies in humans and land animals using prebiotics (nondigestible ingredients of the diet that stimulates the growth of microorganisms) showed their ability to stimulate the activity of probiotic bacteria in the colon [73, 74]. Some commercial aquaculture products included prebiotics in their formulation, such as mannans, glucans, and yucca extract that further increase the beneficial effects of the product [75, 76].

Currently, commercial products are available in liquid or powder presentations, and various technologies have been developed for improvement. on the case of fermentation processes, the interest has been focused on optimizing the fermentation conditions to increase the viability and functionality of probiotics, improving performance [77]. Generally, the production is carried out in batch cultures due to the difficulty of industrial scale operation of continuous systems [69]. More recently, systems have been developed for immobilization of probiotics, especially using microencapsulation. Microbial cells at high density are encapsulated in a colloidal matrix using alginate, chitosan, carboxymethylcellulose, or pectin to physically and chemically protect the microorganisms. The methods commonly used for microencapsulation of probiotics are the emulsion, extrusion, spray drying, and adhesion to starch [78]. Focused on the application to aquaculture, Rosas et al. [79] have effectively encapsulated cells of Shewanella putrefaciens in calcium alginate, demonstrating the survival of encapsulated probiotic cells through the gastrointestinal tract of sole (Solea senegalensis). Encapsulation in alginate matrices protects bacteria from low pH and digestive enzymes; this protection helps to release the probiotic into the intestine without any significant damage [80]. Currently, the lyophilized commercial preparations have advantages for storage and transport. However, conditions for reconstitution of these preparations such as temperature, degree of hydration, and osmolarity of the solution are vital to ensure the viability of bacteria [81]. It is important to emphasize that these products must provide a health benefit to the host; for this, it is necessary that contained microorganisms have the ability to survive storage conditions, and after that in the digestive tract of aquatic species, remaining viable and stable, and finally improving production [20]. According to the opinion of the producers, these preparations are safe to use and effective in preserving the health of aquatic animals [19].

APPLICATIONS OF PROBIOTICS IN AQUACULTURE

The need for sustainable aquaculture has promoted research into the use of probiotics on aquatic organisms. The initial interest was focused on their use as growth promoters and to improve the health of animals; however, new areas have been found, such as their effect on reproduction or stress tolerance, although this requires a more scientific development.

Growth Promoter

Probiotics have been used in aquaculture to increase the growth of cultivated species, in reality it is not known whether these products increase the appetite, or if, by their nature, improve digestibility. Some people are inclined to think that it could be both factors; furthermore, it would be important to determine whether probiotics actually taste good for aquaculture species [20]. According to Balcázar et al. [13], probiotic microorganisms are able to colonize gastrointestinal tract when administered over a long period of time because they have a higher multiplication rate than the rate of expulsion, so as probiotics constantly added to fish cultures, they adhere to the intestinal mucosa of them, developing and exercising their multiple benefits. This also depends on factors such as hydrobionts species, body temperature, enzyme levels, genetic resistance, and water quality.

The effect of probiotics has been tested on phytoplankton (microalgae), which forms the basis of aquatic food chains, due to its nutrient-producing photosynthetic machinery that in most cases, higher organisms are unable to synthesize such is the case of polyunsaturated fatty acids and vitamins. Within groups of microalgae used in aquaculture are distinguished central diatoms as Chaetoceros spp., which have proven to be a good live food; however, production has limitations due to the complexity of their nutritional requirements [82]. Gómez et al. [83] assessed the growth of Vibrio alginolyticus C7b probiotic in the presence of the microalgaeChaetoceros muelleri, proving that these organisms can be grown together to achieve high density and fed to shrimp.

Rotifers are indispensable as the first live feed for larvae of most cultured aquatic species, due to their small size they are more accessible to larvae, for example, the nauplii of brine shrimp, which is a very common live feed. Planas et al. [84] used lactic acid bacteria to increase the growth of the rotifer Brachionus plicatilis and obtained best results with the addition of Lactococcus casei ssp. casei, Pediococcus acidilactici, and Lactobacillus lactis ssp. lactis.

The use of probiotics as growth promoters of edible fishes has been reported. Diet of Nile tilapia (Oreochromis niloticus) was amended with a probiotic Streptococcus strain, increasing significantly the content of crude protein and crude lipid in the fish, also weight has increased from 0.154 g to 6.164 g in 9 weeks of culture [85]. Due to the commercial importance of this species, the effect of supplementing diet with probiotics produced an increase of 115.3% when commercial formulation was used at a concentration of 2% [70].

Examples of growth improvement of ornamental fishes include swordtail (Xiphophorus helleri, X. maculatus) and guppy, (Poecilia reticulate, P. sphenops), their feed was supplemented with Bacillus subtilis andStreptomyces, finding significative increases in growth and survival of Xiphophorus and Poecilia after 90 and 50 days of administration, respectively [27, 86].

Probiotics also have been tested successfully in shellfish culture. Macey and Coyne [87] isolated two yeasts and one bacterial strain (designated SS1, AY1, and SY9, resp.) from the digestive tract of abalone (Haliotis midae). A diet was formulated with a mixture of the three putative probiotics. Each probiont was added to the feed to achieve a final concentration of approximately 10^7 cells g^{-1} of dry feed. The growth rate of small (20 mm) and large (67 mm) abalone was improved by 8% and 34%, respectively, in eight-month cultures. Furthermore, abalones supplemented with probiotics had a survival rate of 62% to the pathogenic bacteriumVibrio anguillarum compared to 25% survival of untreated animals.

Inhibition of Pathogens

Antibiotics were used for a long time in aquaculture to prevent diseases in the crop. However, this caused various problems such as the presence of antibiotic residues in animal tissues, the generation of bacterial resistance mechanisms, as well as an imbalance in the gastrointestinal microbiota of aquatic species, which affected their health [88]. In fact, the European Union has regulated the use of antibiotics in organisms for human consumption [89]. Today, consumers demand natural products, free of additives such as antibiotics; moreover, there is a tendency for preventing diseases rather than treating them. Thus, the use of probiotics is a viable alternative for the inhibition of pathogens and disease control in aquaculture species.

Probiotic microorganisms have the ability to release chemical substances with bactericidal or bacteriostatic effect on pathogenic bacteria that are in the intestine of the host, thus constituting a barrier against the proliferation of opportunistic pathogens. In general, the antibacterial effect is due to one or more of the following factors: production of antibiotics, bacteriocins, siderophores, enzymes (lysozymes, proteases) and/or hydrogen peroxide, as well as alteration of the intestinal pH due to the generation of organic acids [65].

Taoka et al. [51] showed that viable probiotics administered to tilapia Oreochromis niloticus, increased non-specific immune response, determined by parameters such as lysozyme activity, neutrophile migration, and bactericidal activity, which improved the resistance of fish to infection by Edwardsiella tarda. In turn, Robertson et al. [90] isolated a strain of Carnobacterium sp. from salmon bowel and administered alive to rainbow trout and Atlantic salmon, demonstrating in vitro antagonism against known fish pathogens:Aeromonas hydrophila, A. salmonicida, Flavobacterium psychrophilum, Photobacterium damselae, and Vibriospecies. There is also evidence on the effect of dead probiotic cultures consisting on a mixture of Vibrio fluvialis A3-47S, Aeromonas hydrophila A3-51, and Carnobacterium BA211, in the control of furunculosis in rainbow trout. For this specific case, the number of leukocytes was greater than with live cells, in fact, the data suggest that cellular immunity more than humoral factors was involved in the benefits of these preparations of inactivated bacterial cells [91]. In the case of shrimp, studies have focused on the evaluation of probiotics such as Bacillus cereus, Paenibacillus polymyxa, and Pseudomonas sp. PS-102 as biocontrol agents against pathogens of various Vibrio species [92, 93].

Probiotic strains isolated from the gastrointestinal tract of clownfish (Amphiprion percula) have been used to inactivate several pathogens such as Aeromonas hydrophila and Vibrio alginolyticus among others. It has been observed that probiotics in vivo generate a density such that allow the production of antimicrobial metabolites therefore, the bacteria isolated from adult clownfish have the potential to colonize the intestinal mucus and therefore can be used as prophylactic agent and/or therapeutic [94, 95]. Furthermore, it has been found that concentrations of 10^6 to 10^8 cells g^{-1} of probiotic promote the development of healthy microbiota in the gastrointestinal tract of ornamental fishes from the genera Poecilia and Xiphophorus, decreasing the amount of heterotrophic microorganisms [86].

Gómez et al. [96] reported the use of Vibrio alginolyticus strains as probiotics to increase survival and growth of white shrimp (Litopenaeus vannamei), also by using probiotics in Ecuadorian shrimp hatcheries, production increased by 35%, while with the use of antimicrobials it decreased by 94%.

Improvement in Nutrient Digestion

A study has suggested that probiotics have a beneficial effect on the digestive processes of aquatic animals because probiotic strains synthesize extracellular enzymes such as proteases, amylases, and lipases as well as provide growth factors such as vitamins, fatty acids, and aminoacids [13]. Therefore, nutrients are absorbed more efficiently when the feed is supplemented with probiotics [70]. In this sense, probiotics have been used in edible fishes, as in the case of larvae of European bass (Dicentrarchus labrax). It has been reported that the probiotic yeast Debaryomyces hansenii HF1 has the ability to produce spermine and spermidine, two polyamines involved in the differentiation and maturation of the gastrointestinal tract in mammals. In addition this yeast secretes amylase and trypsin, enzymes that aid digestion in sea bass larvae [97]. Studies in juvenile common dentex Dentex dentex L. showed that when diet is supplemented with 0.5 g of Bacillus cereus strain E kg^{-1} of food, increased fish growth due to more efficient use of the food [98]. In the case of rainbow trout, similar results were obtained using B. subtilis, B. licheniformis, and Enterococcus faecium, when these probiotics were provided for 10 weeks along with the diet of fish [99]. In some trials, diet of European sea bass larvae (Dicentrarchus labrax) has supplemented with probiotic yeast (Saccharomyces cerevisiae strain X2180), assessing fish growth and activity and expression of antioxidative key enzymes (catalase, glutathione peroxidase, and superoxide dismutase), finding differences in enzyme activity and gene expression patterns between probiotic supplemented and nonsupplemented treatments, which was attributed to the presence of the yeast [100].

In white shrimp Litopenaeus vannamei Boone and Fenneropenaeus indicus, various strains of Bacillus have been used as probiotics to increase apparent digestibility of dry matter, crude protein, and phosphorus. Results showed higher sizes when the diet is supplemented with 50 g of probiotic kg^{-1} of food [101]. Other research has suggested the importance of managing the probiotic in all ontogenetic stages of the shrimp to generate a constant effect on the production of digestive enzymes [102].

In guppies (Poecilia reticulata, P. sphenops), and swordtail (Xiphophorus helleri, X. maculatus), the effect of incorporating Bacillus subtilis, isolated from the intestine of Cirrhinus mrigala into their diet has been evaluated. The results show an increase in the length and weight of the ornamental fishes as well as the specific activity of proteases and amylases in the digestive tract [86]. According to Moriarty [103], Bacillus secretes a wide range of exoenzymes that complement the activities of the fish and increases enzymatic digestion. In fact, the bacteria isolated from the digestive tract of aquatic animals have shown chitinases, proteases, cellulases, lipases, and trypsin [67].

Improvement of Water Quality

In several studies, water quality was recorded during the addition of probiotic strains especially of the gram-positive genus Bacillus. Probably since this bacterial group is more efficient than gram-negative in transforming organic matter to CO_2. It is suggested that maintaining high levels of probiotics in production ponds, fish farmers can minimize the accumulation of dissolved and particulate organic carbon during the growing season. In addition, this can balance the production of phytoplankton [13]. However, this hypothesis could not be confirmed on tests carried out during cultivation of shrimps or channel catfish, using one or more species of Bacillus, Nitrobacter, Pseudomonas, Enterobacter, Cellulomonas, and Rhodopseudomonas. Thus published evidence for improving water quality is limited, except for the nitrification [65].

In the case of edible fish, trout production farms generate high concentrations of nitrogen ranging from 0.05–3.3 mg L^{-1} of total Kjeldahl nitrogen and up to 6.4 mg L^{-1} after 7 months of monitoring [104]. For tilapia production in recirculating systems, concentrations of total ammonia (NH_4 + NH_3) increased from 4.73 to 14.87 mg L^{-1} in a 21-day-experiment, while the nitrite concentration increased from 3.75 to 9.77 mg L^{-1} [105]. Due to the high concentrations of produced nitrogen compounds, especially the highly toxic total ammonia; the use of probiotics is recommended, as they may improve water quality. Haroun et al. supplemented the food of Nile tilapia Oreochromis niloticus L. with a commercial probiotic made from Bacillus licheniformisand B. subtilis in 17 weeks of culture. Assessment of water quality parameters showed an acceptable range for fish cultivation: 5.7–6.3 mg L^{-1} for dissolved oxygen concentration, 0.36–0.42 mg L^{-1} for ammonia concentration, and pH between 6.3 and 8.2 [70].

Lalloo et al. [106] isolated several strains of Bacillus from Cyprinus carpio and carried out tests to improve water quality in ornamental fish culture and to inhibit the growth of Aeromonas hydrophila. Three out of nine isolates showed high capacity to inhibit the pathogen in 78 of relative incidence rate; moreover, concentrations of ammonia, nitrate, and phosphate were lowered in rates of 74%, 76% and 72%, respectively. Contradictorily, Queiroz and Boyd [22] tested a commercial probiotic in catfish (Ictalurus punctatus), noting a survival and net fish production significantly higher when the probiotic was applied. However, very little differences were significant for the determined water quality variables (ammonia, chemical oxygen demand, nitrate, soluble reactive phosphorus, and dissolved oxygen) between the treated and control ponds. Taoka et al. [51] studied effects of commercial probiotics formulated from mixed cultures of bacteria and yeast on survival of Japanese flounder Paralichthys olivaceus, and water quality in a closed recirculating system. The probiotics-treated groups showed significantly greater survival rate as compared to the control group at the end of rearing experiment (50 days of culture), and water quality parameters were significantly lower in probiotics diet groups (from 0.24 ± 0.22 to 0.12 ± 0.10 mg L^{-1} of NH_4, from 0.15 ± 0.08 to 0.08 ± 0.08 mg $L^{-1}$of NO_2, and from 13.0 ± 3.9 to 10.2 ± 3.0 mg L^{-1} of PO_4). Meanwhile, Wang et al. showed that a commercial product made from Bacillus sp., Saccharomyces cerevisiae, Nitrosomonas sp., and Nitrobacter sp. had the ability to increase the beneficial bacterial microbiota of Penaeus vannamei shrimp, further reducing the concentrations of inorganic nitrogen from 3.74 to 1.79 mg L^{-1} and phosphate from 0.1105 to 0.0364 mg L^{-1}[107].

Stress Tolerance

Aquaculture practices demand intensive productions in shorter times, causing stress in crop species. For example, it has been reported that chronic stress in zebra fish, Danio rerio, induces a general depression on the synthesis of muscle protein [108]. As a result, it was sought to increase stress tolerance by using probiotics. One of the firsts formal reports on this field studied the supplementation of Lactobacillus delbrueckii ssp. delbrueckii in the diet of European sea bass (Dicentrarchus labrax), at time intervals of 25 to 59 days. In addition to evaluating the growth improvement, hormone cortisol was quantified in fish tissue as stress marker, since it is directly involved in the animal's response to stress. Cortisol levels obtained in the treated fishes were significantly lower than those in the control (3.6 ± 0.36 ng g^{-1} and 5.1 ± 0.47 ng g^{-1}, resp.) [49]. Another way to assess stress in fish involve subjecting them to heat shock, as in the case of Japanese flounder (Paralichthys olivaceus) grown in a recirculating system [72]. The stress tests were carried out until half the population died, thus calculated the mean lethal time (LT_{50}) in the absence and with addition of a commercial probiotic containing Bacillus subtilis, Lactobacillus acidophilus, Clostridium butyricum, andSaccharomyces cerevisiae. The group treated with probiotics showed greater tolerance in the stress test than the control group, the LT_{50} was 40 and 25 min, respectively.

Lactate and plasma glucose levels are considered appropriate indicators of stress as they increase as a secondary response during periods of stress to cover high energy requirements induced by this situation. Therefore, Varela et al. have conducted studies on the gilt-head bream (Sparus auratus); the glycogen and triglycerides reserves in the livers of the control group were significantly decreased in relation to concentrations obtained when the fish feed was supplemented with the probiotic Alteromonas sp. Strain Pdp 11 [50].

Castex et al. [52] evaluated the effect of Pediococcus acidilactici MA 18/5 in the antioxidative response of the shrimp Litopenaeus stylirostris to oxidative stress. The results showed high activities of antioxidant enzymes; superoxide dismutase (283.7 and 153.7 mol min^{-1} in control and treated groups, resp.) and catalase (3.08 and 1.34 mol min^{-1} for the control and probiotic-treated, resp.).

The results obtained so far raise the possibility of preparing the fish in advance with probiotic treatment, for conventional aquacultures practices that create stress in animals, such as transport, change in water temperature, and periodic manipulations [46].

Effect on Reproduction of Aquatic Species

According to Izquierdo et al. [109], breeding aquaculture species have high nutritional requirements, thus reproductive capacity depends on appropriate concentrations of lipids, proteins, fatty acids, vitamins C and E, and carotenoids. Furthermore, the relationship of these components influences reproduction in various processes such as fertility, fertilization, birth and development of larvae. At present, for most cultured fish species, there are commercially available "broodstock diets" that just are larger-sized diets. In practice, many fish hatcheries improve the nutrition of their broodstock by feeding them solely on fresh fish byproducts or in combination with commercial diets. The most common fresh organisms used to feed broodstock fishes include squid, cuttlefish, mussels, krill, and small crustaceans. The use of these unprocessed fish products often do not provide adequate levels of nutrients needed by broodstock fishes, increasing the risk of pathogens transmission to the parents and offspring, including parasites, bacteria, and viruses. Therefore, probiotics added to food or water were used in order to prevent infections and to explore their effect on reproduction.

The pioneer study on the effect of probiotic supplementation on reproductive performance of fish was carried out by Ghosh et al. [53], using a strain of B. subtilis isolated from intestine of Cirrhinus mrigala, incorporated at different concentrations to four species of ornamental fishes: Poecilia reticulata, P. sphenops, Xiphophorus helleri, and X. maculates, in a one-year experiment. The results showed that using B. subtilisconcentrations of 10^6–10^8 cells g^{-1} of food, produced increases in the gonadosomatic index, fecundity, viability, and production of fry from the females of all four species. Furthermore, these authors proposed that complex B vitamins synthesized by the probiotic, especially thiamine (vitamin B1) and vitamin B12, contribute to reduce the number of dead or deformed alevins.

Abasali and Mohamad [55] carried out similar studies with X. helleri, using a commercial probiotic containing Lactobacillus acidophilus, L. casei, Enterococcus faecium, and Bifidobacterium thermophilum. The total production of alevin per female and the relative fecundity were evaluated. Their results showed significant differences between the control and probiotic-treated groups; in the first parameter 105 and 150 alevins were found on average, respectively. While in the second, 28 females were fecundated in the control and 41 for the probiotic treatment.

SAFETY CONSIDERATIONS OF PROBIOTIC

Traditionally, probiotics used in food industry have been deemed safe, in fact, no human risks have been determined, remaining as the best proof of its safety [110]. Theoretically, probiotics may be responsible for four types of side effects in susceptible individuals: systemic infections, deleterious metabolic activities, excessive immune stimulation, and gene transfer. However, no hard evidence has been found.

In practice, there are few reports of bacteremia in humans, where isolation of probiotic bacteria from infections seems to be the result of an opportunistic infection caused by skin lesions, cancer, chronic illness, or a drug-induced abnormality. These conditions lead to a decreased intestinal barrier that promotes the passage of the bacteria through the mucosal epithelium. Subsequently, these microorganisms are transported to the mesenteric lymph nodes and other organs, leading to bacteremia that may progress to septicemia [111]. All reported cases of bacteremia occurred in patients with chronic illness or a weakened immune system [69,112].

In the case of some lactic acid bacteria that are regarded as probiotics, the resistance to antibiotics can be linked to genes on chromosomes, plasmids, or transposons. However, there is insufficient information about the circumstances in which these genetic elements could be mobilized [113]. Moreover, it is recognized that some enterococci may possess virulence characteristics and have the ability to transfer antibiotic resistance elements, so it is recommended that no reference should be made to these organisms as probiotics for human consumption, unless the producer can demonstrate that this strain cannot acquire or transfer antibiotic resistance or induce infection [112].

Regarding safety of aquaculture products, in Asia and more recently in Latin America cultures of Penaeus monodon have been reported with bacterial white spot syndrome (BWSS), in farms with recurrent use of probiotics based on Bacillus subtilis. The spots are similar to those generated in the white spot viral syndrome (WSS), which is a deadly disease that spreads rapidly and causes mass mortalities in shrimp cultures [114,115]. Wang et al. [116] demonstrated in 2000 that BWSS is a nonsystemic infection in P. monodon and lesions usually disappear after molting, under this condition cultures are still active and grow normally without significant mortality. However, it is of great concern because most farmers cannot distinguish BWSS from WSS. Farmers are advised in case of suspicion to send samples to the laboratory for confirmatory diagnosis.

Furthermore, since some aquaculture products are consumed raw or half cooked, has raised the question of whether residual probiotics may cause any infection in the final consumer. Shakibazadeh et al. [117] assessed the potential risk to humans caused by the use of probiotic Shewanella algae in shrimp farms. Studies were performed in mice that were given up to 10^{36} cfu to reach the LD_{50} value for S. algae, proving the safety of using probiotics in mice. Based on their results, these authors state that the use of S. algae is safe for the consumer of shrimps, such as for workers in the processing plants and farms.

Because there was no international consensus to ensure efficiency and safety of probiotics, FAO and WHO recognized the need to create guidelines for a systematic approach for the evaluation of probiotics in food, in order to substantiate their health claims. A working group with experts in the field was formed in order to recommend criteria and methodology for the evaluation of probiotics, based on scientific evidence [118]. As a result the "Guide for the Evaluation of Probiotics in Food" was presented, providing guidelines on the evaluation of health and nutrition properties of probiotics in food. The working group stated that no pathogenic or virulent properties were found in lactobacilli, bifidobacteria, or lactococci, although they acknowledged that under certain conditions, some strains of lactobacilli have been associated with rare cases of bacteremia. However, its incidence does not increase with raising the use of lactobacillus in probiotics. It was also mentioned that enterococci may possess virulence characteristics; therefore, it is not recommended as a probiotic for human consumption [113]. Although the guide is not focused on aquaculture products, it creates a precedent for conducting studies to evaluate the safety of probiotics in this area. To date, the use of animal models including mice, rats, and fish has not revealed specific determinants of virulence or pathogenicity of the studied probiotic microorganisms, suggesting the overall safety of them [112]. However, it is important to continue research using three approaches: (i) analyzing the intrinsic properties of probiotic strains, (ii) studying its pharmacokinetics (survival, activity in the intestine, dose response, and recovery from mucosa), and (iii) understanding the interactions between the microorganism and the host [69].

CONCLUDING REMARKS

The current global food crisis and increasing production costs has put pressure on governments and the international community to ensure sufficient food supply for a growing population. Thus, aquaculture is presented as a way to meet the growing demand for fresh water food or seafood, and to meet current challenges relating to the ongoing globalization of trade, intensification and diversification of aquaculture, progress in technological innovations for food production, changes in ecological systems and human behavior, including a greater awareness to protect biodiversity, public health, and the environment. These challenges will lead to increased attention for improving aquaculture practices, and will become an important alternative to overexploitation and modification of aquatic ecosystems caused by capture fisheries. The use of probiotics can potentiate the benefits of this activity because, as presented in this paper, it offers viable alternatives for the generation of a higher-quality livestock product in terms of size, production time, and health. In the near future, it is necessary to conduct studies relating to probiotics resistance to antibiotics, and the chances of transmission of genetic elements to other microorganisms in the fish GIT, and thus to humans when consuming the aquaculture product.

On the other hand, there is a need to strengthen studies of microbial ecology in aquaculture systems, correlating microbial communities (microorganisms on water and in the GIT of aquatic species) with animal growth and its relationship to the water quality. Nowadays, a variety of probiotic strains present in the GIT of aquatic animals and nitrifying bacteria from biofilters have been isolated and characterized using biochemical, morphological, and molecular techniques [68, 119–121]. The development of molecular techniques such as PCR, FISH (fluorescent in situ hybridization), DGGE (denaturing gradient gel electrophoresis), and generation of genomic libraries have started to unveil the diversity present in aquaculture systems. Currently, next-generation sequencing methodologies offer great potential for phylogenetic identification of probiotic microorganisms without using conventional cultivation techniques.

REFERENCES

1. FAO, The State of World Fisheries and Aquaculture, 2012.
2. M. Timmons, J. Ebeling, F. Wheaton, S. Summerfelt, and B. Vinci, Recirculating Aquaculture Systems, Cayuga Aqua Ventures, 2nd edition, 2002.
3. C. E. Boyd and C. S. Tucker, Pond Aquaculture Water Quality Management, Kluwer, Norwell, Mass, USA, 1998.
4. D. Cressey, "Aquaculture: future fish," Nature, vol. 458, no. 7237, pp. 398–400, 2009.

5. P. G. Amaya and D. F. Castellano, Pesca, Acuicultura e Investigación en México, Edited by Cedrssa, 2006.
6. Y. B. Wang and Z. R. Xu, "Probiotics treatment as method of biocontrol in aquaculture," Feed Research, vol. 12, pp. 42–45, 2004.
7. M. G. Bondad, R. P. Subasinghe, J. R. Arthur et al., "Disease and health management in Asian aquaculture," Veterinary Parasitology, vol. 132, no. 3-4, pp. 249–272, 2005.
8. N. Kautsky, P. Rönnbäck, M. Tedengren, and M. Troell, "Ecosystem perspectives on management of disease in shrimp pond farming," Aquaculture, vol. 191, no. 1–3, pp. 145–161, 2000.
9. F. A. O. /OIE/WHO, "Antimicrobial use in aquaculture and antimicrobial resistance," Report of a Joint. Expert Consultation on Antimicrobial Use in Aquaculture And Antimicrobial Resistance, 2006.
10. K. Nomoto, "Prevention of infections by probiotics," Journal of Bioscience and Bioengineering, vol. 100, no. 6, pp. 583–592, 2005.
11. WHO, "Antimicrobial resistance. Fact sheet N∘ 194," 2012,http://www.who.int/mediacentre/factsheets/fs194/es/index.html.
12. C. S. Lewin, "Mechanisms of resistance development in aquatic microorganisms," in Chemothe-Rapy in Aquaculture: From Theory To Reality, C. Michel and D. Alderman, Eds., pp. 288–301, Office International des Epizooties, Paris, France, 1992.
13. J. L. Balcázar, I. D. Blas, I. Ruiz-Z, D. Cunningham, D. Vendrell, and J. L. Múzquiz, "The role of probiotics in aquaculture," Veterinary Microbiology, vol. 114, no. 3-4, pp. 173–186, 2006.
14. M. Kozasa, "Toyocerin (Bacillus toyoi) as growth promotor for animal feeding," Microbiologie Aliments Nutrition, vol. 4, no. 2, pp. 121–135, 1986.
15. R. S. Porubcan, "Reduction of ammonia nitrogen and nitrite in tanks of Penaeus monodon using floating biofilters containing processed diatomaceous earth media pre-inoculated with nitrifying bacteria," in Proceedings of the Program and Abastracts of the 22nd Annual Conference and Exposition, World Aquaculture Society, Puerto Rico, Spain, June 1991.

16. R. S. Porubcan, "Reduction in chemical oxygen demand and improvement in Penaeus monodon yield in ponds inoculated with aerobic Bacillus bacteria," in Proceedings of the Program and Abastracts of the 22nd Annual Conference and Exposition, World Aquaculture Society, Puerto Rico, Spain, June 1991.
17. G. B. Gómez, A. Roque, and J. F. Turnbull, "The use and selection of probiotic bacteria for use in the culture of larval aquatic organisms," Aquaculture, vol. 191, no. 1–3, pp. 259–270, 2000.
18. D. J. W. Moriarty, "Control of luminous Vibrio species in penaeid aquaculture ponds," Aquaculture, vol. 164, no. 1–4, pp. 351–358, 1998.
19. Y. B. Wang, J. R. Li, and J. Lin, "Probiotics in aquaculture: challenges and outlook," Aquaculture, vol. 281, no. 1–4, pp. 1–4, 2008.
20. A. Irianto and B. Austin, "Probiotics in aquaculture," Journal of Fish Diseases, vol. 25, no. 11, pp. 633–642, 2002.
21. S. Rengpipat, W. Phianphak, S. Piyatiratitivorakul, and P. Menasveta, "Effects of a probiotic bacterium on black tiger shrimp Penaeus monodon survival and growth," Aquaculture, vol. 167, no. 3-4, pp. 301–313, 1998.
22. J. F. Queiroz and C. E. Boyd, "Effects of a bacterial inoculum in channel catfish ponds," Journal of the World Aquaculture Society, vol. 29, no. 1, pp. 67–73, 1998.
23. A. Gildberg, H. Mikkelsen, E. Sandaker, and E. Ringø, "Probiotic effect of lactic acid bacteria in the feed on growth and survival of fry of Atlantic cod (Gadus morhua)," Hydrobiologia, vol. 352, no. 1–3, pp. 279–285, 1997.
24. P. A. Douillet and C. J. Langdon, "Use of a probiotic for the culture of larvae of the Pacific oyster(Crassostrea gigas Thunberg)," Aquaculture, vol. 119, no. 1, pp. 25–40, 1994.
25. F. J. Gatesoupe, "The use of probiotics in aquaculture," Aquaculture, vol. 180, no. 1-2, pp. 147–165, 1999.
26. A. R. S. Harzeveli, H. VanDuffel, P. Dhert, J. Swing, and P. Sorgeloos, "Use of a potential probioticLactococcus lactis AR21 strain for the enhancement of growth in the rotifer Brachionus plicatilis(Muller)," Aquaculture Research, vol. 29, no. 6, pp. 411–417, 1998.

27. S. Dharmaraj and K. Dhevendaran, "Evaluation of Streptomyces as a probiotic feed for the growth of ornamental fish Xiphophorus helleri," Food Technology and Biotechnology, vol. 48, no. 4, pp. 497–504, 2010.
28. L. H. H. Hernandez, T. C. Barrera, J. C. Mejia et al., "Effects of the commercial probiotic Lactobacillus casei on the growth, protein content of skin mucus and stress resistance of juveniles of the Porthole livebearer Poecilopsis gracilis (Poecilidae)," Aquaculture Nutrition, vol. 16, no. 4, pp. 407–411, 2010.
29. M. Rahiman, J. Yousuf, T. Ambat, and M. Hatha, "Probiotic effect of Bacillus NL110 and Vibrio NE17 on the survival, growth performance and immune response of Macrobrachium rosenbergii (de Man),"Aquaculture Research, vol. 41, no. 9, pp. e120–e134, 2010. View at Publisher
30. Lin Sh, Y. Guan, L. Luo, and Y. Pan, "Effects of dietary chitosan oligosaccharides and Bacillus coagulanson growth, innate immunity and resistance of koi (Cyprinus carpio koi)," Aquaculture, vol. 342-343, pp. 36–41, 2012.
31. C. I. Chang and W. Y. Liu, "An evaluation of two probiotic bacterial strains, Enterococcus faecium SF68 and Bacillus toyoi, for reducing edwardsiellosis in cultured European eel, Anguilla anguilla L," Journal of Fish Diseases, vol. 25, no. 5, pp. 311–315, 2002.
32. S. Nikoskelainen, A. Ouwehand, S. Salminen, and G. Bylund, "Protection of rainbow trout (Oncorhynchus mykiss) from furunculosis by Lactobacillus rhamnosus," Aquaculture, vol. 198, no. 3-4, pp. 229–236, 2001.
33. A. Irianto and B. Austin, "Use of probiotics to control furunculosis in rainbow trout, Oncorhynchus mykiss (Walbaum)," Journal of Fish Diseases, vol. 25, no. 6, pp. 333–342, 2002.
34. L. Gram, J. Melchiorsen, B. Spanggaard, I. Huber, and T. F. Nielsen, "Inhibition of Vibrio anguillarumby Pseudomonas fluorescens AH2, a possible probiotic treatment of fish," Applied and Environmental Microbiology, vol. 65, no. 3, pp. 969–973, 1999.
35. L. Gram, T. Løvold, J. Nielsen, J. Melchiorsen, and B. Spanggaard, "In vitro antagonism of the probiontPseudomonas fluorescens strain AH2 against Aeromonas salmonicida does not confer

protection of salmon against furunculosis," Aquaculture, vol. 199, no. 1-2, pp. 1–11, 2001.

36. B. Spanggaard, I. Huber, J. Nielsen et al., "The probiotic potential against vibriosis of the indigenous microflora of rainbow trout," Environmental Microbiology, vol. 3, no. 12, pp. 755–765, 2001.
37. C. Ruiz-Ponte, J. F. Samain, J. L. Sánchez, and J. L. Nicolas, "The benefit of a Roseobacter species on the survival of scallop larvae," Marine Biotechnology, vol. 1, no. 1, pp. 52–59, 1999.
38. U. Scholz, D. G. Garcia, D. Riccque, S. L. E. Cruz, A. F. Vargas, and J. Latchford, "Enhancement of vibriosis resistance in juvenile Penaeus vannamei by supplementation of diets with different yeast products," Aquaculture, vol. 176, no. 3-4, pp. 271–283, 1999.
39. B. Austin, L. F. Stuckey, P. A. W. Robertson, I. Effendi, and D. R. W. Griffith, "A probiotic strain ofVibrio alginolyticus effective in reducing diseases caused by Aeromonas salmonicida, Vibrio anguillarum and Vibrio ordalii," Journal of Fish Diseases, vol. 18, no. 1, pp. 93–96, 1995.
40. B. Austin, E. Baudet, and M. Stobie, "Inhibition of bacterial fish pathogens by Tetraselmis suecica,"Journal of Fish Diseases, vol. 90, pp. 389–392, 1992.
41. Y. Youping, M. Dongdong, L. Shijiang, and W. Zhongkang, "Effects on growth and digestive enzyme activities of the Hepialus gonggaensis larvae caused by introducing probiotics," World Journal of Microbiology and Biotechnology, vol. 27, no. 3, pp. 529–533, 2011.
42. A. M. Abdullah, R. Hashim, and P. M. Aliyu, "Evaluating the use of Lactobacillus acidophilus as a biocontrol agent against common pathogenic bacteria and the effects on the haematology parameters and histopathology in African catfish Clarias gariepinus juveniles," Aquaculture Research, vol. 42, no. 2, pp. 196–209, 2011.
43. S. D. Moreira, S. S. Medeiros, L. L. Pereira, L. A. Romano, W. Wasielesky, and B. E. Cupertino, "The use of probiotics during the nursery rearing or the pink shrimp Farfantepenaeus brasiliensis (Latreille, 1817) in a zero exchange system," Aquaculture Research, pp. 1–10, 2011.

44. S. Zhang, Y. Sing, M. Long, and Z. Wei, "Does dietary administration of Lactococcus lactis modulate the gut microbiota of grouper, Epinephelus coioides," Journal of the World Aquaculture Society, vol. 43, no. 2, pp. 198–207, 2012.
45. A. Dohail, M. Abdullah, H. Roshada, and M. Aliyu, "Effects of the probiotic, Lactobacillus acidophilus, on the growth performance, haematology parameters and immunoglobulin concentration in African Catfish (Clarias gariepinus, Burchell 1822) fingerling," Aquaculture Research, vol. 40, no. 14, pp. 1642–1652, 2009.
46. P. A. Tapia, R. P. Díaz, R. J. León et al., "Use or the probiotic Shewanella putrefaciens Pdp11 on the culture of Senegalenses sole (Solea senegalensis, Kaup 1858) and gilthead seabream (Sparaus aurata L.),"Aquaculture International, vol. 21, pp. 1–15, 2012.
47. X. X. Zhou, Y. B. Wang, and W. F. Li, "Effect of probiotic on larvae shrimp (Penaeus vannamei) based on water quality, survival rate and digestive enzyme activities," Aquaculture, vol. 287, no. 3-4, pp. 349–353, 2009.
48. F. Shishehchian, F. M. Yusoff, and M. Shariff, "The effects of commercial bacterial products on macrobenthos community in shrimp culture ponds," Aquaculture International, vol. 9, no. 5, pp. 429–436, 2001.
49. O. Carnevali, L. de Vivo, R. Sulpizio et al., "Growth improvement by probiotic in European sea bass juveniles (Dicentrarchus labrax, L.), with particular attention to IGF-1, myostatin and cortisol gene expression," Aquaculture, vol. 258, no. 1–4, pp. 430–438, 2006.
50. J. L. Varela, I. Ruíz, L. Vargas et al., "Dietary administration of probiotic Pdp11 promotes growth and improves stress tolerance to high stocking density in gilthead seabream Sparus auratus," Aquaculture, vol. 309, no. 1–4, pp. 265–271, 2010.
51. Y. Taoka, H. Maeda, J. Y. Jo et al., "Growth, stress tolerance and non-specific immune response of Japanese flounder Paralichthys olivaceus to probiotics in a closed recirculating system," Fisheries Science, vol. 72, no. 2, pp. 310–321, 2006.
52. M. Castex, P. Lemaire, N. Wabete, and L. Chim, "Effect of dietary probiotic Pediococcus acidilactici on antioxidant defences and oxidative stress status of shrimp Litopenaeus stylirostris," Aquaculture, vol. 294, no. 3-4, pp. 306–313, 2009.

53. S. Ghosh, A. Sinha, and C. Sahu, "Effect of probiotic on reproductive performance in female livebearing ornamental fish," Aquaculture Research, vol. 38, no. 5, pp. 518–526, 2007.
54. G. Gioacchini, F. Maradonna, F. Lombardo, D. Bizzaro, I. Olivotto, and O. Carnevali, "Increase of fecundity by probiotic administration in zebrafish (Danio rerio)," Reproduction, vol. 140, no. 6, pp. 953–959, 2010.
55. H. Abasali and S. Mohamad, "Effect of dietary supplementation with probiotic on reproductive performance of female livebearing ornamental fish," Research Journal of Animal Sciences, vol. 4, no. 4, pp. 103–107, 2010.
56. J. Schrezenmeir and M. De Vrese, "Probiotics, prebiotics, and synbiotics—approaching a definition,"American Journal of Clinical Nutrition, vol. 73, pp. 361S–364S, 2001.
57. E. Metchnikoff, "Lactic acid as inhibiting intestinal putrefaction," in The Prolongation of Life, Optimistic Studies, pp. 161–183, Mitchell Heinemann, London, UK, 1907.
58. D. M. Lilly and R. H. Stillwell, "Probiotics: growth-promoting factors produced by microorganisms,"Science, vol. 147, no. 3659, pp. 747–748, 1965.
59. G. S. Sperti, Probiotics, Avi Publishing, West Point, Miss, USA, 1971.
60. R. B. Parker, "Probiotics, the other half of the antibiotics story," Animal Nutrition Health, vol. 29, pp. 4–8, 1974.
61. R. Fuller, "Probiotics in man and animals," Journal of Applied Bacteriology, vol. 66, no. 5, pp. 365–378, 1989.
62. R. Havenaar and I. Huis, The Lactic Acid Bacteria in Health and Disease, Volume 1, Edited by B. J. B. Wood, Elsevier, New York, NY, USA, 1992.
63. F. Guarner and G. J. Schaafsma, "Probiotics," International Journal of Food Microbiology, vol. 39, no. 3, pp. 237–238, 1998.
64. D. Myers, "Probiotics," Journal of Exotic Pet Medicine, vol. 16, no. 3, pp. 195–197, 2007.
65. L. Verschuere, G. Rombaut, P. Sorgeloos, and W. Verstraete, "Probiotic bacteria as biological control agents in aquaculture," Microbiology and Molecular Biology Reviews, vol. 64, no. 4, pp. 655–671, 2000.

66. L. Vázquez, R. Hernández, E. Sainz et al., "Cambio en la flora intestinal de ratones por la administración de bifidobacterias y jugo de girasol," Veterinaria México, vol. 27, no. 2, pp. 127–131, 1996.
67. N. G. Vine, W. D. Leukes, and H. Kaiser, "Probiotics in marine larviculture," FEMS Microbiology Reviews, vol. 30, no. 3, pp. 404–427, 2006.
68. G. Burr, D. Gatlin, and S. Ricke, "Microbial ecology of the gastrointestinal tract of fish and the potential application of prebiotics and probiotics in Finnish aquaculture," Journal of the World Aquaculture Society, vol. 36, no. 4, pp. 425–435, 2005.
69. C. Soccol, L. Porto, M. Rigon et al., "The potential of probiotics: a review," Food Technology and Biotechnology, vol. 48, no. 4, pp. 413–434, 2010.
70. E. Haroun, A. Goda, and M. Kabir, "Effect of dietary probiotic Biogen supplementation as a growth promoter on growth performance and feed utilization of Nile tilapia Oreochromis niloticus (L.),"Aquaculture Research, vol. 37, no. 14, pp. 1473–1480, 2006.
71. Y. B. Wang, Z. R. Xu, and M. S. Xia, "The effectiveness of commercial probiotics in northern white shrimp Penaeus vannamei ponds," Fisheries Science, vol. 71, no. 5, pp. 1036–1041, 2005.
72. Y. Taoka, H. Maeda, J. Y. Jo et al., "Use of live and dead probiotic cells in tilapia Oreochromis niloticus,"Fisheries Science, vol. 72, no. 4, pp. 755–766, 2006.
73. C. P. Martínez, L. Mayorga, T. Ponce et al., "Efecto de los fructooligosacáridos en la población bacteriana fecal de un neonato, crecida en cultivo por lote," Revista Mexicana De Ciencias Farmacéuticas, vol. 39, no. 1, pp. 32–37, 2008.
74. K. M. Tuohy, H. M. Probert, C. W. Smejkal, and G. R. Gibson, "Using probiotics and prebiotics to improve gut health," Drug Discovery Today, vol. 8, no. 15, pp. 692–700, 2003.
75. A. Y. Dakar, S. M. Shalaby, and I. P. Saoud, "Assessing the use of a dietary probiotic/prebiotic as an enhancer of spinefoot rabbitfish Siganus rivulatus survival and growth," Aquaculture Nutrition, vol. 13, no. 6, pp. 407–412, 2007.

76. Smart Microbials Inc, "Un universo de microbios inteligentes a su servicio. Technical details on the use of commercial probiotic product Aqua BOOSTER," 2012, http://smartmicrobialsinc.com/aqua.php.
77. C. Lacroix and S. Yildirim, "Fermentation technologies for the production of probiotics with high viability and functionality," Current Opinion in Biotechnology, vol. 18, no. 2, pp. 176–183, 2007.
78. S. Rokka and P. Rantamäki, "Protecting probiotic bacteria by microencapsulation: challenges for industrial applications," European Food Research and Technology, vol. 231, no. 1, pp. 1–12, 2010.
79. P. Rosas-Ledesma, J. M. León-Rubio, F. J. Alarcón, M. A. Moriñigo, and M. C. Balebona, "Calcium alginate capsules for oral administration of fish probiotic bacteria: aassessment of optimal conditions for encapsulation," Aquaculture Research, vol. 43, pp. 106–116, 2012.
80. M. A. Moriñigo, V. Sánchez, and T. F. Martínez, "Encapsulation of a bacterial fish probiiotic in alginate beads: protective effect under in vitro simulations of fish gastric conditions," in Abstracts of the International Conference on Fish Diseases and Fish Immunology, pp. 6–9, Iceland University, Reykjavik, Iceland, 2008.
81. J. A. Muller, R. P. Ross, G. F. Fitzgeralk, and C. Stanton, "Manufacture of Probiotic Bacteria," Prebiotics and Probiotics Science and Technology, pp. 125–759, 2009.
82. R. C. Medina and E. B. Cordero, "Crecimiento y composición bioquímica de la diatomea Chaetoceros muelleri Lemmerman, mantenida en cultivo estático con un medio comercial," Ciencia y Mar, pp. 19–25, 2011.
83. G. Gómez, A. Roque, and B. Velasco, "Culture of Vibrio alginolyticus C7b, a potential probiotic bacterium, with the microalga Chaetoceros muelleri," Aquaculture, vol. 211, no. 1–4, pp. 43–48, 2002.
84. M. Planas, J. Vázquez, J. Marqués, R. Pérez, M. González, and M. Murado, "Enhancement of rotifer (Brachionus plicatilis) growth by using terrestrial lactic acid bacteria," Aquaculture, vol. 240, no. 1–4, pp. 313–329, 2004.

85. F. Lara, N. Olvera, M. Guzmán, and M. López, "Use of the bacteria Streptococcus faecium andLactobacillus acidophilus, and the yeast Saccharomyces cerevisiae as growth promoters in Nile tilapia (Oreochromis niloticus)," Aquaculture, vol. 216, no. 1–4, pp. 193–201, 2003.
86. S. Ghosh, A. Sinha, and C. Sahu, "Dietary probiotic supplementation on growth and health of live-bearing ornamental fishes," Aquaculture Nutrition, vol. 14, no. 4, pp. 289–299, 2008.
87. B. M. Macey and V. E. Coyne, "Improved growth rate and disease resistance in farmed Haliotis midae through probiotic treatment," Aquaculture, vol. 245, no. 1–4, pp. 249–261, 2005.
88. T. Nakano, Microorganism. En dietary supplements for the health and quality of cultured fish, CAB International, London, UK, 2007.
89. P. J. Ronsón and R. Medina, Probióticos en la Acuicultura, Ciencia y Mar Notas, 2002.
90. P. A. W. Robertson, C. O›Dowd, C. Burrells, P. Williams, and B. Austin, "Use of Carnobacterium sp. as a probiotic for Atlantic salmon (Salmo salar L.) and rainbow trout (Oncorhynchus mykiss, Walbaum),"Aquaculture, vol. 185, no. 3-4, pp. 235–243, 2000.
91. A. Irianto and B. Austin, "Use of dead probiotic cells to control furunculosis in rainbow trout,Oncorhynchus mykiss (Walbaum)," Journal of Fish Diseases, vol. 26, no. 1, pp. 59–62, 2003.
92. A. V. Ravi, K. S. Musthafa, G. Jegathammbal, K. Kathiresan, and S. K. Pandian, "Screening and evaluation of probiotics as a biocontrol agent against pathogenic Vibrios in marine aquaculture," Letters in Applied Microbiology, vol. 45, no. 2, pp. 219–223, 2007.
93. K. K. Vijayan, I. S. Bright Singh, N. S. Jayaprakash et al., "A brackishwater isolate of Pseudomonas PS-102, a potential antagonistic bacterium against pathogenic Vibrios in penaeid and non-penaeid rearing systems," Aquaculture, vol. 251, no. 2–4, pp. 192–200, 2006.
94. N. G. Vine, W. D. Leukes, and H. Kaiser, "In vitro growth characteristics of five candidate aquaculture probiotics and two fish pathogens grown in fish intestinal mucus," FEMS Microbiology Letters, vol. 231, no. 1, pp. 145–152, 2004.

95. N. G. Vine, W. D. Leukes, H. Kaiser, S. Daya, J. Baxter, and T. Hecht, "Competition for attachment of aquaculture candidate probiotic and pathogenic bacteria on fish intestinal mucus," Journal of Fish Diseases, vol. 27, no. 6, pp. 319–326, 2004. ·

96. R. G. Gómez, J. L. Balcázar, and M. A. Shen, "Probiotics as control agents in aquaculture," Journal of Ocean University of China, vol. 6, no. 1, pp. 76–79, 2007. ·

97. D. Tovar, J. Zambonino, C. Cahu, F. Gatesoupe, R. Vázquez, and R. Lesel, "Effect of live yeast incorporation in compound diet on digestive enzyme activity in sea bass (Dicentrarchus labrax) larvae,"Aquaculture, vol. 204, no. 1-2, pp. 113–123, 2002. ·

98. M. C. Hidalgo, A. Skalli, E. Abellán, M. Arizcun, and G. Cardenete, "Dietary intake of probiotics and maslinic acid in juvenile dentex (Dentex dentex L.): Effects on growth performance, survival and liver proteolytic activities," Aquaculture Nutrition, vol. 12, no. 4, pp. 256–266, 2006.

99. D. L. Merrifield, G. Bradley, R. T. M. Baker, and S. J. Davies, "Probiotic applications for rainbow trout (Oncorhynchus mykiss Walbaum) II. Effects on growth performance, feed utilization, intestinal microbiota and related health criteria postantibiotic treatment," Aquaculture Nutrition, vol. 16, no. 5, pp. 496–503, 2010.

100. R. Tovar, D. Mazurais, J. Gatesoupe, P. Quazuquel, C. Cahu, and J. Zambonino, "Dietary probiotic live yeast modulates antioxidant enzyme activities and gene expression of sea bass (Dicentrarchus labrax) larvae," Aquaculture, vol. 300, no. 1–4, pp. 142–147, 2010.

101. Z. Heizhao, G. Zhixun, Y. Yingying, Z. Wenhui, and J. Zhuojia, "Effect of dietary probiotics on apparent digestibility coefficients of nutrients of white shrimp Litopenaeus vannamei Boone," Aquaculture Research, vol. 35, no. 15, pp. 1441–1447, 2004.

102. S. Ziaei, M. Habibi, G. Azari, D. Lovett, A. Mirvaghefi, and M. Shakouri, "The effect of Bacillus spp. bacteria used as probiotics on digestive enzyme activity, survival and growth in the Indian white shrimpFenneropenaeus indicus," Aquaculture, vol. 252, no. 2–4, pp. 516–524, 2006.

103. D. J. W. Moriarty, "Probiotics and bioremediation in aquaculture," Asian Shrimp News, vol. 26, article 3, 1996.

104. V. M. Maillard, G. D. Boardman, J. E. Nyland, and D. D. Kuhn, "Water quality and sludge characterization at raceway-system trout farms," Aquacultural Engineering, vol. 33, no. 4, pp. 271–284, 2005.

105. G. Rafiee and C. R. Saad, "Nutrient cycle and sludge production during different stages of red tilapia (Oreochromis sp.) growth in a recirculating aquaculture system," Aquaculture, vol. 244, no. 1–4, pp. 109–118, 2005.

106. R. Lalloo, S. Ramchuran, D. Ramduth, J. Görgens, and N. Gardiner, "Isolation and selection of Bacillusspp. as potential biological agents for enhancement of water quality in culture of ornamental fish,"Journal of Applied Microbiology, vol. 103, no. 5, pp. 1471–1479, 2007.

107. L. Jiqiu, T. Beiping, M. Kangsen et al., "Comparative study between probiotic bacterium ArthrobacterXE-7 and chloramphenicol on protection of Penaeus chinensis post-larvae from pathogenic Vibrios,"Aquaculture, vol. 253, no. 1–4, pp. 140–147, 2006.

108. S. Vianello, L. Brazzoduro, V. Dalla, P. Belvedere, and L. Colombo, "Myostatin expression during development and chronic stress in zebrafish (Danio rerio)," Journal of Endocrinology, vol. 176, no. 1, pp. 47–59, 2003.

109. M. Izquierdo, H. Palacios, and A. Tacon, "Effect of broodstock nutrition on reproductive performance of fish," Aquaculture, vol. 197, no. 1–4, pp. 25–42, 2001.

110. M. Saxelin, H. Rautelin, S. Salminen, and P. H. Makela, "Safety of commercial products with viableLactobacillus strains," Infectious Diseases in Clinical Practice, vol. 5, no. 5, pp. 331–335, 1996.

111. N. Ishibashi and S. Yamazaki, "Probiotics and safety," American Journal of Clinical Nutrition, vol. 73, no. 2, pp. 465S–470S, 2001.

112. S. J. Lahtinen, R. J. Boyle, A. Margolles, R. Frías, and M. Gueimonde, "Safety assessment of probiotics,"Prebiotics and Probiotics Science and Technology, pp. 1193–1235, 2009.

113. FAO/WHO, Guidelines for the Evaluation of Probiotics in Food, 2006.

114. H. Y. Chou, X. Y. Huang, C. H. Wang, H. C. Chiang, and C. F. Lo, "Pathogenicity of a baculovirus infection causing white spot syndrome in cultured penaeid shrimp in Taiwan," Diseases of

Aquatic Organisms, vol. 23, no. 3, pp. 165–173, 1995.

115. Y. G. Wang, M. D. Hassan, M. Shariff, S. M. Zamri, and X. Chen, "Histopathology and cytopathology of white spot syndrome virus (WSSV) in cultured Penaeus monodon from peninsular Malaysia with emphasis on pathogenesis and the mechanism of white spot formation," Diseases of Aquatic Organisms, vol. 39, no. 1, pp. 1–11, 1999.
116. Y. G. Wang, K. L. Lee, M. Najiah, M. Shariff, and M. D. Hassan, "A new bacterial white spot syndrome (BWSS) in cultured tiger shrimp Penaeus monodon and its comparison with white spot syndrome (WSS) caused by virus," Diseases of Aquatic Organisms, vol. 41, no. 1, pp. 9–18, 2000.
117. S. Shakibazadeh, C. R. Saad, A. Christianus, M. S. Kamarudin, K. Sijam, and P. Sinaian, "Assessment of possible human risk of probiotic application in shrimp farming," International Food Research Journal, vol. 18, pp. 433–437, 2011.
118. M. Pineiro and C. Stanton, "Probiotic bacteria: Legislative framework—requirements to evidence basis," Journal of Nutrition, vol. 137, pp. 850S–835S, 2007.
119. A. D. Schulze, O. A. Abayomi, S. A. Tattersall, and K. M. Miller, "Bacterial diversity in a marine hatchery: balance between pathogenic and potentially probiotic bacterial strains," Aquaculture, vol. 256, no. 1–4, pp. 50–73, 2006.
120. H. Sugita, H. Mizuki, and S. Itoi, "Diversity of siderophore-producing bacteria isolated from the intestinal tracts of fish along the Japanese coast," Aquaculture Research, vol. 43, no. 4, pp. 481–488, 2012.
121. Y. H. Ling, S. Y. Shang, M. R. Long, and Y. J. Dan, "PCR-DGGE analysis of the autochthonous gut microbiota of grouper Ephinephelus coioides following probiotic Bacillus clausii administration,"Aquaculture Research, vol. 43, no. 4, pp. 489–497, 2012.

Chapter 4

Alterations in Histopathological Features and Brain Acetylcholinesterase Activity in Stinging Catfish Heteropneustes Fossilis Exposed to Polluted River Water

Sharmin Ferdewsi Rakhi[1], Abdul Hakim Mohammad Mohsinul Reza[1], Mohammad Shafaet Hossen[1], and Zakir Hossain1,[2]

[1]Department of Fisheries Biology and Genetics, Bangladesh Agricultural University, Mymensingh, 2202, Bangladesh

[2]Richardson Center for Functional Foods and Nutraceutical, Department of Human Nutritional Sciences, Manitoba University Winnipeg, Winnipeg, MB, R3T 2N2, Canada

ABSTRACT

Responses of stinging catfish (*Heteropneustes fossilis*) to pollution were studied in three freshwater rivers, namely Buriganga, Turag, and Shitalakkhya (Dhaka, Bangladesh), which are potentially affected by anthropogenic pollution originating from industrial and sewage dumping. Partial parameters about water quality (temperature, dissolved oxygen, and pH) and seasonal plankton fluctuation were recorded at wet and dry seasons. Histopathology and acetylcholinesterase (AChE) activity were used as biomarkers to assess water toxic effects in 7-and 10-day exposures of *H. fossilis*to three rivers waters, respectively. The lowest level of dissolved oxygen was recorded as 0.7 ± 0.1 mg/l, and the lowest count of plankton genera was 21 at lean period. Furthermore, the 7-day exposure of fish to polluted water abruptly altered the normal structure of various organs. Major structural damages were partial and total epidermal loss, dermis and muscle separation, melanin pigment and vacuole in skin muscle; missing of lamellae, clubbing, fungal granuloma, hyperplasia and hemorrhage in gills; hyperplasia, hemorrhage, pyknosis, vacuole, necrosis, nuclear alteration, fatty degeneration, lipid droplets in liver; degenerating glomerular and tubule, hemorrhage, pyknosis and vacuole in kidneys; and scattered spermatozoa and prominent interstitial space in the testis. After subsequent exposure to polluted water, a significant ($P<0.05$) inhibition of AChE activity in the fish brain was observed with the following order of potency: 102.00 ± 5.00 nmol/min/mg protein (Turag) $\geq 104.00 \pm 5.00$ nmol/min/mg protein (Buriganga) $> 130.67 \pm 3.51$ nmol/min/mg protein (Shitalakkhya). This study confirmed the utility of biomarkers in biomonitoring studies and reflected the potential hazards of pollution to aquatic biota.

BACKGROUND

River pollution is one of the recently focused environmental issues where the most attention is drawn to the rivers and canal systems surrounding Dhaka, Bangladesh. Rapid and unplanned urbanization and industrialization centering this area are increasing at an alarming rate. Due to this situation, the major three rivers, Buriganga, Turag, and Shitalakkhya, surrounding Dhaka have been steadily experiencing complicated problems of pollution and encroachment that have almost suffocated these valuable lifelines of the city. The presence of pollutants in the environment is partially due to natural processes but mainly as a result of industrial waste. The polluting industries surrounding the capital are mainly concentrated at Hazaribag and Lalbag (Old

Dhaka), Tongi (Gazipur), and Demra (Narayangang) that dispose their huge untreated effluents directly into these three rivers. These rivers specially the Buriganga are also loaded by sewage pollution. However, high concentration of suspended and dissolved solids has also been reported; they previously occurred at low concentration and are now found in high concentrations (Zakir et al. 2006; Mohiuddin et al. 2011).

Occurrence of potential toxicants in aquatic ecosystem causes a reduction in the quality of the aquatic environment that results in impaired level of dissolved oxygen (DO), pH, temperature, biological oxygen demand, and chemical oxygen demand (Roberts 2001). Adverse water quality, moreover, makes the aquatic habitat biologically dead. Availability of a plankton community is an indicator of water quality. Ferdous and Muktadir (2009) described the high potentialities of zooplankton as a bioindicator. However, evaluations on reduced bioavailability of plankton that resulted from pollution have been made earlier (Begum and Khanam 2009; Shah et al. 2008; Begum 2008; Solomon et al.2009; Sharma et al. 2010).

Though chemical monitoring of water and sediment is a common and reliable measure to describe the degree of contamination, it is not the case for the overall assessment for evaluating the effects of pollution on the environment as toxic or biological effects on organisms cannot be obtained by this method. Recently, different types of biomarkers have been studied and evaluated for their acceptability to detect the biological effects as a biomonitoring tool (Amiard et al. 2006; Magni et al.2006; Nigro et al. 2006).

Histopathological assessment is a sensitive biomonitoring tool in toxicant impact assessment to indicate the effect of toxicants on fish health in polluted aquatic ecosystems. Histopathological assessment of fish tissue allows for early warning signs of disease and detection of long-term injury in cells, tissues, or organs. Structural changes in various tissues into the polluted ecosystem have also been acknowledged (Peuranen et al. 2000; Marchand et al. 2009). Earlier histopathological assessments of fish exposed to a variety of pollutants reveal the potency of this biomarker against pollution.

Acetylcholinesterase (AChE) is the main cholinesterasic form in all invertebrate and vertebrate tissues such as the brain (Rodrigues et al. 2011), muscles, blood cells, and liver (Valbonesi et al. 2011). This enzyme is found at neuromuscular junctions and cholinergic nervous system where its activity serves to terminate synaptic transmission. It degrades (through its hydrolytic activity) the neurotransmitter acetylcholine, producing choline and an acetate group in both vertebrates and invertebrates (Varo et al. 2008). Cholinesterase inhibitors such as organophosphate and carbamate block the function of AChE and thus provoke excess acetylcholine accumulation in the synaptic cleft that eventually causes neuromuscular paralysis, leading to death by asphyxiation (Nunes et al. 2003; Purves et al. 2008; Xuereb et al. 2009). Recent studies have shown that AChE is a very useful biomarker of pollution stress under a variety of environmental factors and chemical mixtures in different geographical regions (Baršienė et al. 2006; Kopecka et al. 2006; Schiedek et al. 2006).

In spite of having a lot of deleterious effects of pollution, a limited number of research were conducted in Bangladesh to ascertain their effects on fish at cellular and molecular level. To our knowledge, limited investigations have been made till now to assess the neurotoxic effects (in terms of AChE inhibition) of river pollutants on fish, thus indicating the need for due attention on this matter. Thus, the purpose of the present study is to assess the cellular and neurotoxic effects of river pollution on *Heteropneustes fossilis* through the determination of potency of two biomarkers against pollution.

METHODS

Study Area

Buriganga (near Lalbag, Dhaka), Turag (near Tongi Bridge, Gazipur), and Shitalakkhya (near Demra, Narayangang) are supposed to derive massive pollutant loadings from sewage and industrial effluents directly as industries, textiles, pharmaceuticals, and tanneries have clustered here. During the rainy season, the water quality improves moderately, but on the advent of the dry season, pollution concentration increases abruptly because the water level of the rivers reduces a lot at this time, but the rate of pollutants released into the rivers remains identical. Location of the three rivers and sampling sites are shown in Figure 1.

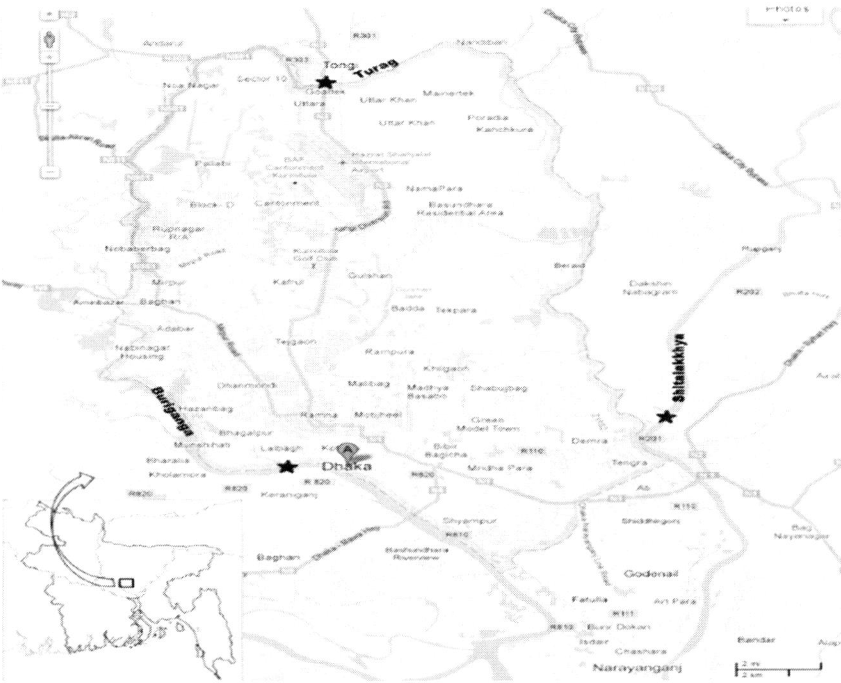

Figure 1: Location of the three rivers, Buriganga, Turag, and Shitalakkhya. Black star (★) indicates the sampling sites (image was taken from Google map).

Water Quality Parameter Measurements

Some water quality parameters were measured from the three rivers at two different seasons (early September 2010 and early March 2011). A mercury centigrade thermometer was used to measure the water temperature; pH and DO were measured by a pH meter (HI 98127, HANNA Instruments, Beijing, China) and a dissolved oxygen meter (DO-5509, Tyner, Dongguan City Electronic Technology Co., Ltd., Guangzhou, China), respectively. Each parameter was recorded at two different points with three replications in the same river.

Plankton Collection and Identification

With a view to record the seasonal plankton availability, samples were collected in early September 2010 and early March 2011. Planktons were collected randomly from the three rivers by plankton net towing. Collected samples were immediately preserved with 5% buffered formalin in separate tagged plastic bottles. For species identification, the bottle containing plankton samples was gently shaken to resuspend all materials, was poured on water a petri dish, and was allowed to settle for a minute. Two drops of water were placed on a glass slide and covered with a cover slip. The planktons were then identified up to genus level under a compound microscope (OPTIKA B-350, OPTIKA Microscopes, Ponteranica, Bergamo, Italy) according to APHA (1992), Bellinger (1992), and Palmer (1980).

Histopathological Study

To assess the effects of polluted water exposure to fish, water samples were separately collected from Buriganga, Turag, and Shitalakkhya rivers in six plastic containers (30 l) and were carried out to the wet laboratory of the Faculty of Fisheries, Bangladesh Agricultural University, Mymensingh. Experiments were conducted in nine aquaria of size $48 \times 26 \times 30$ cm^3. Water samples from the three rivers were kept in three different aquaria, each having two replications, whereas one aquarium was kept as control. *H. fossilis* with average size and weight of 12 ± 1.4 cm and 10.5 ± 1.2 g, respectively, were collected from a local fish market in live condition. Forty-five fishes (five fishes in each aquarium) were exposed to three river water samples for a period of 7 days with continuous aeration. After the 7-day exposure, two fishes were taken from each aquarium and sacrificed. Gills, skin muscle, liver, kidney, and gonads were collected and preserved in 10% neutral-buffered formalin, while gonads were preserved in Bouin's fluid. The preserved samples were then dehydrated, cleaned and infiltrated in an automatic tissue processor (ThermoFisher Scientific, Waltham, MA, USA), embedded in melted paraffin wax, and sectioned (5 μm) with a microtome machine (Leica Junc 2035, Leica Microsystems Srl, Milan, Italy). Thereafter, the sections were stained with hematoxylin and eosin (H and E) stains. After staining, the sections were mounted with Canada balsam and kept overnight for the permanent slide. Photomicrography of the stained samples was done using a photomicroscope (OPTIKA B-350). The extent of alteration was scored as severe (+++), moderate (++), mild (+), and not found (−). When a pathology occurred in >50%

cell or area in maximum investigated slides, it scored severe (+++), followed by >25% for moderate (++), and <25% for mild (+).

AChE Activity Measurement

x`For the analysis of AChE activity, *H. fossilis* was exposed to river water in glass aquaria for 10 days. Fish exposed to pollutant-free water was kept as control. Following exposure, three fishes were taken from each aquarium ($n = 9$) for each river. The whole brain was dissected out by sacrificing the fish and was placed in ice-cold 0.1-M sodium phosphate buffer (pH 8.0). In this study, where brain sample was used similarly with teleost, AChE is maximally distributed in the brain (Kopecka et al. 2004; Ferenczy et al. 1997). Tissues were then weighted and homogenized using a glass-Teflon homogenizer in a homogenization buffer (0.1-M sodium phosphate buffer, 0.1% Triton X-100, and pH 8.0) to achieve the final concentration of 20 mg tissue/ml phosphate buffer. Tissue homogenate was centrifuged at $10{,}000 \times g$ for 15 min at 4°C, and the supernatant was removed. An aliquot of supernatant was then removed and measured for protein according to the method of Lowry et al. (1951) using bovine serum albumin in homogenization buffer as a standard.

AChE activity in the fish brain was measured according to the method of Ellman et al. (1961), as optimized by Habig et al. (1988) and Sandahl and Jenkins (2002). Tissue homogenate (50 μl) was added to 900 μl of cold sodium phosphate buffer (0.1 M containing 0.1% Triton X-100, pH 8.0) and 50 μl of 5,5-dithiobis (2-nitrobenzoic acid) (6 mM), then vortexed, and allowed to stand at room temperature for 10 min. Aliquots of 200 μl in triplicate were then placed into microtiter plate wells. The reaction was started with the addition of 50 μl of acetylthiocholine iodide (15 mM) specific for fish (Jash et al. 1982). Changes in absorbance were measured with a microplate reader (SpectraMax 340PC^{384}, Molecular Devices LLC, and Sunnyvale, CA, USA) at 412 nm for 10 min at 12-s intervals. AChE activity is expressed as nanomole per minute per milligram protein.

Statistical Analysis

Data were analyzed using one way analysis of variance and expressed as mean ± SD. A *post hoc* Waller Duncan multiple test range was performed which considered a 5% significant level using SPSS ver. 11.5 computer software program.

RESULTS AND DISCUSSION

Water Quality Parameters

Water quality parameters of the three rivers in two different seasons are presented in Table 1. The temperature in the wet season ranged from 22.5°C to 24.5°C where it increased to 29°C to 31.5°C in the dry season. Significant reduction in DO level was observed in dry season where Turag River had the lowest DO level (0.7 mg/l). No wide fluctuation in pH level was observed at two different seasons that ranged from 6.9 to 7.2.

Table 1: List of water quality parameters of the three rivers at two different seasons

River	Season	Water quality parameters		
		Temperature (°C)	**DO (mg/l)**	**pH**
Buriganga	Wet	24.0 ± 1.0	6.8 ± 0.1	7.2 ± 0.2
	Dry	29.5 ± 1.0	1.5 ± 0.2	7.1 ± 0.1
Turag	Wet	24.5 ± 2.0	5.1 ± 0.1	7.1 ± 0.1
	Dry	31.5 ± 0.5	0.7 ± 0.1	6.9 ± 0.1
Shitalakkhya	Wet	22.5 ± 1.0	7.2 ± 0.1	7.2 ± 0.1
	Dry	29.0 ± 1.2	1.9 ± 0.2	7.1 ± 0.1

Data are presented as mean ± SD.

Rakhi *et al.*

Rakhi *et al. International Aquatic Research* 2013 **5**:7, doi: 10.1186/2008-6970-5-7

Variation in water quality parameters is mainly due to seasonal environmental factors. Increased temperature in the dry season affects the DO level as they are inversely correlated. In the study, very low DO levels (0.7 to 1.9 mg/l) were recorded in the dry season where >5 mg/l is recommended for biological organisms. This anoxic condition especially in Turag reflects the breakdown of untreated organic waste principally received from domestic sewage and chemical residues from various industries surrounding Dhaka (The World Bank 2006). A similar phenomenon was previously reported from these rivers (Begum 2008; Begum and Khanam 2009; The World Bank 2006; Saha et al. 2009).

Plankton Composition

The plankton communities of the three rivers were identified at rainy and dry seasons. A total of 33, 26, and 35 genera were identified from Buriganga, Turag, and Shitalakkhya rivers, respectively in the rainy season, whereas, in the dry season, a lesser number of genera were recorded: 21, 19, and 26, from Buriganga, Turag, and Shitalakkhya rivers, respectively (Table 2). Among the recorded phytoplankton groups, Bacillariophyceae were found in both seasons in the respective rivers, and Chlorophyceae were recorded more only in the wet season. However, among the recorded zooplankton groups, Cladocera occurred more frequently in the wet season than in the dry season. Frequent abundance of Copepoda represented by two genera was observed from the three rivers in both seasons. Rotifera were recorded low, but the lowest count was made in the dry season; no genera were even found in the dry season from Turag River.

Table 2: List of plankton recorded from Buriganga, Turag, and Shitalakkhya rivers at wet and dry seasons

Plankton	Class	Species	Wet season			Dry season		
			Buriganga	**Turag**	**Shitalakkhya**	**Buriganga**	**Turag**	**Shitalakkhya**
Phytop-lankton	Bacillari-ophyceae	*Fragilaria* sp.	✓	×	✓	×	×	✓
		Cyclotella sp.	✓	✓	✓	✓	×	×
		Cymbella sp.	✓	✓	✓	✓	✓	✓
		Gomphonema sp.	✓	✓	✓	✓	✓	✓
		Gyrosigma sp.	✓	✓	✓	✓	✓	✓
		Melosira sp.	×	×	✓	✓	×	✓
		Navicula sp.	✓	✓	✓	✓	✓	✓
		Nitzschia sp.	✓	✓	✓	✓	✓	✓
		Synedra sp.	×	×	✓	×	×	✓
	Chloro-phyceae	*Ankistrodesmus*sp.	✓	×	✓	×	×	×
		Chara sp.	×	✓	×	×	×	×
		*Chlamydomonas*sp.	✓	✓	✓	×	×	×
		Chlorella sp.	×	✓	✓	×	✓	×
		Chlorogonium sp.	✓	✓	×	×	×	×
		Cosmarium sp.	✓	×	×	✓	×	×
		Eudorina sp.	×	×	✓	×	×	×
		Microspora sp.	×	×	×	×	×	✓
		Oedogonium sp.	×	✓	✓	×	×	×
		Pediastrum sp.	✓	×	×	×	×	×
		Pyrobotrys sp.	×	×	×	×	✓	×
		Scenedesmus sp.	✓	×	✓	×	✓	×
		Spirogyra sp.	✓	✓	✓	✓	✓	✓
		Spirulina sp.	✓	✓	✓	✓	✓	✓
		Ulothrix sp.	✓	✓	×	×	×	×
		Volvox sp.	✓	✓	✓	✓	✓	✓
		Zygnema sp.	×	×	×	✓	×	✓
	Cryptop-hyceae	*Cryptomonas* sp.	✓	×	×	×	×	×
	Chrysop-hyceae	*Mallomonas* sp.	×	×	×	×	×	✓
	Cyano-phyceae	*Anabaena* sp.	×	✓	✓	×	×	✓
		*Aphanizomenon*sp.	×	×	×	×	✓	×
		Chlococcus sp.	×	×	×	✓	×	✓
		*Gomphosphaeria*sp.	×	✓	✓	✓	×	×
		Microcystis sp.	×	×	✓	×	×	×
		Oscillatoria sp.	×	✓	✓	×	✓	✓
		Phormidium sp.	×	✓	×	✓	✓	×
	Euglenop-hyceae	*Euglena* sp.	✓	×	✓	✓	×	✓
		Phacus sp.	✓	×	✓	×	×	✓
		*Trachelomonas*sp.	×	×	✓	×	×	×

Zoo-plankton	Cladocera	*Bosmina* sp.	✓	×	×	×	×	×
		Daphnia sp.	✓	✓	×	✓	✓	×
		*Diaphanosoma*sp.	×	✓	×	×	×	×
		Moina sp.	✓	✓	×	✓	✓	×
		Nauplius	✓	✓	×	×	✓	×
	Copepoda	*Cyclops* sp.	✓	✓	×	✓	✓	×
		Diaptomus sp.	✓	✓	×	✓	✓	×
	Rotifera	*Brachionus* sp.	✓	×	×	✓	×	×
		Filinia sp.	×	×	×	×	×	×
		Keratella sp.	✓	×	×	×	×	×
Total			33	26	35	21	19	26

Rakhi *et al.*

Rakhi *et al. International Aquatic Research* 2013 **5**:7, doi: 10.1186/2008-6970-5-7

Seasonal variations in plankton are related to a variety of environmental factors in aquatic environments where temperature has been claimed to be the major determining factor in phytoplankton growth and development (Çetin and Şen 2004; Baquero et al. 2006). The less abundance of plankton communities in the dry season mainly due to high temperature and low DO. The occurrence of Chlorophyceae only in the wet season and Bacillariophyceae in both two seasons indicates that Chlorophyceae are more sensitive to pollutant discharge, whereas Bacillariophyceae seem to be very well adapted to polluted zone (Begum and Khanam 2009; Shah et al. 2008). Among the zooplankton, the members of Cladocera occurred in lower number in the dry season because Cladocera are highly responsive against pollutants; they even react against low concentration of contaminants (Ferdous and Muktadir 2009). Copepoda were represented by two genera and appeared all year round as this group is much more tolerant to O_2 deficiency. On the contrary, lower representation by the members Rotifera in the dry season and no genera in Turag is opposed to the studies of Solomon et al. (Solomon et al. 2009) and Sharma et al. (2010) who reported the dominance of Rotifera among all zooplankton. This is because the frequency of that group is lower in polluted water than in unpolluted or lower polluted zones (Eloranta 1980).

Histopathological Observations

After subsequent exposure of *H. fossilis* to Buriganga, Turag, and Shitalakkhya river water samples, histopathological assessment of skin muscle, gills, liver, kidney, and testis was made by comparing them with the control. Mild to severe alterations in the different organs were assessed (Table 3).

Table 3: Histopathological effects on *H. fossilis* after 7-day exposure to Buriganga, Turag, and Shitalakkhya river water

Histopathological alterations in organ Buriganga		Extent of alteration		
		Turag	Shitalakkhya	
Skin muscle	Melanin pigment	+++	+	+
	Vacuoles	–	++	+
	Epidermal loss	+	++	+++
	Muscle separation	++	+	+++
Gill	Hemorrhage	+++	+++	++
	Necrosis	++	–	–
	Gill clubbing	++	++	++
	Fungal granuloma	+++	+++	+
	Missing of secondary gill lamellae	+++	++	++
	Hyperplasia and hypertrophy	++	++	+
Liver	Hemorrhage	+++	+++	+
	Pyknosis	++	++	+
	Vacuole	+	+	++
	Necrosis	+	++	+
	Fatty degeneration	++	++	+
	Lipid droplet	–	++	–
	Nuclear alteration	–	–	+
	Hyperplasia and hypertrophy	–	–	+

Kidney	Degenerated kidney tubule	+	+	+
	Hemorrhage	+	+	−
	Vacuole	++	++	−
	Degenerated glomerular tubule	−	+	−
Testis	Scattered spermatozoa	++	+	+
	Vacuole	++	+	++
	Testis interstitial space	+++	+++	++

Extent of alteration: severe (+++), moderate (++), mild (+), not found (−).

Rakhi *et al.*

Rakhi *et al. International Aquatic Research* 2013 **5**:7, doi: 10.1186/2008-6970-5-7

The skin muscle of the control group was in a systemic arrangement of epidermis, dermis, and muscle (Figure 2a). The major pathological signs observed in skin muscle of fish exposed to the water of three different rivers were partial loss of epidermis, totally missing epidermis, separation of dermis from epidermis, separation of muscle from dermis, melanin pigment, and vacuole in muscle and dermis (Figure 2b,c,d). As skin muscle is the primary site of exposure, pollutants affected the epidermis abruptly. Melanin pigment is a prominent feature of chronic inflammatory response.

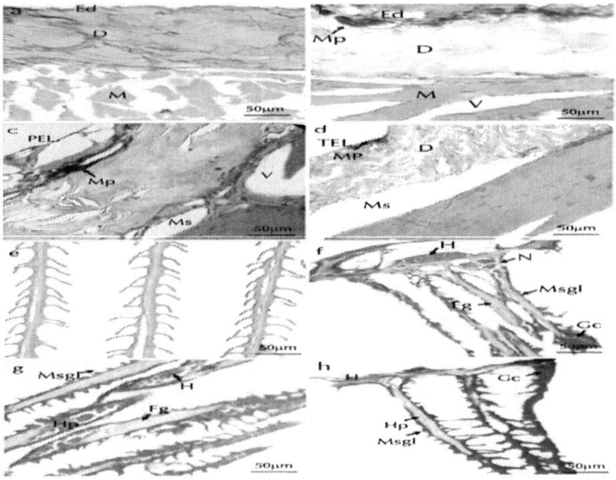

Figure 2: Photomicrograph of skin muscle and gills of *H. fossilis* from control and from the three rivers. Photomicrograph of skin muscle from (a) control, (b) Buriganga, (c) Turag, and (d) Shitalakkhya. Photomicrograph of gills from (e) control, (f) Buriganga, (g) Turag, and (h) Shitalakkhya. Ed, epidermis; D, dermis; M, muscle; Mp, melanin pigment; V, vacuole; PEL, partial epidermal loss; TEL, total epidermal loss; Ms, muscle separation; H, hemorrhage; N, necrosis; Gc, gill clubbing; Fg, fungal granuloma; Msgl, missing of secondary gill lamellae; HP, hyperplasia and hypertrophy (H and E × 430).

Gills are the primary site for any histological alteration as it is directly exposed to polluted water. In our present study, the structure of gills in the control group was almost normal. Primary and secondary gill lamellae were found with no pathology (Figure 2e). Moderate to severe structural changes with mentionable pathological signs were observed in the gills of treated fish including missing secondary gill lamellae, hemorrhage, necrosis, hyperplasia and hypertrophy, gill clubbing, and fungal granuloma (Figure 2f,g,h). Disruption in gill structure and function possibly due to various environmental factors, pH, ion concentration, heavy metals, and other pollutants were previously described (Tkatcheva et al.2004; Peuranen et al. 2000; Playle 1998). Thickening and lifting of the secondary lamellar epithelium due to hypertrophy are the first signs that gills have been exposed to hazardous chemicals, or physical agents may have been a response to increase the diffusion distance between DO and blood, which accordingly was related to hypoxia in fish (Liu et al. 2010). Gill clubbing is due to excess mucus production. In the presence of pollutants, the epithelium of the secondary lamellae has a tendency to increase the number of mucus cell. Excess mucus from mucus cell causes the fusion of secondary gill lamellae resulting in impaired respiration.

Alteration in the liver structure may be used as a biomarker indicating prior exposure to environmental stressors. A constant exposure to toxicants may cause damage to the liver tissue (Nero et al. 2005). In the present study, hepatocytes and other cells were systematically arranged and no structural alteration was assessed in the liver of the control group (Figure 3a) where the treated group revealed a normal liver tissue structure with severe alterations like deposition of body fat, hypertrophy and hyperplasia of hepatocytes, rupture of blood vessel resulting in hemorrhagic area and necrosis, nuclear alteration, pyknosis, vacuoles, and fatty degeneration (Figure 3b,c,d). A similar assessment was made by Liao et al. (2007) who additionally found basophilic cytoplasm but no lipid droplets in the hepatocytes of medaka (*Oryzias latipes*) exposed to single mercury and single selenium. Farag et al. (2006) observed lipid droplets in the liver of Chinook salmon (*Oncorhynchus tshawytscha*) after chronic chromium exposure, whereas livers of the control group had no hepatocellular lipids. Liver necrosis was found in Nile tilapia (*Oreochromis niloticus*) after exposure to sediment containing a variety of organic chemicals (Perez et al. 2000). Shaw and Handy (2006) found marked hepatic lipidosis (increased intracellular fat stores) in Nile tilapia (*O. niloticus*). Histopathological alterations in the liver of *Clarias gariepinus* from polluted aquatic systems were also found by Marchand et al. (2009).

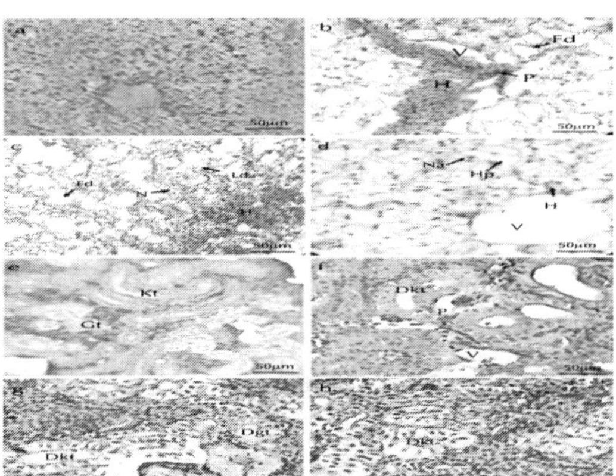

Figure 3: Photomicrograph of liver and kidney of *H. fossilis* from control and from the three rivers. Photomicrograph of liver from (a) control, (b) Buriganga,

(c) Turag, and (d) Shitalakkhya. Photomicrograph of kidney from (e) control, (f) Buriganga, (g) Turag, and (h) Shitalakkhya. H, hemorrhage; Fd, fatty degeneration; Ld, lipid droplet; N, necrosis; P, pyknosis; Na, nuclear alteration; Hp, hyperplasia and hypertrophy; Kt, kidney tubule; Gt, glomerular tubule; Dkt, degenerating kidney tubule; Dgt, degenerating glomerular tubule; V, vacuole (H and E × 430).

This could be expected as the liver is the main detoxification organ involved in the metabolism and excretion of heavy metals. It is therefore a target organ of various toxic substances. Pollutants cause alterations in the liver, lysis of hepatocytes resulting in necrosis, breakdown of blood vessel resulting in a hemorrhagic area, cirrhosis, and ultimately death. Hepatic lipid accumulation is influenced by toxins and environmental stress factors (Tanaka et al. 2002; Xu et al. 2009).

The kidney is a major organ involved in fluid and ionic balance of fish. In the present study, the normal structures of the kidney tubule, glomerulus, and other hematopoietic cells of kidney were found in a reference group (Figure 3e). Mild structural changes were observed including vacuolation, necrosis, mild pyknosis, and mild tubular degeneration from the kidney of fish exposed to different river water (Figure 3f,g,h). However, necrosis, fibrosis (scarring) and dilation of tubular lumina, and lipid peroxidation were observed in affected kidneys as a result of chromium exposure, but not in reference kidneys (Farag et al. 2006) as the exposure time was longer (105 days). The appearance of vacuoles and tubular degeneration might be a result of a general metabolic disturbance leading to an intensified reabsorption of amino acids and small proteins from the ultrafiltrate (1993). Necrosis that resulted from accumulation of granules is due to karyolysis and vacuolation in the cytoplasm (Rangsayatorn et al. 2004).

The immature testes of the control fish possess a normal arrangement of spermatocytes in the testicular lumen and a smaller testis interstitial space (Figure 4a). Some structural alterations were observed in the testes of treated fish such as the appearance of some vacuoles, scattered spermatocytes in the testicular lumen, and larger testis interstitial space (Figure 4b, c, d). Similar findings, except for vacuoles and scattered spermatocytes, were also made earlier by Schultz et al. (2011) in male fathead minnows exposed to antidepressant pharmaceuticals. Intersex gonads were recorded in several species exposed to estrogen-polluted water source (Barnhoorn et al. 2004Barnhoorn et al. 2010). However, no intersex testis was observed in the present study. This may be due to less exposure time and sexual immaturity of the fish. A larger testis interstitial space from all treated groups indicated the presence of toxicants in the three Reference Rivers. These prominent spaces are due to the accumulation of testis interstitial fluid which interrupts the normal functioning of luteinizing hormone.

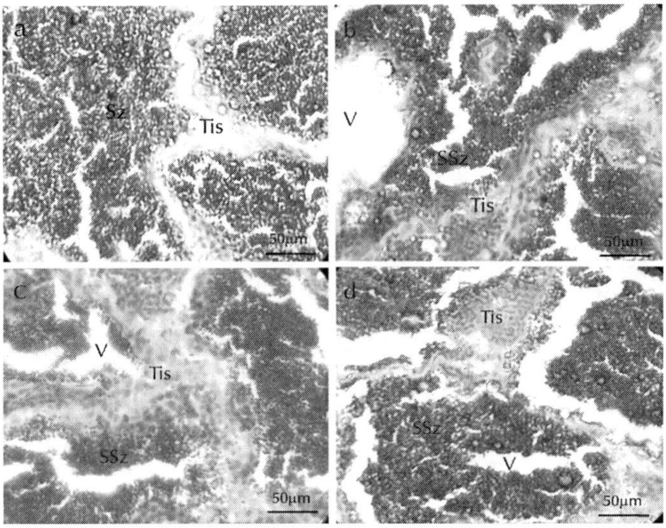

Figure 4: Photomicrograph of the testis of *H. fossilis* from control and from the three rivers. (a) Control, (b) Buriganga, (c) Turag, and (d) Shitalakkhya. V, vacuole; Sz, spermatozoa; Ssz, scattered spermatozoa; Tis, testis interstitial space (H and E × 430).

AChE Activity of *h. Fossilis* Exposed to Three River Water

H. fossilis were exposed to polluted water collected from Buriganga, Turag, and Shitalakkhya for 10 days. After 10 days of exposure time, the AChE activities in the fish brain were determined. In the present study, a steady decrease of AChE activity in the fish brain was found in the case of *H. fossilis*exposed to water samples of the three rivers (Figure 5). In the control fish, AChE activities were measured as 202.67 ± 6.51 nmol/min/mg proteins. Furthermore, AChE activities in the brain of *H. fossilis* exposed to water samples of Buriganga, Turag, and Shitalakkhya rivers were 104.00 ± 5.00, 102.00 ± 5.00, and 130.67 ± 3.51 nmol/min/mg protein, respectively. Significant inhibition of AChE activity ($P < 0.05$) was observed from all river water samples compared to the control. In this study, it was observed that due to polluted water exposure, AChE activity decreased values were 48.78%, 49.63%, and 35.56% from Buriganga, Turag, and Shitalakkhya river water samples, respectively.

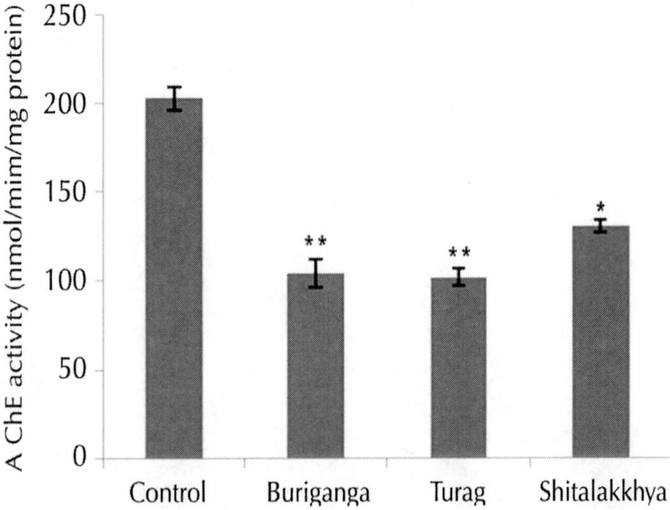

Figure 5: AChE activity measured in *H. fossilis* exposed to three different river water for 10 days. Data presented as mean ± SD. *$P < 0.05$, **$P < 0.01$.

AChE activity in vertebrates and invertebrates is a widely used biomarker of neurotoxicity. Moreover, fish AChE activity has been utilized as a highly sensitive biomarker response of freshwater pollution (de la Torre et al. 2002). A significant decrease in this cholinesterase activity in fish indicates the presence of neurotoxic pollutants in the aquatic ecosystem. In the present study, *H. fossilis* were exposed to polluted water collected from Buriganga, Turag, and Shitalakkhya for 10 days. After 10 days of exposure time, the AChE activities in the fish brain were determined. In the present study, a steady decrease of AChE activity in the fish brain was found in the case of *H. fossilis* exposed to water samples of the three rivers (Figure 5). In the control fish, the AChE activities were measured as 202.67 ± 6.51 nmol/min/mg proteins. Furthermore, AChE activities in the brain of *H. fossilis* exposed to water samples of Buriganga, Turag, and Shitalakkhya were 104.00 ± 5.00, 102.00 ± 5.00, and 130.67 ± 3.51 nmol/min/mg proteins, respectively. Significant inhibition of AChE activity ($P < 0.05$)

was observed from all river water samples compared to the control. In this study, it was observed that due to polluted water exposure, AChE activity decreased values were 48.78%, 49.63%, and 35.56% from Buriganga, Turag and Shitalakkhya river water samples, respectively. However, the larger decline of cholinesterase activity in the water samples of Turag and Buriganga than that of Shitalakkhya compared to the control suggests that Turag and Buriganga rivers are more highly polluted with neurotoxic compounds. The extent of AChE depression required to cause death in aquatic organisms. In fish, most estimates lie in the range of 70% to 85% AChE reduction. Eel (*Anguilla anguilla*), over a 96-h exposure period to pesticide, were able to survive up to 57% reduction in AChE activity (Sancho and Andreu 1998).

Rank et al. (2007) noted a responding change in AChE activity to pollution in native and transplanted mussels in the areas close to coastal chemical dumping sites with some interpretation due to seasonal fluctuation in exposure situation. According to Forget et al. (2003), neurotoxic contaminants brought by rivers caused a 70% to 80% AChE inhibition in copepods from an estuary in comparison with those from upstream. An ascending order of AChE inhibition with the increased concentration of arsenic in*Channa punctatus* was mentioned by Roy et al. (2006). In contrast, the ameliorative potential of selenium on arsenic-mediated inhibition of AChE activity was also described. Combined *in vivo* and *in vitro* effects of cadmium and aluminum like heavy metal on AChE inhibition have also been reported (Carageorgiou et al. 2004; Kohila et al. 2004).

CONCLUSIONS

This study showed that in dry season, DO of the three rivers existed below the standard level (≥5 mg/l) and were extremely intolerable for plankton community that eventually resulted in the lowest plankton count. Furthermore, structural damage in fish organs and significant inhibition of AChE in the fish brain suggest the potency of the two biomarkers against pollution. The biomarker data from this study can, in the future, be used to evaluate the effects of management actions. With a view to minimize the devastating effects of pollutants, effluent treatment plants are recommended to establish corporately near the major industrial zone to treat industrial effluents before disposal.

AUTHORS' CONTRIBUTIONS

SFR participated in the design of the study, performed the statistical analysis, and drafted the manuscript. AHMMR has made substantial contributions to the concept and design, acquisition, and interpretation of data. MSH helped in the design of the study and in collection of data. ZH supervised the group to coordinate the research, revised the manuscript critically for important intellectual content, and had given the final approval of the version to be submitted. All authors read and approved the final manuscript.

ACKNOWLEDGMENTS

This work is funded by Bangladesh Agricultural University Research System (BAURES). The authors are indebted to Professor Dr. Mohammad Shamsuddin of the Department of Surgery and Obstetrics, Faculty of Veterinary Science, Bangladesh Agricultural University for facilitating Field Fertility Clinic Laboratory.

REFERENCES

1. Amiard JC, Amiard-Triquet C, Barka S, Pellerin J, Rainbow PS (2006) Metallothioneins in aquatic invertebrates: their role in metal detoxification and their use as biomarkers. Aquat Toxicol. 76:160–202
2. APHA (1992) Standard methods for the examination of water and wastewater American Public Health Association, Washington DC
3. Baquero MR, Carrillo P, Arco BJ, Martinez PC, Argaiz VM (2006) Climate-driven change on phytoplankton-zooplankton coupling and nutrient availability in high mountain lakes of Southern Europe. Freshwater Biol. 51:989–998
4. Barnhoorn IEJ, Bornman MS, Pieterse GM, Van Vuren JHJ (2004) Histological evidence of intersex in feral sharptooth catfish (*Clarias gariepinus*) from an estrogen-polluted water source in Gauteng, South Africa. Environ Toxicol. 19:603–608

5. Barnhoorn IEJ, Vandyk JC, Pieterse GM, Bornman MS (2010) Intersex in feral indigenous freshwater*Oreochromis mossambicus*, from various parts in the Luvuvhu River, Limpopo Province, South Africa. Ecotoxicol Environ Saf. 73:1537–1542
6. Baršienė J, Lehtonen KK, Koehler A, Broeg K, Vourinen PJ, Lang T, Pempkowiak J, Šyvokienė J, Dedonytė V, Rybakovas A, Repečka R, Vountisjarvi H, Kopecka J (2006) Biomarker responses in flounder (*Platichthys flesus*) and mussel (*Mytilus edulis*) in the Klaipėda-Būtingė area (Baltic Sea). Mar Pollut Bull. 53:422–436
7. Begum ZNT (2008) A taxonomic account on the phytoplankton of a pond receiving textile industrial effluents. Bang J Plant Tax 15:129–139
8. Begum ZNT, Khanam D (2009) Physicochemical aspects and phytoplankton of the river Shitalakhya receiving pharmaceutical effluents. Bang J Bot 38:77–85
9. Bellinger EG (1992) A key to common algae: freshwater, estuarine and some coastal species The Institution of Water and Environmental Management, London p 138
10. Bucher F, Hofer R (1993) The effects of treated domestic sewage on three organs (gills, kidney, liver) of brown trout (*Salmo trutta*). Water Res. 27:255–261
11. Carageorgiou H, Tzotzes V, Pantos C, Mourouzis C, Zorros A, Tsakiris S (2004) *In vivo* and *in vitro*effects of cadmium on adult rat brain total antioxidant status, acetylcholinesterase, (Na+, K+)-ATPase and Mg2 + −ATPase activities: protection by L-cysteine. Pharmacol Toxicol 94:112–118
12. Çetin AK, Şen B (2004) Seasonal distribution of phytoplankton in Orduzu Dam Lake (Malatya, Turkey). Turk J Bot 28:279–285
13. de la Torre FR, Ferrari L, Salibián A (2002) Freshwater pollution biomarker: response of brain acetylcholinesterase activity in two fish species. Pharmacol Toxicol 131:271–280
14. Ellman GL, Courtney KD, Andres VJ, Featherstone RM (1961) A new and rapid colorimetric determination of acetylcholinesterase activity. Biochem Pharmacol. 7:88–95
15. Eloranta P (1980) Zooplankton in a watercourse polluted by sulphite pulp mill. Ann Zoo Fennici 17:261–267

16. Farag AM, May T, Marty GD, Easton M, Harper DD, Little EE, Cleveland L (2006) The effect of chronic chromium exposure on the health of Chinook salmon (*Oncorhynchus tshawytscha*). Aquat Toxicol. 76:246–257
17. Ferdous Z, Muktadir AKM (2009) A review: potentiality of zooplankton as bioindicator. Am J App Sci 6:1815–1819
18. Ferenczy J, Szegletes T, Bálint T, Ábrahám M, Nemcsók J (1997) Characterization of acetylcholinesterase and its molecular forms in organs of five freshwater teleosts. Fish Physiol Biochem. 16:515–529
19. Forget J, Beliaeff B, Bocquené G (2003) Acetylcholinesterase activity in copepods (*Tigriopus brevicornis*) from the Vilaine River estuary, France, as a biomarker of neurotoxic contaminants. Aquat Toxicol. 62:195–204
20. Habig C, Di Giulio RT, Abou-Donia MB (1988) Comparative properties of channel catfish (*Ictalurus punctatus*) and blue crab (*Callinectes sapidus*) acetylcholinesterases. Comp Biochem Physiol C Toxicol Pharmacol 91:293–300
21. Jash NB, Chatterjee S, Bhattacharya S (1982) Role of acetylcholine in the recovery of brain acetylcholinesterase in *Channa punctatus* (Bloch) exposed to furadan. Comp Physiol Ecol 7:56–58
22. Kohila T, Parkkonen E, Tähti H (2004) Evaluation of the effects of aluminium, ethanol and their combination on rat brain synaptosomal integral proteins *in vitro* and after 90-day oral exposure. Arch Toxicol. 78:276–282
23. Kopecka J, Rybakowas A, Baršiene J, Pempkowiak J (2004) AChE levels in mussels and fish collected off Lithuania and Poland (southern Baltic). Oceanologica 46:405–418
24. Kopecka J, Lehtonen KK, Baršiene J, Broeg K, Vuorinen PJ, Gercken J, Pempkowiak J (2006) Measurements of biomarker levels in flounder (*Platichthys flesus*) and blue mussel (*Mytilus trossulus*) from the Gulf of GdaDsk (southern Baltic). Mar Pollut Bull. 53:406–421
25. Liao CY, Zhou QF, Fu JJ, Shi JB, Yuan CG, Jiang GB (2007) Interaction of methylmercury and selenium on the bioaccumulation and histopathology in medaka (*Oryzias latipes*). Environ Toxicol. 22:69–77

26. Liu XJ, Luo Z, Xiong BX, Liu X, Zhao YH, Hua GF, Lv GJ (2010) Effect of waterborne copper exposure on growth, hepatic enzyme activities and histology in *Synechogobius hasta*. Ecotoxicol Environ Saf. 73:1286–1291
27. Lowry OH, Rosebrough NJ, Farr AL, Randall RJ (1951) Protein measurement with the Folin phenol reagent. J Biol Chem. 193:265–275
28. Magni P, De Falco G, Falugi C, Franzoni M, Monteverde M, Perrone E, Sgro M, Bolognesi C (2006) Genotoxicity biomarkers and acetylcholinesterase activity in natural populations of *Mytilus galloprovincialis* along a pollution gradient in the Gulf of Oristano (Sardinia, western Mediterranean). Environ Poll. 142:65–72
29. Marchand MJ, Van Dyk JC, Pieterse GM, Barnhoorn IE, Bornman MS (2009) Histopathological alterations in the liver of the sharptooth catfish*Clarias gariepinus* from polluted aquatic systems in South Africa. Environ Toxicol. 24:133–147
30. Mohiuddin KM, OgawaY ZHM, Otomo K, Shikazono N (2011) Heavy metals contamination in water and sediments of an urban river in a developing country. Int J Environ Sci Technol 8:723–736
31. Nero V, Farwell A, Lister A, Van der Kraak G, Lee LE, Van Meer T, MacKinnon MD, Dixon DG (2005) Gill and liver histopathological changes in yellow perch (*Perca flavescens*) and goldfish (*Carrasius auratus*) exposed to oil sands process affected water. Ecotoxicol Environ Saf. 63:365–377
32. Nigro M, Falleni A, Del Barga I, Scarcelli V, Lucchesi P, Regoli F, Frenzilli G (2006) Cellular biomarkers for monitoring estuarine environments: transplanted versus native mussels. Aquat Toxicol. 77:339–347
33. Nunes B, Carvalho F, Guilhermino L (2003) Characterization of total head cholinesterases of *Gambusia holbrooki* (mosquito fish) and the assessment of effects induced by two environmental contaminants. J Vet Pharmacol Ther 26:260–261
34. Palmer CM (1980) Algae and Water Pollution Cambridge Printers Limited, England p 123
35. Perez ZO, Alvarez SR, Barroso EN, Güemes J, Bouchot GG, Ortega A, Medina AA (2000) Toxicity of sediments from Bahia de Chetumal, Mexico, as assessed by hepatic EROD induction and

histology in Nile tilapia *Oreochromis niloticus*. Mar Environ Res. 50:385–391

36. Peuranen S (2000) The effects of aluminium and iron on fish gills Academic dissertation, Helsinki pp 8–30
37. Playle RC (1998) Modelling metal interactions at fish gills. Sci Total Environ. 219:147–163
38. Purves D, Augustine GJ, Fitzpatrick D, Hall WC, LaMantia AS, McNamara JO, White LE (2008) Synaptic transmission Sinauer Associates, Sunderland MA pp 121–122
39. Rangsayatorn N, Kruatrachue M, Pokethitiyook P, Upatham ES, Lanza GR, Singhakaew S (2004) Ultrastructural changes in various organs of the fish *Puntius gonionotus* fed cadmium-enriched cyanobacteria. Environ Toxicol. 19:585–593
40. Rank J, Lehtonen KK, Strand J, Laursen M (2007) DNA damage, acetylcholinesterase activity and lysosomal stability in native and transplanted mussels (*Mytilus edulis*) in areas close to coastal chemical dumping sites in Denmark. Aquat Toxicol. 84:50–61
41. Roberts RJ (ed) (2001) Fish Pathology Saunders WB, Philadelphia
42. Rodrigues SR, Caldeira C, Castro BB, Gonçalves F, Nunes B, Antunes SC (2011) Cholinesterase (ChE) inhibition in pumpkinseed (*Lepomis gibbosus*) as environmental biomarker: ChE characterization and potential neurotoxic effects of xenobiotics. Pestic Biochem Physiol. 99:181–188
43. Roy S, Chattoraj A, Bhattacharya S (2006) Arsenic-induced changes in optic tectal histoarchitecture and acetylcholinesterase–acetylcholine profile in *Channa punctatus*: amelioration by selenium. Comp Biochem Physiol C Toxicol Pharmacol. 144:16–24
44. Saha ML, Khan MR, Ali M, Haque S (2009) Bacterial load and pollution level of the river Buriganga, Dhaka, Bangladesh. Bang J Bot 38:87–91
45. Sancho FMD, Andreu E (1998) *In vivo* inhibition of AChE activity in the European eel *Anguilla anguilla*exposed to technical grade fenitrothion. Comp. Biochem. Physiol. Part C 120:389–395
46. Sandahl J, Jenkins JJ (2002) Pacific steelhead (*Oncorhynchus mykiss*) exposed to chlorpyrifos: benchmark concentration

estimates for acetylcholinesterase inhibition. Environ Toxicol Chem. 21:2452–2458

47. Schiedek D, Broeg K, Barsiene J, Lehtonen KK, Gercken J, Pfiefer S, Vuontisjärvi H, Vuorinen PJ, Dedonyte V, Koehler A, Balk L, Schneider R (2006) Biomarker responses as indication of contaminant effects in blue mussel *(Mytilus edulis)* and female eelpout *(Zoarcesviviparus)* from the southwestern Baltic Sea. Mar Pollut Bull. 53:387–405
48. Schultz MM, Painter MM, Bartell SE, Logue A, Furlong ET, Werner SL, Schoenfuss HL (2011) Selective uptake and biological consequences of environmentally relevant antidepressant pharmaceutical exposures on male fathead minnows. Aquat Toxicol. 104:38–47
49. Shah MMR, Hossain MY, Begum M, Ahmed ZF, Ohtomi J, Rahman MM, Alam MJ, Islam MA, Fulanda B (2008) Seasonal variations of phytoplanktonic community structure and production in relation to environmental factors of the southwest coastal waters of Bangladesh. J Fish Aquat Sci 3:102–113
50. Sharma S, Siddique A, Singh K, Chouhan M, Vyas A, Solnki CM, Sharma D, Nair S, Sengupta T (2010) Population dynamics and seasonal abundance of zooplankton community in Narmada River (India). Research 2:1–9
51. Shaw BJ, Handy RD (2006) Dietary copper exposure and recovery in Nile tilapia *Oreochromis niloticus*. Aquat Toxicol. 76:111–121
52. Solomon SG, Atagub GA, Baiyewunmi AS (2009) Study of dry season zooplankton of Lower River Benue at Makurdi, Nigeria. J Anim Plant Sci 1:42–50
53. Tanaka RY, Higo T, Shibata N, Suzuki H, Hatate H, Nagayama K, Nakamura T (2002) Accumulation of hydroxy lipids in live fish infected with fish diseases. Aquaculture. 211:341–351
54. TheWorldBank(2006)Bangladeshcountryenvironmentalanalysis. TheWorld Bank, Washington, DC. http://siteresources. worldbank. org/BANGLADESHEXTN/Resources/2957591173922647418/ complete pdf
55. Tkatcheva V, Hyvärinen H, Kukkonen J, Ryzhkov LP, Holopainen IJ (2004) Toxic effects of mining effluents on fish gills in a subarctic lake system in NW Russia. Ecotoxicol Environ Saf. 57:278–289

56. Valbonesi P, Brunelli F, Mattioli M, Rossi T, Fabbri E (2011) Cholinesterase activities and sensitivity to pesticides in different tissues of silver European eel, *Anguilla anguilla*. Comp Biochem Physiol C Toxicol Pharmacol. 154:353–359
57. Varo I, Amat F, Navarro JC (2008) Acute toxicity of dichlorvos to *Aphanius iberus* (Cuvier & Valenciennes, 1846) and its anti-cholinesterase effects on this species. Aquat Toxicol. 88:53–61
58. Xu WN, Liu WB, Liu ZP (2009) Trichlorfon-induced apoptosis in hepatocyte primary cultures of*Carassius auratus gibelio*. Chemosphere. 77:895–901
59. Xuereb B, Chaumot A, Mons R, Garric J, Geffard O (2009) Acetylcholinesterase activity in *Gammarus fossarum* (Crustacea Amphipoda): intrinsic variability, reference levels, and a reliable tool for field surveys. Aquat Toxicol. 93:225–233
60. Zakir HM, Sharmin S, Shikazono N (2006) Heavy metal pollution assessment in water and sediments of Turag River at Tongi area in Bangladesh. Int J LakRiv 1:85–96

Chapter 5

How Do Small-Scale Fishers Adapt to Environmental Variability? Lessons from Baja California, Sur, Mexico

Leila Sievanen

Joint Institute for Marine and Atmospheric Research, 1845 Wasp Blvd, Honolulu 96818, HI, USA

Brown University, Institute for the Study of Environment and Society, 85 Waterman St., Providence 02912, RI, USA

ABSTRACT

Many fisheries stocks and the livelihoods of those who make their living from fishing are in decline, and these declines are exacerbated by uncertainties associated with increased climate variability and change. Social scientists have long documented the importance of mobility and diversification in reducing the risk and uncertainty associated with climate variability, particularly in the context of small-scale fishing. However, it is unclear how these traditional mechanisms are buffering fishers against the varied stressors they currently face, including those associated with environmental variability. This paper examines how fishers on the southern gulf coast of the Mexican state of Baja California Sur perceive and respond to stressors associated with normal environmental variability, how their ability to adapt is spatially distributed, and what threats they perceive to their continued ability to adapt. Understanding the adaptation strategies and everyday vulnerabilities that fishers face can elucidate problems associated with current fisheries management and the underlying factors that cause vulnerability, and also help decision makers, including fishers themselves, develop more effective adaptation strategies in the face of climate change.

RESEARCH

Small-scale fisheries are a major source of livelihood for people living in the Mexican state of Baja California Sur. Nevertheless, as in many parts of the world, small-scale fishers in Mexico face many challenges like competition with coastal tourism and other fishing sectors, declines in fish stocks, climate variability, and market fluctuations. Sustaining small-scale fisheries has only recently been prioritized in fisheries management and development policy (Cudney-Bueno et al. [2009], Villanueva-Aznar et al. [2012]). A key question is how well fishing communities are able to adapt to environmental and institutional variability, both now and in the future.

The focus on adaptation has a long history in anthropology (e.g., McCay [1978]). Now, it is commonly used to examine how people adjust to and cope with environmental change and uncertainty, with linkages to ideas of risk, vulnerability, exposure and sensitivity (Head[2010]). The Intergovernmental Panel on Climate Change (IPCC) defines adaptation as "adjustments in natural or human systems in response to actual or expected climatic stimuli or their effects, which moderates harm or exploits beneficial opportunities" (Intergovernmental Panel on Climate Change IPCC [2007]a). As people are often not reacting specifically to climate change, a more general definition is a change in a system allowing it to better cope with or adjust to a particular change or stressor. Fishers continuously confront multiple environmental and social stressors that necessitate changes in their behavior. In this paper, I focus on how individuals and households on the southern gulf coast of Baja California Sur adapt to stressors associated with seasonal changes that affect fisheries, and how these stressors interact with other drivers of change, including shifts in marine management and associated regulations.

Early work on fisheries and climate change focused on documenting trends in fish abundance and distribution (Glantz [1992], Cushing [1982]). Syntheses of responses of fishing communities to change highlight several common short-term strategies: intensification and diversification of fishing, migration or mobility, and practices like seeking employment in other sectors, relying on social networks, and waiting for fisheries to improve (e.g., Perry et al.[2011]). In this paper, I focus on two strategies fishers use to buffer uncertainty: mobility and diversification (e.g., Löfgren [1972], Andersen [1974], Allison and Ellis [2001]). Mobility refers to movement by fishers to new fishing grounds, which often follows seasonal fish movements, enabling more continuous income generation. Diversification is the process by which a household increases its number of income-generating activities, both inside and outside of fisheries (Ellis [2000]). Often studied in association with adaptation, diversification is a household risk management strategy used to spread risk, smooth the effects of temporal variations in access to resources, and reduce vulnerability (Allison and Ellis [2001], Hoorweg et al. [2008]). For example, in the Pacífico Norte area of Baja California Sur, during and after El Niño events, some cooperatives diversified from lobster and abalone to include other taxa such as finfish, whelk, sea cucumber, and sea urchin (McCay et al. [2011]).

On the southern gulf coast of Baja California Sur, most research on fisheries and environmental variability has focused on documenting fluctuations in fish abundance and distribution (e.g., Aburto-Oropeza et al. [2007], [2010]). In other parts of the Gulf and Pacific coast, scholars have investigated adaptation strategies and vulnerability of fishing communities to climate change (e.g., McGuire and Greenberg [1993], Vásquez-León [1994],[2002], McCay et al. [2011], [2013], Morzaria-Luna et al. [2014]). Vulnerability is often described in the climate change literature as a function of the exposure and sensitivity to a stressor and adaptive capacity, or the ability to respond (e.g., Smit and Wandel [2006]). Most individuals and communities can cope with small deviations from average environmental conditions, but they may not be able to adapt to conditions outside of a certain threshold. Peoples' ability to modify or change behavior to cope better with an external stressor will vary among individuals and households within a community (Adger et al. [2003]) and even between neighboring communities (Cinner et al. [2013]). Vulnerability has both social and ecological dimensions (e.g., Perry et al. [2011], Cinner et al. [2013]); changes in ecological systems affect fishing communities and vice versa. Some cases examining community responses to environmental change focus on major shocks like coral bleaching (e, g., Cinner et al. [2013]) or large ENSO (El Niño-Southern Oscillation) events (e. g., Broad [2000]). In other cases such as this one, impacts are more subtle and fishers may not even perceive the effects of environmental change when compounded by other stressors like declines in fish stocks, new fishing regulations, and market fluctuations. In this paper, I rely on qualitative methods and directed analysis at the local scale to understand how fishers describe their own adaptation strategies and vulnerabilities to normal seasonal variation. Understanding how local fishers are already adapting to changes along with their current concerns can shed light on the broader social, economic, and political context in which they live and work. By identifying problems they associate with current fisheries management, we can work towards reducing fisheries' vulnerability to both climate variability and change.

In the Global South, the state generally does not play a direct role in developing climate change adaptation strategies, and communities have developed bottom-up, local-scale practices. In Mexican fisheries in particular, while state economic and policy changes influence local-level decisions, these are often indirect effects (e. g., Young [2001], Cinti et al.[2010], Basurto et al. [2013]). While it is unclear in many cases how climate change will affect fisheries, it is possible to understand stressors associated with normal environmental variability that local people face and how they modify their behavior to adapt to these stressors. Climatic conditions are inherently variable, on annual and decadal time periods. Thus, adaptation to climate change will necessarily include the ability to cope with variability (Katz and Brown [1992], Smithers and Smit [1997], Smit et al. [1999]). Focusing on how local people change their behavior to cope with normal environmental variability rather than rarer large-scale events also can help elucidate current problems with fisheries management and the underlying factors that cause vulnerability (Coulthard [2008]).

Southern Baja California Sur provides a good setting in which to study adaptation strategies. It is flanked by the Gulf of California (hereafter, "the Gulf") to the east, which is one of the most significant fisheries regions in Mexico, and the Pacific Ocean to the west. The gulf region produces approximately 71% of fisheries landings by volume and 57% by value in a given year (Organisation for Economic Co-operation and Development OECD [2006]). Small-scale fishing (or *pesca ribereña*) is one of the region's most important activities: nearly 18,000 small boats operate in the region (Cisneros-Mata [2010]). In some areas, 90% of the landings correspond to small-scale fisheries (Erisman et al. [2011]). Most fishing cooperatives on the gulf coast are not involved in fisheries co-management. A few cooperatives in the La Paz area are able to influence the fishing practices of their members, especially related to size selection and the use of specific fishing gear in particular habitats (Reddy et al. [2013]). However, as they lack rights to particular species or areas, none actively patrol fishing areas.

Environmental variability, particularly ENSO events, impact key fisheries species in the Gulf (Aburto-Oropeza et al. [2007], [2010]), as well as fishers' decisionmaking (Micheli et al.[2012]. A recent UNFCCC report (UNFCCC [2007]) noted that Mexico is at risk for extreme weather events and sea level rise associated with climate change. And it is not only climate change that coastal communities are facing. Like many coastal areas around the world, since the 1970s the economy has steadily been transitioning away from agriculture and fishing and towards tourism and service (Lauterio and Arizpe [2012], Gamez and Angeles [2010]). In the 1990s, the region also was recognized as a biodiversity hotspot, and conservation tools such as marine protected areas began to be implemented (Cudney-Bueno et al. [2009], Álvarez-Romero et al. [2013]). It is unclear how these changes will affect fisheries in this area or how individuals and groups will respond.

This paper examines the strategies that fishing communities in southern Baja California Sur use to adapt to environmental variability. I answer four questions: 1. How do fishers perceive seasonal variability? 2. How do fishers adapt to this variability? 3. How is the ability to adapt distributed spatially? 3. What threats do fishers perceive to their continued ability to adapt?

APPROACH

Data informing this paper come from 60 household surveys (of the approximately 500 households that depend on fishing in the focal communities) and 30 interviews with community leaders and government officials that investigate the vulnerability and adaptive capacity of fishers in the face of environmental variability and institutional, political, and economic changes in the Mexican state of Baja California Sur (Figure 1). This study was undertaken as part of a 2-year postdoctoral project in association with a broader Coupled Human and Natural Systems NSF project (GEO 1114964). Combining anthropology, ecology, and economics, this project integrated social and ecological data to understand social and ecological responses to environmental and institutional changes in southern Baja California Sur, particularly those related to small-scale fisheries. It also draws from participant observation over the course of four visits over a total of five months between 2011 and 2012.

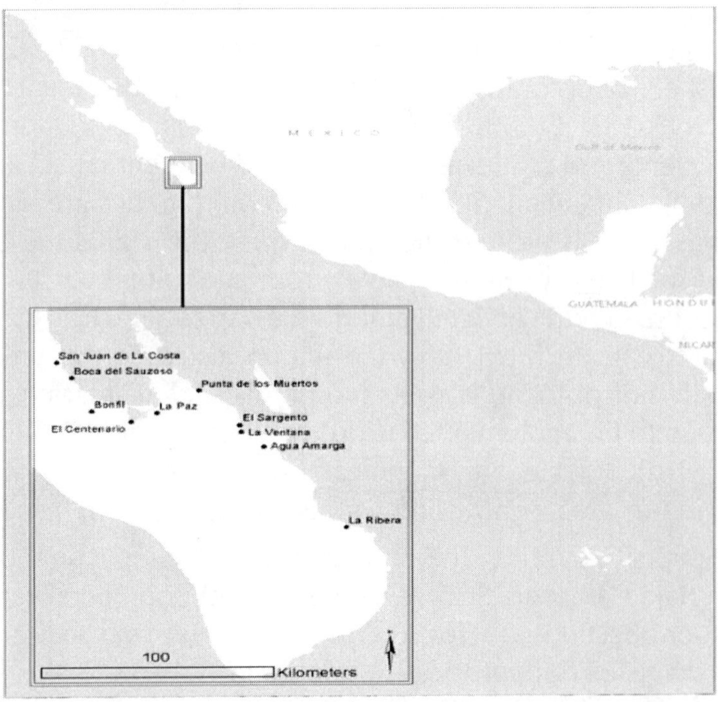

Figure 1: Household survey sites (Map credit: Miguel Castrence).

When I first began the study, I intended to speak with fishers about inter-annual variation to better understand their perceptions and responses to the changes in fish abundance and distribution that biologists had found to be associated with ENSO events. However, while fishers on the gulf coast of Baja California Sur said that they had not seen impacts of the large 1998 ENSO event and did not note any clear inter-annual patterns in fish abundance or distribution, they spoke about intra-annual climate variation. We adapted our research plan accordingly.

Themes covered in the surveys include basic demographics, information about fishing activities and patterns, perceived changes in fisheries, organizational strategies, adaptive capacity, and perceptions and use of marine protected areas. This study focuses primarily on adaptation practices and vulnerabilities. Specifically, how do fishers cope when fishing locally is not a viable option? What other kinds of income-generating activities do household members engage in? What is the seasonality of these activities? Can non-fishing work be alternated with fishing or is it full-time? Does non-fishing work require moving to another location?

I pre-tested household surveys with 15 fishers in La Paz and El Sargento. Households with active fishers over 18 years of age were randomly selected in the city of La Paz (pop. 215,000), four rural towns of 900–5,000 people (El Sargento, El Centenario, San Juan de la Costa, La Ribera), and five very rural communities of 50–400 people (La Ventana, Boca del Sauzoso, Punta de los Muertos, Alfredo V. Bonfil, Agua Amarga) (Table 1). These locations were chosen to encompass a range of community types, from urban to very rural. As a list of active fishermen was not available for any of the locations, I worked with community leaders to identify fishing households. I then selected every third household. In the case of La Paz, I randomly selected areas in the town, and selected every third household where fishing gear (boats, nets, etc.) was visible in the yard and a fisher was at home and available to be interviewed.

Table 1: Key characteristics of study communities

	Type	Population*	No. of fishers(est)**	Cooperatives***	Pangas (est)**	[redacted]
La Paz	Urban	215,178	400-600	23	300-400	12
El Centenario	Rural	4,696	10-30	0	5-10	3
La Ribera	Rural	2,050	80-150	3	30-50	9
El Sargento	Rural	958	50-80	2	10-30	15
San Juan de la Costa	Rural	902	10-30	1	5-10	2
Agua Amarga	Very rural	382	50-80	1	50-100	4
Bonfil	Very rural	300	5-10	1	1-2	1
La Ventana	Very rural	255	20-40	1	30-60	9
Boca del Sauzoso	Very rural	40	10-15	1	10-20	4
Punta de los Muertos	Very rural	5	3	0	1-2	1

*2010 Census data (http://www.inegi.org.mx/ webcite).

** Estimated based on interviews with community fisheries experts and 2010 CONAPESCA data. A range is given, because of the presence of unregistered fishers.

***2012 unpublished CONAPESCA data.

Sievanen

Sievanen *Maritime Studies* 2014 13:9 doi: 10.1186/s40152-014-0009-2

I conducted surveys with a local research assistant for two months in 2011-2012. In most cases, I interviewed the fisher alone, but sometimes other fishers or his family were present I also conducted semi-structured interviews with fishers, fishing cooperative presidents, nongovernmental organization workers, and government fisheries managers associated with the federal agencies like CONAPESCA and SEMARNAT during all four visits in 2011–2012. All interviews and surveys were conducted in Spanish.

I then entered the surveys into an SPSS database for analysis. I audio recorded the interviews, transcribed them, and coded them using the qualitative data analysis software NVIVO 10. The general approach to transcript analysis was grounded theory (Glaser [1992]), whereby interview transcript data were coded and categorized into themes that arose from the text, rather than based on a preconceived coding scheme. The themes that arose in the transcripts and explored in this paper include those related to inter-annual climate variations, fisher mobility, livelihood diversification, and fishers' perceived threats to their continued ability to adapt to variation associated with both environmental and regulatory change.

Study Region

The study region encompasses ten fishing communities located in the southern portion of the Baja California Peninsula, in and around the city of La Paz, in the state of Baja California Sur, Mexico. La Paz is by far the largest city in the otherwise sparsely populated state. Baja California Sur is made up of five municipalities: Mulege, Loreto, Comondu, Los Cabos, and La Paz. The latter two municipalities make up the southern end of the peninsula and represent the major population center in the region. They are also sites of mass tourism development and have experienced a great deal of coastal land use change in the past 30 years (Gamez and Angeles [2010]).

In the 1950s tourism in Baja California Sur mainly consisted of people from the United States visiting Los Cabos to charter fish and Mexicans from the mainland visiting La Paz for duty free shopping (Gamez and Angeles [2010]). It has grown substantially and diversified since this time. Approximately 40% of the regional economy is now dependent on tourism, which employs about 30% of the state's inhabitants (Gamez and Angeles [2010]). Tourism investors in the area are mostly foreign. While La Paz has a more diversified economic base than Los Cabos, tourism has risen in importance over the past ten years. There are many impacts of tourism across the region. Resorts, second homes owned by Americans and Canadians, and golf courses are growing in number on the gulf coast (Gamez and Angeles [2010]). As tourism growth is closely linked to the US market, it fluctuates depending on the US economy and perceptions of safety in Mexico. The number of international arrivals to Baja has decreased since 2008, but is beginning to rise again (Global Hospitality Resources, Inc [2013]).

Fishers in the Baja California peninsula are of relatively recent origin. Early populations were efficiently utilizing the region's inshore marine resources at least 10,000 years ago (Carmean[1994]). However, by the 1800s, native groups had either been decimated by disease brought by Europeans, or had migrated or intermarried (Aschmann [1959]). Beginning in the 1500s, La Paz and the surrounding area hosted a world-renowned pearl fishery that lasted until the early 1900s (Gerhard [1956]). This fishery was linked to Spanish colonization efforts; the Spanish initially came to the region in search of pearls. After the pearl fishery declined, commercial marine harvest focused on sea turtles and shark to sell to merchant ships from the US and for trade with inland communities (Chenaut [1985]). Largely due to state subsidies and policies encouraging migration from the Mexican mainland, numbers of fishers in the Gulf rose from about 10,000 in 1945 (Higgins Industries Inc [1949]) to around 120,000 in 2009 (unpublished INAPESCA data).

Today Baja California Sur's more than 2000 km of coastline supports a diverse fishery (Robadue [2002], Enriquez-Andrade et al. [2005]). In the area surrounding La Paz, small-scale fishers targeted 55 taxa in 2010. These taxa include particular species like Pacific red snapper or *huachinango* (*Lutjanus peru*) and broader taxonomic groups like sharks (*Elasmobrachii*). Of these 55 taxa, 20 comprised approximately 90% of the biomass and the value created by small-scale fishers (based on 2010 CONAPESCA data). However, the top 20 taxa vary markedly in their landed price per kg (Leslie, HM, et al. Operationalizing the social-ecological systems framework to assess sustainability. Submitted). Fishermen are paid more than 150 pesos (12 USD) per kg for lobsters, for example, whereas most other taxa bring less than 13 pesos (1 USD) per kg (Leslie et al., unpublished data). Taxa landed by La Paz fishers include both coastal and offshore species, and inhabit a wide range of marine habitats. Some, like the chocolate clam (*Megapitaria squalida*), inhabit shallow sandy estuaries, whereas others, like the snappers (*Lutjanidae*), groupers (*Serranidae*), spiny lobsters (*Panulirus inflatus*), and triggerfish (*Balistes polylepis*), are more closely associated with rocky reefs (Leslie, HM, et al. Operationalizing the social-ecological systems framework to assess sustainability. Submitted). Still others are pelagic species, including yellowtail (*Seriola lalandi*), ocean whitefish (*Caulolatilus princeps*) and Spanish mackerel (*Scomberomorus concolor*).

These species have different life histories and habitat preferences, which require that fishers be knowledgeable and adept in multiple fishing techniques. Many fishers use more than one gear type depending on their target. However, their ability to use different gear types is often constrained by the permit. While many fishers in this area are very proud of using hook and line, there are several other common gear types: gillnets or lured lines to catch pelagic fish like pacific sierra (*Scomberomorus spp*), longlines for sharks and other pelagic species, and diving with hookah (connected to a surface air supply in shallow waters for sedentary species like sea cucumbers and clams) (Arreguín-Sánchez et al. [2004]). Many fishers in this region also participate in the charter boat or sportsfishing sector mainly targeting dorado (*Coryphaena hippurus*), marlin (*Tetrapturus audax*), and sailfish (*Istiophorus platypterus*).

The majority of fishers in Baja California Sur are small-scale, involving small catches and boats (7–9 meter outboard motor boats, or *pangas*) (Figure 2). Small-scale fisheries make up about 40% of the total national catch (Arreguín-Sánchez et al. [2004]). Nevertheless, small-scale fisheries have received little attention from the federal government when compared to the industrial fisheries targeting shrimp and small pelagics like anchoveta and sardines (Cinti et al. [2010]).

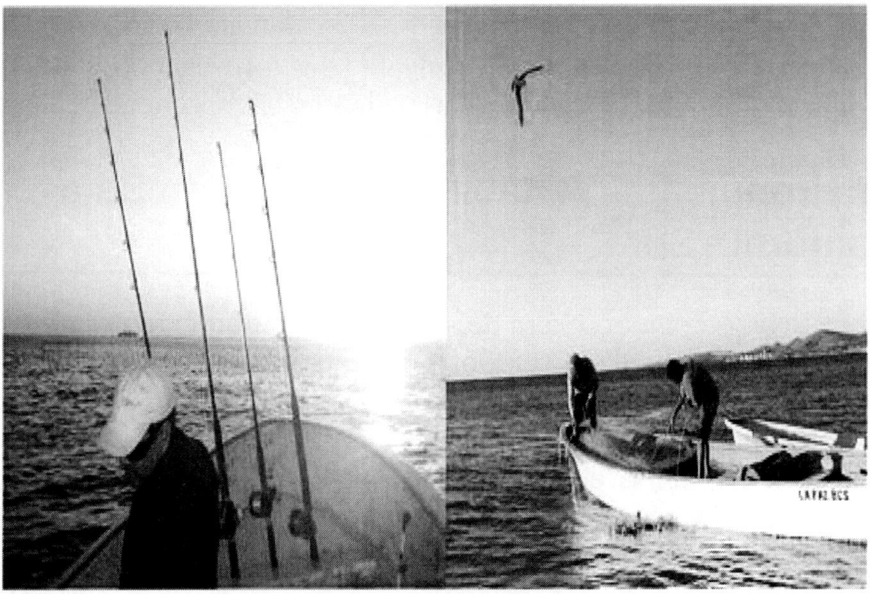

Figure 2: Small-scale fishers using hook and line (left) and gillnet (right) in La Paz.

Since the early 2000s, two federal agencies have been charged with regulating fisheries in Mexico: SAGARPA (via CONAPESCA, the National Fisheries Commission) and SEMARNAT (which regulates the use of species listed under special protection). Fishing permits have been the most common management tool used to regulate access to marine resources. Permits designate specific species (e. g., octopus, clams) or groups of species (e. g.,*escama*, which includes 271 species of finfish, or shark, which includes 46 species of elasmobranchs) to be harvested within a delineated region. It is likely that these permits that allow for catching multiple species are allowing fishers to diversify. See (Leslie, HM, et al. Operationalizing the social-ecological systems framework to assess sustainability. Submitted) for more information on the social organization and governance of fisheries in this region.

Despite management efforts such as marine protected areas, area-based concessions, and permitting, scientists have documented a downward trend in the abundances of many marine species in the Gulf (e. g., Sala et al. [2004], Sáenz-Arroyo et al. [2006], Cudney-Bueno et al.[2009]). There is also a high degree of illegal activity that occurs, often an unintentional result of externally-imposed regulations (Vásquez-León [1994], Cinti et al. [2010]). It is within this context of little management of small-scale fisheries and increasing scientific and community concern that I conducted this investigation in order to understand how fishers perceive and adapt to environmental change.

Environmental Variability in Southern Baja California Sur

People living on the southern tip of the Baja California peninsula have traditionally adapted to seasonal changes in resource availability. There is archaeological evidence dating back at least 10,000 years that points to coastal communities diversifying resource exploitation through seasonal movement (Carmean [1994], Des Lauriers [2011]).

Environmental variability occurs on both intra-annual and inter-annual cycles. Over the course of the year, the region experiences two main seasons. During summer months (June through September) weak winds blow from the southeast, while in the winter (November through February) strong northwest winds (locally known as *las collas nortes*) blow for several days at a time. Water temperature also varies seasonally between winter and summer in the Gulf. In the La Paz area, sea temperatures in the summer average 28.4 degrees C and 22.5 degrees C in the winter (Lluch-Cota et al. [2007]). While some species are available to fishers year round, others migrate seasonally. Catch data confirm seasonal variation.

ENSO is the most significant inter-annual signal in the region (Herrera-Cervantes et al.[2007], Lluch-Cota et al. [2010]). ENSO events occur every two to seven years and are associated with large-scale changes in wind, rainfall, sea surface temperature, and surface pressure. Scientists have found that fish species respond very differently to these changes. With warmer water temperatures, slower upwelling, and increased rainfall associated with a strong El Niño event, some may have their growth delayed, others may fail to reproduce, and some may change their distribution patterns (Lluch-Cota [2004]). For example, using landing statistics from the southern Gulf over 11 years, Aburto-Oropeza et al. ([2007], [2010]) show that fisheries landings of two economically significant species of reef fish, leopard grouper (*Mycteroperca rosacea*) and yellow snapper (*Lutjanus argentiventris*), are related to ENSO events, and particularly climatic conditions at the time of settlement. Leopard grouper larvae settle in shallow sargassum seaweed beds. However, because ENSO events affect the fishes' recruitment, there is a lag time of four years for yellow snapper and seven years for leopard grouper between the event and when effects are observed in the fishery.

RESULTS

How Do Fishers Perceive Seasonal Variability?

When asked about variation in fish abundance, no fisher connected these changes to a clear inter-annual pattern, such as an ENSO event. When asked specifically if El Niño events had any effect on the abundance of particular species (such as leopard grouper or yellow snapper) no fisher stated that they did and most responded that El Niño events were not important to Gulf fisheries. Most stated that they didn't use the term El Niño with each other and mainly associated it with scientists. One fisher explained, "we talk more about wind here [than temperature] as affecting fishing."

Fishers did recognize intra-annual variability. They distinguish between the cold winter months (*tiempo de frío*) and warm summer months (*tiempo de calor*). While some species are widely recognized to stay near La Paz all year (e. g., mullets (*Mugil spp*) and red snappers (*Lutjanus peru*)), other migratory species (*especies de corrida*) (e. g., marlin (*Tetrapturus audax*) and sharks (*Elasmobranchii*)) are present for several months and then move elsewhere. Fishers who target migratory fish (mainly charter boat operators and those who occasionally pursue squid (*Dosidicus gigas*) commercially) explained that marlin are present locally when water temperature is warm and squid are present in cold temperatures. And divers discussed that when it is unusually warm, the waters become nutrient poor and clams die.

However, just because fishery species are present does not mean that they can be easily caught. Even resident fisheries species are known to have their seasons (*temporada*); fishers had explanations for why they are not caught during other times of the year. Some explained that there are months when a particular species bites and months when it does not (*"hay meses cuando jalan y cuando no jalan"*). A few suggested that this could be because the fish are not hungry all the time, and shared stories about pulling up nets and finding red snappers, which are normally caught with hook and line, and finding the fishes' stomachs full of jellyfish. Fishers also tended to differentiate between the size classes of fish found during cold and warm seasons. For example, some said that in February only medium size red snappers are biting and that big red snappers either go deep or migrate when the water is cold. The wind was explained as another differentiating factor between winter and summer. Talking to fishers in January and February, it was difficult for them not to discuss the northwest winds and large swells (*marejadas*) that prohibited them from fishing on some days. One fisher elaborated, "those bad times are now – November, December, January –because of the wind."

How Do Fishers Adapt to Seasonal Variability?

Fishers have a range of adaptation strategies when fishing locally is not a viable option. I focus on two of the main strategies fishers use to cope with seasonal changes in Baja California Sur: moving to a new fishing spot and livelihood diversification.

Many fishers move to a different fishing spot, often to target particular species. Sometimes this involves taking their pangas to another location within their municipality and sometimes they need to temporarily relocate to other municipalities. During the winter months, many fishers go to the Pacific coast to fish. One cooperative leader explained, "In the Gulf, fish naturally make their own closed season. When it's cold and windy like it is now (January), we do not fish. We go to the Pacific where it's calmer."

He explained that during the winter the majority of *pescado de primera* (fish sold for the highest price) comes from the Pacific. On the Pacific coast there are a number of fishing camps that exist specifically for these seasonal trips; fishers go for days to even several months at a time. Fishers frequent spots around Bahia Magdelena and Los Cabos. Several fishers also said that they go to Loreto and Santa Rosalia on the Gulf side during the winter (Figure 3).

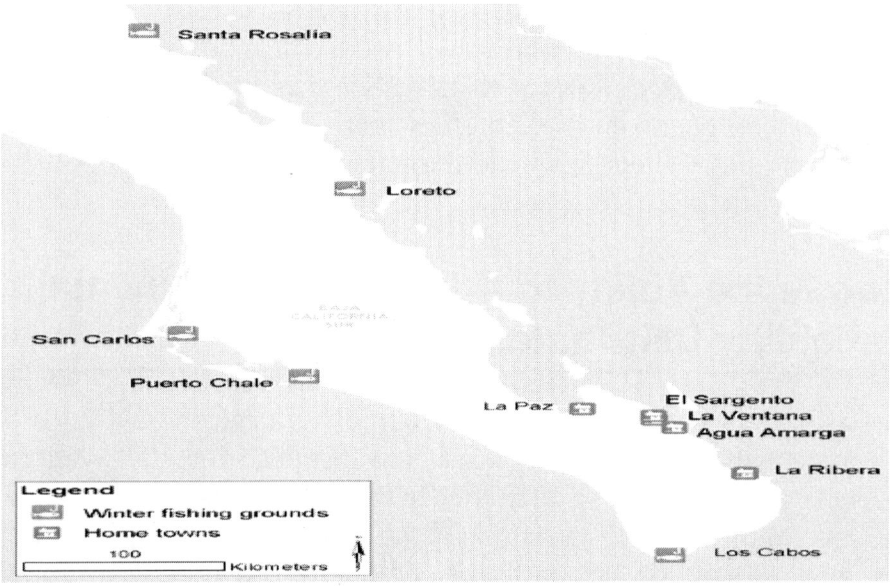

Figure 3: Typically from November to February, fishers in the La Paz area travel to either the Pacific coast (San Carlos, Puerto Chale or the Los Cabos area), or less frequently, to Loreto and Santa Rosalia on the gulf coast (Map credit: Miguel Castrence).

One motivation to move fishing sites, besides the lack of fish nearby, is that fishers can make more money. Fishers tend to work longer hours when not at home and also occasionally target higher value species. For example, Don Felix in El Sargento is a 50 year old fisher who spends three months out of the year fishing pescado de primera in San Carlos. His father traveled to fish in San Carlos and as a young man he began to travel there as well. He earns between 10–40,000 pesos per month (~800-3,000 USD) in the Pacific compared to 6–8,000 (~460-614 USD) around El Sargento.

Other strategies involve diversifying fisheries and occupations. Being a member of a cooperative that holds multiple permits allows fishers to fish for multiple taxa, and potentially in a more diverse set of locations. Multi-species permits for finfish and shark also allow them to fish for multiple taxa. Finfish is the most commonly held permit in the La Paz municipality, with over 50% of cooperatives holding it. Sixty-five percent (N=39) of fishers surveyed had multiple occupations in their households. One fisher described these additional occupations as "trabajo del flojo" (work of the lazy, due to their not requiring a full-time commitment). Amongst younger fishers, several said that they added another job onto fishing when they needed a more stable income, often due to marriage or a new baby. Some older fishers stated that they switched occupations when they were no longer physically able to fish full-time. Others sought additional income when an opportunity arose.

How is the Ability to Adapt to Environmental Variability Distributed Spatially?

Not all fishers utilize the above adaptation strategies equally. Of the two major strategies, moving to a new fishing spot and livelihood diversification, there was a difference between fishers living in urbanized vs. very rural areas. In La Paz and the four towns with populations between 900–5000, 75% of fishers still traveled over 100 km to fish. In the towns with populations of 50–400, there were no fishers who traveled more than 100 km to fish. However, even amongst fishers who travel, some mentioned that they do not go to as many places as they did in the past. For example, in La Ventana, out of nine fishers surveyed, four did not go as many places as they used to go because they have lost access to the permits that enabled them to access other geographic areas, beyond their home municipality. Many of the people who no longer travel at all to fish cited old age, health problems, isolation, and families that required them to remain nearby. In the rural village of Bonfil, that requires a four-wheel drive to access, only one household still fishes. Don Guadalupe and his two son's fish while his wife runs a restaurant situated on the main highway. They no longer travel to other areas to fish because they do not have anyone with whom to share gas costs. Similarly, fishers in more populated areas tended to have more diverse livelihoods. In the city of La Paz, 80% of households included members who engaged in more than one occupation. In the four towns with populations between 900–5000, 58% of households had more than one occupation. And in the three towns with populations between 50–400, 29% of households had more than one occupation. In other words, fishers living in the city of La Paz are less dependent on fishing than those in rural areas.

What Threats do Fishers Perceive to their Continued Ability to Adapt?

Many fishers explained that a number of relatively recent events were challenging the ways they have traditionally adapted to environmental variability, making it harder to make a living from fishing. Specifically, fishers cited a combination of declines in fish catch and difficulties in access to fisheries.

Ninety percent (N=54) of fishers surveyed stated that their catch had declined since they began fishing. The main reasons given for this decline were both a reduction in the total number of fish available as well as loss of access to fish. Over half of the fishers surveyed stated that unsustainable fishing practices by other groups such as industrial shrimpers, nighttime spearfishers, gillnetters, those who use sophisticated equipment like sonar, and charter boat operators who practice catch and release were responsible for the decline. As discussed above in the section on seasonal variability, some fishers stated that overall fish abundance has not decreased but that the fish are not biting anymore (*"la pesca no jala"*).

Another explanation for reductions in fish catch involved the loss of access to fish. Many lamented that it has recently become more difficult to diversify the species they target or to move to new fishing spots. This is due to both difficulties in accessing permits and more spatial and temporal restrictions on small-scale commercial fishing. Many older fishers remember a time when they could fish anywhere they desired. For example, in La Paz, I spoke with Don Enrique in his comfortable home office about changes in the fishery. Don Enrique was in his 60s and had been fishing since he was a child. 30 years ago he started a fishing cooperative so that his four sons could better access state subsidies, fishing equipment and permits. He described, "now our permits are only good for the municipality. If we go to Laguna de San Ignacio, they [other fishers] will chase us out..." Currently, even though permits can be issued for more than one municipality, in approximately 84% of cases observed in the 2010 CONAPESCA data for the state of Baja California Sur, fishers only had a permit for one municipality (Leslie, HM, et al. Operationalizing the social-ecological systems framework to assess sustainability. Submitted). Permits also specify a smaller fishing area than in the past.

In addition to concerns about reduced access to fish is a perception that the state is privileging other sectors over small-scale commercial fishing. Don Enrique described "now there are a lot of marine parks and restrictions for sport fishing and diving; areas for commercial fishing are getting smaller..." He also said that the rules are not enforced for charter boat fishers in the same way that they, as small-scale commercial fishers, experience enforcement. One of his sons explained, "All the power is with tourism ... the fisheries inspector lets charter fishing boats with tourists catch 20–30 marlin but if I catch more sandbass (*Paralabrax spp*) than I am permitted, I am fined." Marlin (*Tetrapturus audax*), swordfish (*Xiphias gladius*), rooster fish (*Nematistius pectoralis*), dorado (*Coryphaena hippurus*), and sailfish (*Istiophorus platypterus*) are species exclusively dedicated to sport fishing within inshore waters (NOM 017-pesc, art 0.3). There is a common perception that local differences in power and resources allow for differential access to marine resources. Many fishers feel that the poor suffer the rules, or risk their lives breaking the law, while the wealthy can still access restricted resources.

Additionally, there is a perception that non-fishing work is increasingly difficult to find. In most towns, fishers said that work is scarce. Fishers mostly compete for low- level jobs because their education levels tend to be low. Of the 60 fishers surveyed, only two had university degrees and the vast majority had only attended elementary school. The most common jobs for small-scale commercial fishers to have are as carpenters, painters, maintenance workers, and in the tourism sector (e.g., as sport fishing operators and tour guides). Some said that a decline in the number of tourists over the past several years has made tourism jobs more difficult to find. Also, at least two fishing cooperatives in the La Paz region have benefited from state and non-governmental programs that encourage engagement in ecotourism through capacity building and subsidizing the high entrance costs to this sector. However, those who work as tour guides state that in addition to there being fewer tourists, they find it hard to compete with resorts that offer packages that tourists can purchase online. There is a perception that the state would like fishers to move into tourism, however many feel that there are not enough jobs in tourism for everyone to be gainfully employed. They also associate this drop in tourists with a decreased demand (presumably by restaurants) for particular fish like grouper (see Reddy et al. [2013] for an example of how fisheries-related ecological and economic outcomes in this area are mediated by tourist demand).

On the other hand, some mentioned that it is now easier for the younger generation to pursue other opportunities in addition to fishing. Many older fishers stated that education was a barrier for them in gaining alternative employment, but education opportunities have increased in recent years. The two fishers who had university degrees were both in their early 20s. While many fishers have children who are not involved in fishing, most younger fishers surveyed stated that they fish because they love it. Thus, there are still younger people entering fishing, but education opportunities are providing alternatives for some.

DISCUSSION

Kenneth Broad ([2000]) suggested that El Niño events provide opportunities for anthropologists to study societal responses and vulnerability to environmental change. Equipped with information on how several fish species responded to the large 1998 ENSO event that biologists on our research team had collected, I originally set out to examine how small-scale fishers on the southern gulf coast of Baja California Sur perceive and adapt to ENSO events. On my scoping trip to the region in 2011, I found that fishers did not associate the changes they noted in fisheries abundance and distribution with inter-annual variability. Furthermore, they said that they had not witnessed effects of the large 1998 ENSO event.

Studies in other parts of the world (e.g., Glantz [1992]) as well as Mexico's Gulf of California and Pacific coast have shown that fishers often connect El Niño events to changes in the fishery. Fishers in the upper Gulf associate El Niño events with increases in freshwater from the Colorado River (McGuire and Greenberg [1993]). Scientists and fishers in this area believe that fish catch has declined because of the discontinuation of river flow. (McCay et al. [2011],[2013]) have also documented how fishing cooperatives in the Pacífico Norte area of Baja California Sur have perceived and successfully adapted to El Niño events. They showed that when an El Niño event depressed the lobster and abalone stocks that fishing communities in the Pacífico Norte area of Baja California Sur relied on, fishers developed rules and practices aimed at sustaining these resources (McCay et al. [2011], Micheli et al. [2012]). In each of these cases, El Niño events were directly associated with a relatively rapid change in fish abundance and distribution. In the La Paz area, on the other hand, there are time lags between the event and when the effects are felt in the fishery. Additionally, signals may be obscured by the diversity of taxa targeted by small-scale fishers. Thus, I adapted this research to focus on the intra-annual changes that the fishers reported.

As in many parts of the world, fishing-based livelihoods in Baja California Sur are adapted to deal with a certain degree of environmental variability. I focused on mobility and diversification as two components of fishers' livelihood strategies: they enable fishers to spread risk, smooth variability in access to resources, and reduce vulnerability. However, fishers perceive that a variety of political, economic and ecological factors are reducing their ability to deal with normal seasonal changes. One of the factors that fishers identified as influencing their ability to respond to seasonal changes is a decline in species on which they have historically depended. While biologists have documented fisheries declines in the Gulf due to overexploitation (e.g., Sala et al. [2004], Sáenz-Arroyo et al. [2006]), for fishers, declines in catch are also related to loss of access to fishing grounds due to economic development and regulatory shifts (such as MPAs and the regionalization of permits). For many, the concern about the loss of access to fish is exacerbated by perceptions that rules are unequally enforced.

In the literature there are markedly different perspectives regarding the vulnerability of coastal fishing communities (Bailey and Pomeroy [1996], Pomeroy et al. [2006]). Pomeroy et al. ([2006], 7) portray coastal communities in a way that evokes Tawney's ([1966]) metaphor of a "man standing permanently up to the neck in water, so that even a ripple is sufficient to drown him." Others have emphasized the inherent resilience of coastal fishing communities (Bailey and Pomeroy [1996], Fauzi and Anna [2010]). Bailey and Pomeroy argue that coastal communities' dependence on not just a single fish stock but an entire ecosystem reduces fishers' vulnerability to economic downturns and other instabilities. Fauzi and Anna ([2010]) argue that fishers employ a variety of techniques such as temporal and seasonal migration and income diversification to cope with uncertainty. However, the ability to adapt to change is not evenly distributed amongst communities or even individuals within a community (Adger et al.[2003], Cinner et al. [2013]).

Knowledge has been shown to be an important resource that allows small-scale fishers to adapt to variability in the Gulf of California and Pacific. Vásquez-León ([1994]) found that small-scale shrimp fishers in the Gulf of California and the Pacific Coast of Mexico who are from traditional fishing families have access to knowledge that allows them to diversify when shrimp become scarce. Less knowledgeable fishers were more dependent on shrimp (Vásquez-León [1994]). As few fishers in the La Paz region are dependent on a single species, and many are from multi-generational fishing families, knowledge likely plays less of a role in facilitating diversification, however, is still important in moving to new fishing areas, switching gear types, and procuring non-fishing jobs.

Figure 4 provides an empirically grounded summary of how adaptation occurs among the small-scale fishers of the La Paz region of Baja California Sur. Fishers' capacity to cope and adapt to environmental variability depends on their knowledge and perceptions, institutions, and individual and community-level characteristics. Furthermore, environmental variability affects associated human communities within a particular ecological, cultural, political, and economic context (McCay [2002]). Fishers are not only responding to environmental variability but a host of other stressors. While other scholars recognize the importance of some of these factors over others (Adger et al. [2003], Cinner et al. [2013]), this framework emphasizes that institutions, knowledge and perceptions, and larger contextual variables are key determinants of how fishers are able to respond in this region. Fishers' responses include strategies like moving fishing locations or diversifying fisheries or occupations, such as on the gulf coast, or developing rules to better manage fisheries. In turn, these responses influence social and ecological outcomes which provide feedbacks and influence the adaptation process.

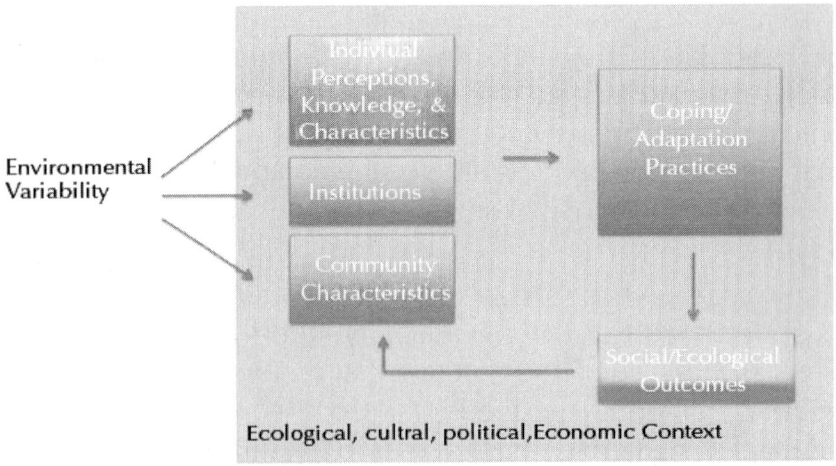

Figure 4: Conceptual framework illustrating how fishers adapt to environmental variability on the southern gulf coast of Baja California Sur. Please see text for details.

Some individual and community-level characteristics that fishers in Baja California Sur identified match those in the literature such as access to credit, occupational mobility, occupational multiplicity, social capital, material style of life, gear diversity, community infrastructure, trust, capacity to change, and debt (Cinner et al. [2013]). Fishers also identified factors like age and isolation. There are also broader considerations that influence how fishers are able to adapt. Fishers living in the city of La Paz are less dependent on fishing than those in rural areas and have more access to non-fishing work. In rural areas fishers identify a lack of available jobs and few other fishers with whom to share the gas costs required to move to new fishing areas as factors that affect their ability to cope with seasonal changes. We would expect that those currently less able to adapt to the stressors associated with the changes brought about by normal variation would face the greatest difficulties adapting to larger stressors that may be associated with climate change. Fishers also talked about the broader scale contextual variables that influence their capacity to deal with change such as changes in fisheries regulations, declines in fish stocks, and economic downturns that impact tourism and job growth in the area.

Investigating the everyday vulnerabilities that fishing households experience can elucidate broader scale contextual variables that likely influence fishers' ability to adapt to geographically extensive shocks, whether they are environmentally or institutionally mediated. The approach I took in Baja can also shed light on fishers' perceptions of environmental variability and change, particularly whether they believe a problem exists and whether they feel capable of doing something about it (McCay [2002]). On the gulf coast of Baja California Sur, fishers perceive that catch has declined but expressed little optimism that they can do something to improve their situation. Institutions, defined as both informal and formal rules for fisheries management, also influence fishers' choices. Few fishers on the gulf coast feel that they have any influence over how fisheries are managed. Many describe feeling helpless in the face of unsustainable fishing practices and often upset that while they are paying the costs, coastal users that are operating illegally are reaping the benefits. Furthermore, there is a common feeling that traditional mechanisms of coping with change such as mobility and diversification are being undermined by new regulations that have led to reduced availability of permits and restrictions in fishing area.

In order to reduce vulnerability of fishing households, we must confront these basic problems of fisheries management and the underlying factors that contribute to fishers' vulnerability. Encouraging policies that enhance fishers' mobility and ability to diversify is key. For example, offering grouped permits that allow for traditional strategies such as switching target species and fishing grounds could allow for greater flexibility. Whether this is already occurring amongst those who possess multi-species finfish and shark permits is a topic of ongoing investigation. Moreover, any new policy should recognize the multiple approaches and benefits of enhancing social and ecological resilience

(Leslie and Kinzig [2009], Basurto and Coleman [2010]). Currently in the La Paz area most fishers do not actively participate in management decisions and there is little incentive to conserve resources in the face of illegal fishing and little ability to exclude others from using the same resource. Facilitating long-term adaptive responses by fishing communities will require creating institutions that provide incentives for sustainable use.

CONCLUSIONS

It remains unclear how climate change will impact fisheries in Baja California Sur or how communities will respond. As environmental variability impacts fisheries and in turn, the well-being of associated human communities, understanding vulnerability to future climate impacts will require research on the vulnerability of fish species and their habitats as well as associated human communities.

Historically, small-scale fishers have needed to deal with uncertainty so there is an expectation of change and a stock of knowledge and experience in coping with it. Until quite recently however, temporal and spatial variability in fish catch in southern Baja California Sur was described by fishers as somewhat normal and not problematic. Patchy seasonal variability has traditionally been a part of life for fishers in the region, and in response they have devised a variety of coping mechanisms. Despite evidence that marine resources were more abundant in the past, there is no archaeological evidence that communities have ever solely relied on these resources. Recently, however, a number of factors have caused fishers to become concerned about their continued ability to adapt to the suite of changes that are occurring.

Predicting how small-scale fishers may respond to future environmental and institutional change can be informed by an understanding of their current adaptation strategies and vulnerabilities. Pressures from coastal development, declines in fish stocks, and changing societal expectations and allocation of marine resources are issues facing small-scale fishers in many parts of the world (Jentoft and Eide [2011]). Understanding how these changes interact with fishers' ability to respond to their already uncertain environment may provide insight useful for planning efforts. Adapting to climate change will require addressing some of the fundamental problems of fisheries management and ameliorating factors currently causing vulnerability. Policies that incorporate lessons about fishers' adaptation strategies in response to past and current environmental stressors can mitigate future impacts by ensuring continued flexibility.

ACKNOWLEDGEMENTS

This research was conducted while I was a postdoctoral scholar at Brown University and supported by the Coupled and Natural Systems (CNH) program of the US National Science Foundation (GEO 1114964). Thank you to community members in the La Paz area who agreed to be interviewed for this research. Thank you to Heather Leslie for comments on earlier drafts of this paper and related fisheries data analysis, based on CONAPESCA data synthesized by Octavio Aburto and colleagues from Scripps Institute of Oceanography and the Center for Marine Biodiversity and Conservation in La Paz. I also thank my mentors and collaborators on the broader NSF project: Heather Leslie, Sriniketh Nagavarapu, Sheila Walsh Reddy, Octavio Aburto-Oropeza, and Gustavo Hinajosa, Manuel Calderon Parra, Alexandra Sánchez, Juan José Cota, and Dalia Sarabia; and particularly Xavier Basurto and Mateja Nenadovic for their valuable comments on this paper and collaboration. Additional support was provided by the David and Lucile Packard Foundation (grant to Heather Leslie) and Brown University's Environmental Change Initiative (grant to Leila Sievanen and Heather Leslie). The paper greatly benefited from feedback from three anonymous reviewers

REFERENCES

1. Aburto-Oropeza, O, E Sala, G Paredes, A Mendoza, and E Ballesteros. 2007. Predictability of reef fish recruitment in a highly variable nursery habitat. Ecology 88: 2220–2228.
2. Aburto-Oropeza, O, G Paredes, I Mascareas Osorio, and E Sala. 2010. Climatic influence on reef fish recruitment and fisheries. Marine Ecology Progress Series 410: 283–287.

3. Adger, WN, S Huq, K Brown, D Conway, and M Hulme. 2003. Adaptation to climate change in the developing world. Progress in Development Studies 3 (3): 179–195.
4. Allison, EH, and F Ellis. 2001. The livelihoods approach and management of small- scale fisheries. Marine Policy 25 (5): 377–88.
5. Álvarez-Romero, JG, RL Pressey, NC Ban, J Toree-Cosío, and O Aburto-Oropeza. 2013. Marine conservation planning in practice: lessons learned from the Gulf of California. Aquatic Conservation 23 (4): 483–505.
6. Andersen, R. 1974. North Atlantic fishing adaptations: origins and directions. In Fisheries conflicts in the North Atlantic, ed. Pontecorvo G, 15–33. Ballinger, Cambridge, MA.
7. Arreguín-Sánchez, F, A Hernández-Herrera, M Ramírez-Rodríguez, and H Pérez- España. 2004. Optimal management scenarios for the artisanal fisheries in the ecosystem of La Paz Bay, Baja California Sur, Mexico. Ecological Modelling 172 (2–4): 373–382.
8. Aschmann, H. 1959. The central desert of Baja California: demography and ecology. University of California Press, Berkeley. Bailey, C, and C Pomeroy. 1996. Resource dependency and development options in coastal Southeast Asia. Society and Natural Resources 9: 191–99.
9. Basurto, X, and E Coleman. 2010. Institutional and ecological interplay for successful self- governance of community-based fisheries. Ecological Economics 69: 1094–1103.
10. Basurto, XA, A Bennett, AH Weaver, S Rodriguez-Van Dyck, and J Aceves-Bueno. 2013. Cooperative and non-cooperative strategies for small-scale fisheries self- governance in the globalization era: implications for social-ecological fit and resource stewardship. Ecology and Society 18 (4): 38.
11. Broad, K. 2000. El Niño and the anthropological opportunity. Practicing Anthropology 22 (4): 20–23.
12. Carmean, K. 1994. Archaeological investigations in the Cape Region's Cañon de San Dionisio. Pacific Coast Archaeological Society Quarterly 30 (1): 25–51.

13. Chenaut, V. 1985. Los Pescadores De Baja California. MNCP-UAP, Mexico.
14. Cinner, JE, C Huchery, ES Darling, AT Humphries, NAJ Graham, CC Hicks, N Marshall, and TR McClanahan. 2013. Evaluating social and ecological vulnerability of coral reef fisheries to climate change. PLOS One 8 (9): e74321.
15. Cinti, A, W Shaw, R Cudney-Bueno, and M Rojo. 2010. The unintended consequences of formal fisheries policies: social disparities and resource overuse in a major fishing community in the Gulf of California, Mexico. Marine Policy 34 (2): 328–339.
16. Cisneros-Mata, MÁ. 2010. The importance of fisheries in the Gulf of California and ecosystem-based sustainable co-management for conservation. In The Gulf of California: biodiversity and conservation, ed. Brusca RC, 119–134. The University of Arizona Press, Tucson.
17. Coulthard, S. 2008. Adapting to environmental change in artisanal fisheries – insights from a South Indian lagoon. Global Environmental Change 18 (3): 479–489.
18. Cudney-Bueno, R, L Bourillón, A Sáenz-Arroyo, J Torre-Cosío, P Turk-Boyer, and WW Shaw. 2009. Governance and effects of marine reserves in the Gulf of California, Mexico. Ocean and Coastal Management 52 (3–4): 207–218.
19. Cushing, DH. 1982. Climate and fisheries. Academic Press, London.
20. Des Lauriers, MR. 2011. Of clams and clovis: paleocoastal archaeology on Isla Cedros, Baja California. In Trekking the shore: changing coastlines and the antiquity of coastal settlement, ed. Bicho N, Haws J, Davis L, 161–177. Springer Press, New York.
21. Ellis, F. 2000. Rural livelihoods and diversity in developing countries. Oxford University Press, Oxford.
22. Enriquez-Andrade, R, G Anaya-Reyna, JC Barrera-Guevara, MA Carvajal-Moreno, ME Martínez-Delgado, J Vaca- Rodríguez, and C Valdés-Casilllas. 2005. An analysis of critical areas for biodiversity conservation in the Gulf of California region. Ocean and Coastal Management 48: 31–50.
23. Erisman, BE, GA Paredes, T Plomozo-Lugo, JJ Cota-Nieto, PA Hastings, and O Aburto-Oropeza. 2011. Spatial structure of

commercial marine fisheries in Northwest Mexico. ICES Journal of Marine Science 68: 564–571.

24. Fauzi, A, and Z Anna. 2010. Social resilience and uncertainties: the case of small-scale fishing households in the north coast of Central Java. MAST 9 (2): 55–64.
25. Gamez, A, and M Angeles. 2010. Borders within: tourism growth, migration and regional polarization in Baja California Sur (Mexico). Journal of Borderland Studies 25 (1): 1–18.
26. Gerhard, P. 1956. Pearl diving in lower California, 1533–1830. Pacific Historical Review 25 (3): 239–249.
27. Glantz, MH. 1992. Climate variability, climate change and fisheries. Cambridge University Press, Cambridge.
28. Glaser, B. 1992. Basics of grounded theory analysis. Sociology Press, Mill Valley, CA.
29. Global Hospitality Resources, Inc. 2013. San Diego California: Accessed 20 April 2014.
30. Head, L. 2010. Cultural ecology: adaptation-retrofitting a concept? Progress in Human Geography 35: 686–695.
31. Herrera-Cervantes, H, DB Lluch-Cota, SE Lluch-Cota, and GS Gutiérrez-de-Velasco. 2007. The ENSO signature in sea-surface temperature in the Gulf of California. Journal of Marine Research 65 (5): 589–605.
32. 1949. Estudio sobre Mexico. Economia-Transportes-Navegacion. Monografias Industriales de Banco de Mexico, SA.
33. Hoorweg, JC, B Wangila, and A Degen. 2008. Livelihoods and income diversification among artisanal fishers on the Kenyan coast. In Inside poverty and development in Africa: critical reflections on pro-poor policies, ed. Rutten M, Leliveld A, Foeken D, Brill, Leiden.
34. 2007. Climate change 2007: Synthesis report. Fourth assessment report of the Intergovernmental Panel on Climate Change. Cambridge University Press, Cambridge.
35. Jentoft, S, and AH Eide. 2011. Poverty mosaics: realities and prospects in small-scale fisheries. Springer, London.
36. Katz, R, and B Brown. 1992. Extreme events in a changing climate: variability is more important than averages. Climatic Change 21: 289–302.

37. Lauterio, C, and JUO Arizpe. 2012. Proposing strategies for a sustainable tourism: a case study of El Sargento and La Ventana, BCS, Mexico. In Sustainable tourism V, ed. Pineda FD, Brebbia CA, WIT Press, Massachusetts.
38. Leslie, HM, and AP Kinzig. 2009. Resilience science. In Ecosystem-based management for the oceans, ed. McLeod KL, Leslie HM, Island Press, Washington DC.
39. Lluch-Cota, SE. 2004. Climate change and fisheries. In Water interactions with energy, environment, food, and agriculture, ed. Donoso MC, Eolss Publishers, Encyclopedia of life support systems (EOLSS), UNESCO, Oxford.
40. Lluch-Cota, SE, EA Aragón-Noriega, F Arreguín-Sánchez, D Aurioles-Gamboa, JJ Bautista-Romero, RC Brusca, R Cervantes-Duarte, R Cortés-Altamirano, P Del-Monte-Luna, A Esquivel-Herrera, G Fernández, ME Hendrickx, S Hernández-Vázquez, H Herrera-Cervantes, M Kahru, M Lavín, D Lluch-Belda, DB Lluch-Cota, J López-Martinez, SG Marinone, MO Nevárez-Martínez, S Ortega-García, E Palacios-Castro, A Parés-Sierra, G Ponce-Díaz, M Ramírez-Rodríguez, CA Salinas-Zavala, RA Schwartzlose, and AP Sierra-Beltrán. 2007. The Gulf of California: review of ecosystem status and sustainability. Progress in Oceanography 73 (1): 1–26.
41. Lluch-Cota, SE, A Parés-Sierra, VO Magaña-Rueda, F Arreguín-Sánchez, G Bazzino, H Herrera-Cervantes, and D Lluch-Belda. 2010. Changing climate in the Gulf of California. Progress in Oceanography 87 (1–4): 114–126.
42. Löfgren, O. 1972. Resource management and family firms: Swedish west coast fishermen. In North Atlantic fishermen, ed. Andersen R, Wadel C, 82–103. Memorial University, St John's.
43. McCay, BJ. 1978. Systems ecology, people ecology, and the anthropology of fishing communities. Human Ecology 6 (4): 397–422.
44. McCay, BJ. 2002. Emergence of institutions for the commons: contexts, situations, and events. In The drama of the commons, ed. Ostrom E, Dietz T, Dolak N, Stern PC, Stonich S, Weber EU, 361–402. National Academy Press, Washington, DC.
45. McCay, BJ, W Weisman, and CF Creed. 2011. Coping with environmental change: systemic responses and the roles of

property and community in three fisheries. In World fisheries: a social-ecological analysis, ed. Ommer R, Perry I, Cury P, Cochrane K, Wiley-Blackwell, Oxford.

46. McCay, BJ, F Micheli, G Ponce-Díaz, G Murray, G Shester, S Ramirez-Sanchez, and W Weisman. 2013. Cooperatives, concessions, and co-management on the Pacific coast of Mexico. Marine Policy. In Press.
47. McGuire, T, and J Greenberg. 1993. Maritime community and biosphere reserve: crisis and response in the upper Gulf of California, Occasional Paper No.2 Bureau of Applied Research in Anthropology. University of Arizona, Tucson.
48. Micheli, F, A Sáenz-Arroyo, A Greenley, L Vazquez, JA Espinoza Montes, M Rossetto, and GA De Leo. 2012. Evidence that marine reserves enhance resilience to climatic impacts. Plos One 7 (7): e40832.
49. Morzaria-Luna, HN, P Turk-Boyer, and M Moreno-Baez. 2014. Social indicators of vulnerability for fishing communities in the Northern Gulf of California, Mexico: implications for climate change. Marine Policy 45: 182–193.
50. 2006. Agricultural and Fisheries Policies in Mexico. Recent achievements, continuing the reform agenda. OECD Publishing, Paris.
51. Perry, RI, RE Ommer, M Barange, S Jentoft, B Neis, and UR Sumaila. 2011. Marine social-ecological responses to environmental change and the impacts of globalization. Fish and Fisheries 12 (4): 427–450.
52. Pomeroy, RS, BD Ratner, SJ Hall, J Pimoljinda, andV Vivekanandan. 2006. Coping with disaster: rehabilitating coastal livelihoods and communities. Marine Policy 30: 786–793.
53. Reddy, SMW, A Wentz, O Aburto-Oropeza, M Maxey, S Nagavarapu, and HM Leslie. 2013. Evidence of market-driven size-selective fishing and the mediating effects of biological and institutional factors. Ecological Applications 23 (4): 726–741.
54. Robadue, D. 2002. An overview of governance of the Gulf of California. Coastal Resources Center, University of Rhode Island, Narragansett, Rhode Island.

55. Sáenz-Arroyo, A, CM Roberts, J Torre, M Cariño-Olvera, and JP Hawkins. 2006. The value of evidence about past abundance: marine fauna of the Gulf of California through the eyes of 16th to 19th century travelers. Fish and Fisheries 7 (2): 128–146.
56. Sala, E, O Aburto-Oropeza, G Paredes, M Reza, and L Lopez-Lemus. 2004. Fishing down coastal food webs in the Gulf of California. Fisheries 29: 19–25.
57. Smit, B, and J Wandel. 2006. Adaptation, adaptive capacity and vulnerability. Global Environmental Change 16 (3): 282–292.
58. Smit, B, I Burton, RJT Klein, and R Street. 1999. The science of adaptation: a framework for assessment. Mitigation and Adaptation Strategies for Global Change 4: 199–213.
59. Smithers, J, and B Smit. 1997. Human adaptation to climatic variability and change. Global Environmental Change 7 (2): 129–146.
60. Tawney, RH. 1966. Land and labor in China. Beacon Press, Boston.
61. 2007. Climate change: impacts, vulnerability, and adaptation in developing countries. A report by the United Nations Framework Convention on Climate Change.
62. Vásquez-León, M. 1994. Avoidance strategies and governmental rigidity: the case of the small-scale shrimp fishery in two Mexican communities. Journal of Political Ecology 1: 67–81.
63. Vásquez-León, M. 2002. Assessing vulnerability to climate risk: the case of small-scale fishing in the Gulf of California, Mexico. Investigaciones Marinas 30 (1): 204–205.
64. Villanueva-Aznar, C, HM Leslie, and L Sievanen. 2012. Artisanal fisheries of the northern Gulf of California, Mexico: environment and society project (PANGAS), a case study of marine ecosystem-based management. Univ of Michigan and Brown & Duke Universities. Marine Ecosystem-Based Management in Practice. . Accessed 20 August 2013.
65. Young, E. 2001. State intervention and abuse of the commons: fisheries development in Baja California Sur, Mexico. Annals of the Association of American Geographers 91 (2): 283–306.

Chapter 6

Negotiating Risk and Poverty in Mangrove Fishing Communities of the Bangladesh Sundarbans

Mohammad Mahmudul Islam[1] and Ratana Chuenpagdee[2]

[1]Bremen International Graduate School for Marine Sciences (GLOMAR), Research Center for Sustainability Studies (artec), University of Bremen, Bremen 28359, Germany

[2]International Coastal Network, Department of Geography, Memorial University of Newfoundland, St. John's, NL A1B 3X9, Canada

ABSTRACT

Small-scale fishers in Bangladesh face substantial risks due to their occupation and their geographical setting. Without any effective buffer against crises, recurring shocks and on-going risk exposure are major factors pushing fishers into poverty. Not all fishers experience these events in the same way, however, with some of them showing higher capacity to negotiate risks. In this study, we ask how fishers cope with shock, what factors differentiate them in their risk negotiations, and what implications these factors may have on poverty alleviation policy.

On the basis of the study's findings, we posit that poverty alleviation in small-scale fishing communities in Bangladesh requires interventions that target not only risk minimization, but also the endowment of fishers with socio-economic capitals to help them handle varying degrees of risk and shocks. Such policies as, for instance, providing employment for fisherwomen or providing a basic social safety net will increase the overall resilience and well-being of fisher communities.

BACKGROUND

Sea fishing has long been considered a risky profession due to natural hazards and technological failures (Smith 1998). High occupational hazards such as accidents while hauling in nets (Lincoln et al. 2002), health risks such as those from disease (Kissling *et al.* 2005), substantial variability in catch and consequent uncertainty in financial return (Salas et al. 2011), market risks such as increases in fuel price (Andrade and Midré 2011; Edvardsson et al. 2011), and political and security risks such as theft and conflicts (Béné and Friend 2009) reinforce this claim. The situation is likely to be further accentuated in the future by climate-related risks (Allison et al. 2009; Chuenpagdee and Juntarashote 2011). Poor fishers and their families in less developed and developing countries are more affected by most of these risks than those in developed countries because they have fewer means to cope with shocks and the aftermath of exposure to multiple risks (cf. Sinha et al. 2002; Fafchamps 1999).

Cashdan (1985: 455) refers to risk as the probability that "an unpredictable loss will occur." Shock, on the other hand, is the "manifestation of risk" (Hoogeveen et al. 2004: 4), or the "adverse events that lead to a loss of household income, a reduction in consumption and/or a loss of productive assets." (Dercon et al. 2005: 563). In Bangladesh, risks and subsequent shocks are perceived to be ubiquitous in the livelihoods of the coastal poor, but surprisingly few researchers have examined them. As argued by Hoddinott and Quisumbing (2010), the understanding of risks, shocks and their consequences is a necessary, though not sufficient, step in the design of immediate interventions and short-term programs to minimize their impacts. Dercon (2010) further posits that such understanding has crucial implications for appropriate long-term policy responses, like building social safety nets for the poor. An investigation of the role that risks and shocks play in inducing vulnerability and poverty in people's livelihoods, and of the complexity of their risk negotiations, is therefore needed in order to fine-tune policies and interventions.

A study of risks and shocks in the context of small-scale fisheries in the Sundarbans mangrove forest is highly relevant because of the dangerous and insecure natural environment and the fact that nearly everyone is dependent on fishing as the main, if not the only, basis for livelihood. Seasonality is a phenomenon that the fishing people need to navigate on a regular basis, while facing recurring natural disasters. Markets function poorly and social safety nets (such as the Vulnerable Group Feeding program[a]), even though present for a few, are not able to guarantee support when needed. Our early field observations of the fishing communities in this area revealed, however, that not all members in the fishing communities are exposed to risk and experience shocks in the same way. They also vary in how they can negotiate risks. Using a case study approach, we conducted in-depth research in the Sundarbans mangrove forest from November 2009 to April 2010, with a follow-up field visit in August 2011 to examine the following topics: i) the risks and shocks faced by the various members of the fishing communities in the Sundarbans; ii) the consequences these events have on their well-being; iii) how fishing households cope with risks and shocks; iv) the factors that foster coping mechanisms of some groups but inhibit those of others; and v) what can be done to enhance the coping capacity of the latter groups and to mitigate overall impacts due to risk exposure and subsequent shocks.

[a]The Vulnerable Group Feeding (VGF) program in Bangladesh is a relief program that is usually initiated during or after a disaster to support the affected people who are vulnerable to hunger.

The paper is structured as follows. First, we conceptualize risks and shocks in the context of the well-being of individuals and households. Next, we describe data collection methods and the study areas. This is followed in section three by an overview of the fisheries practiced in the Sundarbans mangrove forest and the socio economic features of the resource users of the forest. Subsequently, we present the empirical data to describe different shock exposure and coping strategies and factors that foster or inhibit coping mechanisms. We conclude with a discussion of ways to enhance fishers' coping abilities and the policy implications of our research.

CONCEPTS OF RISK AND SHOCK

Risk is generally understood as the "presence of a potentially large number of different possible circumstances that may materialize at a particular moment in time in the future" (Dercon 2010:15). Following Tingley et al. (2010: 1249), we consider risk as "multidimensional and subjective concept", where a particular risk event has different meanings for different people (The Royal Society 1992as cited in Tingley et al. 2010). While our study focuses on risk exposure, we note that not all events result in risks, and that shocks can stem from both risk and non-risk events. Non-risk events, like slight price fluctuations of food grains, can also create a shock, such as to poor households who are net buyers of food. Uninsured risks and unmitigated 'shocking' experience of these risks can lead to adverse welfare outcomes and can cause poverty (Dercon et al. 2005).

Risk can be covariate or idiosyncratic. Covariate risk is an aggregated risk such as a flood that affects everybody in a particular community or area. Idiosyncratic risk, on the other hand, only affects a particular individual in the community such as a health shock (Dercon 2002; Takasaki et al. 2004). Chambers (2006: 33) exemplifies this using the vulnerability framework, which has two sides: "an external side of risks, shocks, and stress to which an individual or household is subject; and an internal side which is defencelessness, meaning a lack of means to cope without damaging loss." This framework helps to understand the relationships between risk management and vulnerability to poverty of rural households in developing countries (Webb and Harinarayan 1999; Tai et al. 2010). We note that vulnerability is not synonymous with risk. While risk is about exposure to external hazards over which people have no or limited control, vulnerability conceptually includes also the capacity to manage such risks without suffering damaging or socially unacceptable loss of well-being (Dercon 2006; Chambers 2006; Hoogeveen et al. 2004; UNDP 2007).

Households generally try to negotiate risk through a range of strategies, which may be *ex ante* (i.e. before shocks occur) or *ex post* (i.e. after shocks occur) (Dercon 2010Dercon 2002; Morduch1995Morduch 1999). These responses have further implications. For instance, among the *ex-post*coping strategies, selling of assets can deplete the scarce resources of households, thus reducing their earning potential and pushing their productivity into a downward spiral. This situation is particularly evident if shocks are recurrent and are continued for longer periods that provide little prospect to household to rebuild their assets (Mendoza 2009).

Risk can be insured. Once risk is insured, it ceases to be a concern as subsequent shocks will not affect welfare outcomes. Both market-based insurance and self-insurance systems can avert negative welfare consequences in the event of risk exposure (Hoogeveen et al. 2004). Uninsured risks lead to poverty in two ways (Dercon 2010). First, as previously stated, risks, and shocks, are costly to individuals and households as they directly result in income loss. Second, a household or households' response to risk for some additional protection against shocks may come at the cost of income gains (Dercon 2002). For instance, for the fear of total investment loss, poor households may choose to invest in lower risk and lower return choices, and forego risky but higher return production choices (Dercon 2005; Chaudhuri et al. 2002; Morduch 1999). Finally shocks may directly lead to loss of assets (such as death of livestock) that contribute to further poverty (Dercon 2010).

Exposure to risk and resulting shock can also increase entrenched social inequality (Rosenzweig and Binswanger 1993; Dercon 2002). As Mosley and Verschoor (2005: 60) put in "if the poor do not invest and the rich do, gains in enterprise income will be restricted to the rich, with the implication of growing inequality over time." Women and children, particularly girls, are particularly susceptible to shocks. Women usually act as 'shock absorbers' for the household by reducing their food consumption to leave more for other members, notably their children and earning members (Mendoza 2009; Quisumbing et al. 2008). They also supplement household income through multiple jobs, limit spending, and collect foods and fuel from nature to meet the basic needs of their households (Mendoza 2009; Hossain 2009; WFP 2009as cited in Mendoza 2009). Shocks can cause severe harm to children since families may cut spending and investments on nutrition and education. Poor nutrition in early childhood can lead to long term harm in the forms of stunting and lower cognitive capacity and other persistent health impacts. Adverse health impacts and lack of education can cause intergenerational transmission of poverty (Mendoza 2009; Dercon 2006).

STUDY AREAS AND METHODS

The Sundarbans is the largest single tract mangrove forest in the world. It was declared a reserve forest under the forest act of 1855. The Forest Department (FD) of the Ministry of Environment and Forest of Bangladesh Government controls fishing activities by issuing fishing permits to fishers (Hoq2007). Fishing activities in the Sundarbans are predominantly undertaken by small-scale fisheries. These are labour intensive, low in capital investment, and are pursued for subsistence and commercial purposes or both (Hoq 2007; Rouf and Jensen 2001). Fishing gears and crafts are mostly traditional. Gears include different types of gillnets (such as drift, large mesh, fixed, and bottom set), estuarine set bag nets, trammel nets, beach seines, push nets, drag nets, and many different types of hand-operated gears and traps (Rouf and Jensen 2001; Hoq 2007). Shrimp and prawn postlarvae collection for stocking in local coastal aquaculture ponds can be considered as the largest fishing activity in terms of number of people involved. About 70–75 percent of the households living along the rivers and creeks of the Sundarbans are engaged in this activity. Mixed species of white fish, crab (*Scylla serrata*), Hilsha (*Tenualosa illisha*), and *Golda* (*Macrobrachium rosenbergii*) are the most economically important species (Rouf and Jensen 2001). The Sundarbans provide a major source of livelihoods for about 200,000 fishers (Hoq 2007).

The livelihoods of resource harvesters of the Sundarbans are characterized by high levels of income poverty and human development poverty. Most of them have limited access to basic social services, such as safe drinking water and healthcare. They also lack knowledge of health and sanitation practices. Most of them suffer long term debt bondage and face exploitative relations with moneylenders. They generally lack organizational skills, do not have professional memberships, and have a muted voice in decision making. Infrastructure is poorly developed and access to markets is restricted. Women are particularly underprivileged and marginalized, with minimum access to income, livelihood opportunities, education, and healthcare. Moreover, there is no mobilization and organization of the Sundarbans resource extractors in order for them to be recognized as stakeholders in the management of the Sundarbans (Mitra 2000; Asian Development Bank 1998). Large income inequality between better off and poor households is another feature. Incomes of the richest households are six times higher than those of the poorest groups. Agricultural land ownership is extremely skewed, with only 51 percent of the population owning land. The average household size in the impact zone is 6.3 persons and the literacy rate is 36.5 percent (all data in the preceding sentences from Mitra 2000).

The study was conducted in the three fishing communities (Figure 1) of Mothurapur, Chandipur and Dumuria villages in the edge of the Sundarbans mangrove forest within Shymnagar sub-district of Satkhira. The fishing village in Mothurapur is located in Munshigonj Union[b] on the coastal embankment bordering the river that separates coastal land from Sundarbans forest. It consists of lower caste Hindus of 53 fishing households. Infrastructure in the Mothurapur village is poorly developed, with no electricity and an inadequate sanitary system. Fishermen are mostly involved in beach and shore seine net fishing, whereas fisherwomen collect postlarvae of shrimp and prawn. Some women also do labour work, such as digging land for soil and using the soil for nearby road preparation and maintenance. The fishing hamlet Chandipur is situated in Buri Goalini Union. The community has 36 lower caste Hindu fishing households and is situated close to a paved road that leads to the district headquarters. Most fishermen are involved in beach seine and shore seine net fishing, but some fishermen also collect crabs. A number of fishers engage in marketing activities. Women are housewives but some do the same labour work as fisherwomen in Mothurapur. The fishing hamlet Dumuria is situated in Gabura Union, which was badly affected by cyclone Aila in May 2009. The first phase of the study was conducted soon after the cyclone and all households were largely dependent on food and water rations as food sources and health and sanitation facilities were almost totally destroyed. We interviewed 30 Muslim fishing households in Dumuria. Fishers in this area collect shrimp and prawn postlarvae, and are also involved in crab collection.

[b]Union Council is the lowest tier of the three-tiered local administration in Bangladesh.

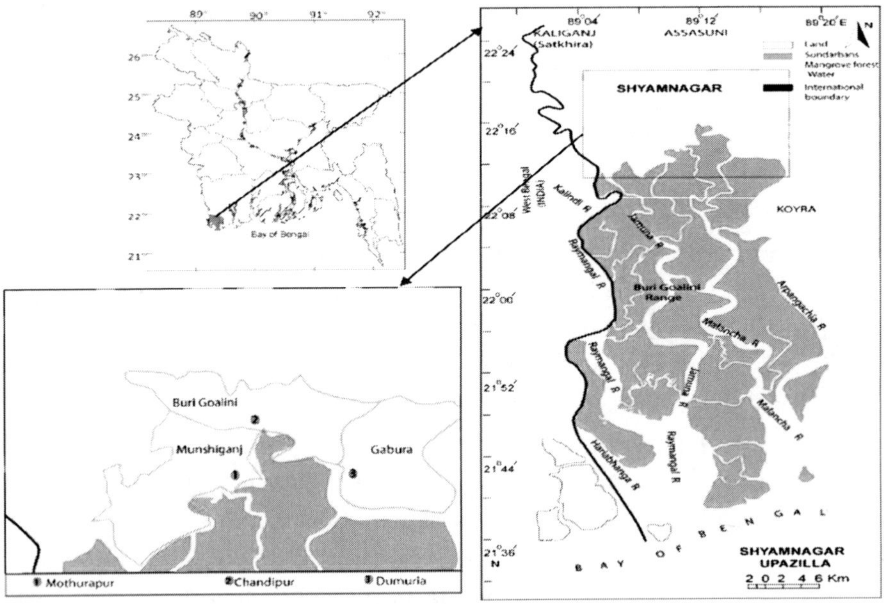

Figure 1: Map of the three study areas in the Sundarbans in Bangladesh.

Data were collected through individual and key informant interviews, as well as participatory observation from November 2009 to April 2010, with a follow-up field visit in August, 2011. Interviews were done using a semi-structured questionnaire, consisting of questions regarding household characteristics, possessions and productive assets, target species and gear used, risk perception, risks and shocks faced during fishing and in daily life, and coping strategies. In total, ninety five interviews were conducted, eighty of which were with fishers (both men and women). The rest were with people involved in post-harvest activities and credit markets, some forest officials and non-governmental organization (NGO) officials. Each individual interview lasted about 45 minutes on average. As fishers felt uncomfortable with tape recording, the responses were hand-written by a research assistant. In Mothurapur, the majority of the interviewees were women, while in Chandipur, both men and women were interviewed. In the case of Dumuria, the interviewees were all males from 30 households who had taken temporary shelter on coastal embankments after their village was devastated by the cyclone. Additionally, twenty key informant and in-depth interviews were conducted with some knowledgeable and interested persons who wanted to give more information. Supplementary to the interviews, we reviewed secondary data sources, mainly daily newspapers and reports published by NGOs. This secondary data was particularly helpful in providing information about rehabilitation activities after cyclone Aila, and about illegal and unlawful activities that take place in the Sundarbans. Hand-written data were transcribed with the help of a research assistant. After transcription, content was analyzed and classified into different themes for theoretically-guided analysis.

RESULTS

Shock-Ridden Fishing Communities in the Sundarbans

"We have crocodiles in the water, tigers on the land and dacoits[c] on the boat but nobody is there to heed our grief."

A Fisherman from Chandipur

This section utilizes empirical data gathered by our research to describe the livelihoods of the fishers of the Sundarbans with an emphasis on the events that create shock exposure and on the factors that mediate shock impacts. These events and factors are presented in Table 1.We also provide examples to illustrate the consequences of risks and shocks on the fishing livelihoods of the Sundarbans. Fishing activities in the Sundarbans are characterized by a peak week (*goon*) of good harvest, followed by a lean week (*bhati*) of poor harvest, caused respectively by spring tide and neap tide cycle. Fishers normally do not go out to the forest during lean weeks, thus fishing is limited to two weeks in a month. Most fishers go out once a day for only three to four hours because of tidal variation. Shrimp and prawn postlarvae collectors, on the other hand, fish twice a day. Extending the fishing period is not possible as high tidal water may damage the fishing gear and wash away the harvest. In addition, fishers are susceptible to natural fluctuations in catch. One fisher from Mothurapur described the situation:

Fishing is like a lottery- catch varies from day to day, one week to another. Maybe in one day you get bumper catch, but on subsequent days you may suffer poor or even no catch.

[c]A member of a land-based robber gang.

Table 1: Events that create shocks, factors that mediate shock exposure, and strategies to address shock impacts (Based on interviews with fishers and participant observation in the Sundarbans)

Events that create shock exposure	Factors that mediate impacts of shock	Strategies to address shock impacts
Risk events		
i.Cyclones and other extreme climatic events	i.Ownership of land and other productive assets, such as fishing gear and craft	i.Adjusting labour supply and using children as labour
ii.Physical accidents during fishing	ii.Gender differences in family headship	ii.Shifting to non-fishing occupations
iii.Tiger attacks	iii.Demographic characteristics of family and dependency ratio	iii.Diversification of fishing occupations
iv.Attacks by criminal gangs	iv.Diversification of target species, fishing gears and fishing methods	iv.Changes in target species and fishing gear
v.Illegal rent seeking (ransoms, bribes)	v.Access to information networks and alliances with powerful individuals	v.Illegal and or unsustainable extraction of fisheries and other wood and non-wood forest resources

vi.Food insecurity and drinking water crises	vi.Risk perception	vi.Family cooperation and consumption adjustment
vii.Illness and health problems	vii.Type of risk	vii.Taking loans from neighbours and network
viii.Legal procedures after breach of regulations		viii.Informal mutual supports and mutual insurance
ix.Social exclusion due to tiger widowhood		i.Trust, reciprocity and kinship
		ii.Occasional migration
		iii.Rituals and beliefs
Non-risk events		
i.Price fluctuations of fish and food		
ii.Seasonality and harvest failure of fish catch		
iii.Credit inaccessibility		
iv.Changes in land usage pattern (e.g. aquaculture)		
v.Costs due to marriage and dowry		
vi.Resettlement		

Islam and Chuenpagdee

Islam and Chuenpagdee *Maritime Studies* 2013 12:7, doi:10.1186/2212-9790-12-7

Unexpectedly poor catches or harvest failure in a single peak fishing week is a blow to the income of the fishing households. The shock becomes severe when poor harvests are recurrent for more than one peak period, or when fishers are forced to discontinue fishing due to the number of other reasons such as bad weather or tidal surges in the monsoon season.

Income from fishing may be further dissipated by illicit acts, such as ransom by dacoits and bribery by forest officials. Dacoits rob collected fish and crab, nets and even boats, and often kidnap fishers or physically attack them. At least 20,000 BDT (about 245 US$) is claimed as ransom for each kidnapped fisher. Some fishers are killed by dacoits each year; numerous fishers are wounded, and their families become bankrupt as a consequence. A number of ex-fishers said they left fishing because of dacoits and are now doing van[d] pulling. With respect to bribery, fishers have to pay a certain fee for getting permits to fish in the forest. This management rule allegedly involves corruption, as fishers claim that they need to pay ten to fifteen times the amount of the actual fees for the permit. They may also need to bribe forest officials at different checkpoints when staying in the forest longer than the permitted period. Khuda (2008: 6) estimates that forest officials in the Sundarbans extort around 2.3 million BDT (about 28,400 US$) per year from fishers. The different forms of rent dissipation are explained by a fisher in Mothurapur as follows:

[d]This three wheeled human hauler (different than a rickshaw) is a widely used means of transportation in the study areas for passengers and goods.

Income from fishing in the Sundarbans goes to seven[e] families. You have to give bribes to forest officials to secure a permit for fishing, extortion or ransom money goes to dacoits, weightier (a person who weighs catch at landing sites) and commission agents will demand extra money at the fish landing centre, then *mohajan* (money lenders) may come to the scene to claim money.

[e]Seven is the symbolic number for many.

To recover these additional expenses, fishers usually resort to illegal fishing, as well as illegal logging, creating thus a vicious circle of overexploitation and corruption. When fines are given to fishers for illegal activities, they add another shock to household's income. Fishing permits may be revoked and fishers have to take frequent trips to the district headquarters to pursue legal procedures, all of which involve money and time, and increase exposure to bureaucratic harassment.

For most of the interviewed households, the collection of shrimp and prawn postlarvae is a very important income supplementing activity for fishing families. The price of these products depends, however, on the cycle of shrimp aquaculture. During the off-peak season, demand for postlarvae is less, and the price may drop to about half of that received during the peak season. Thus their daily income maybe lowered from two American dollars to one dollar. Despite the regularity and predictability of these price fluctuations, they pose a shock to marginal fishers with very low income. Since most of them are net buyers of food and other daily necessities except fish, fluctuations in food prices also have profoundly negative impacts on family consumption, thus raising their food insecurity (cf. Mendoza 2009). The dilemma of price declines and food buying is complex. One may question why fishers need to buy food rather than consuming more of the fish that they catch. In this particular case, it is not only that shrimp and prawn postlarvae are non-consumable fish products, but it is also rice, not fish, that is their staple food. Price instability of necessary daily commodities is an added ingredient to their vulnerability. Fishing households in our study areas spend more than sixty percent of their daily income on food. This situation drastically reduces their capacity to invest or save for future needs. After exposure to different shocks, fishers are in dire need of money to keep their families afloat. The formal credit market is poorly supplied, and in most instances excludes small-scale fishers from benefiting due to absent or insufficient collateral in the form of assets. Taking loans from money lenders is also risky because failure to repay the loan may force the sale of remaining productive assets, such as boats and nets. As our study reveals, several fishers absconded in order to avoid or delay repayment of loans from NGOs and money lenders.

Fishing activities in the Sundarbans take place mainly in narrow canals and tributaries where territorial use of space often creates conflicts and tension. This is particularly the case with estuarine setbag nets for shrimp and prawn postlarvae collection, where theft or destruction of gear by other users takes place. Additionally, small-scale fishers compete for space with coastal aquaculture. Canals and water-logged agriculture fields in the rainy season, earlier used by poor fishers for their livelihood activities, have been turned into shrimp ponds. Discharge of farm effluents containing hazardous substances together with overfishing by shrimp and prawn postlarvae collectors has drastically reduced fisheries productivity in the remaining freshwater bodies (Islam and Wahab 2005). Much*khas*, or government-owned land around coastal embankments, which had been used by the poor for their settlements, now has become the private property of aquaculture entrepreneurs. The expansion of shrimp aquaculture has thus removed a buffer for the livelihoods of many marginal fishers. One fisherwoman from Mothurapur recalled:

Even by digging up holes made by rats in paddy fields, we could collect the remains of paddy that ensured our food security for at least two months. We worked in the paddy field during harvest seasons and payment of the labour was in grains rather than in cash and that was positive for our food security. We could even use collected paddy chaff for fuel, for thatch or food for cattle. Now we have to travel long distances inland to find a paddy field to work on, because all farm land nearby has been converted into aquaculture ponds.

Another issue related to shrimp farming is environmental quality. In Dumuria, a number of fishers mentioned that before shrimp aquaculture was initiated, they could drink groundwater and cultivate vegetables and fruits in their home yards. Now, one fisher from Dumuria said:

Only in the rainy season can we drink rain-harvested fresh water, the rest of the year we have to drink water from ponds after purification or buy water, because ground water is too saline to drink.

Health problems often constitute a significant shock in fishing communities. Women and children who use drag nets to collect shrimp and prawn postlarvae, need to spend five to six hours per day in the water. These uncomfortable working conditions affect their health. Skin diseases and gynecological problems are reported for women and young girls who work as collectors. Many fishermen are distressed by infestations of mosquitoes. One fisherman from Chandipur said that:

Mosquito bites in the forest are so harsh and acute that sometime I feel that begging on land is better than fishing in the forest.

Moreover, village settlements are highly congested and sanitation facilities are poorly developed. Many households still lack sanitary toilets, exposing them to risk of water borne disease. Illness of a family head and main income earner is one of the most cited causes of shock. Although almost all members in fishing households contribute to family income, illness of one earning member can put them in a situation where they are unable to meet the costs of treatment. Their welfare is highly affected because they usually have little or no savings to fall back on. Even for some better off households, they risk becoming bankrupt, as they have to sell assets to meet high treatment costs. Many fishing households are living in the condition that Krishna (2010:17) describes as "only one illness away from poverty".

A number of shocks also emanate from extreme natural events. Fishers are killed each year in the seas adjacent to the mangrove forest due to hostile weather conditions. In Dumuria, during cyclone Aila, coastal embankments protecting the island from tidal water were destroyed and washed away, along with vast swaths of agricultural land, shrimp farms, and homes. Many better off households were able to leave the island, while the rest stayed in temporary tents on the remaining wrecked coastal embankments. After more than one year, they went back to their homes but torrential rain in 2011 again flooded their village. In our study areas, some households needed to shift their houses four times due to erosion. With a very limited asset base, a onetime shift of settlement is already beyond their coping capacity. The accompanying loss of livestock, paddy fields, and other food sources seriously worsens local food security. In this particular circumstance, a vicious circle occurs as the non-fishing families, or non-fishing members of fishing families are pushed into fishing due to limited income generation options elsewhere. Going to the forests for maintaining livelihoods is often considered an activity of last resort, as a local proverb says:

Nirdhon? Jao Bon- no Assets? Then Go to the Forest

One key informant noted that since cyclone Aila the number of men entering and working in the forests has constantly increased. The Government of Bangladesh, after cyclone Aila, put a ban on wood collection in the Sundarbans to enable mangrove regeneration. For this reason, many former wood collectors enter into fisheries, thereby increasing pressure on the fisheries resources.

The Royal Bengal tigers that roam the Sundarbans are an impending risk for resource harvesters. In the last thirty years, 14 people have been killed in Chandipur and 10 people in Mothurapur study areas. According to the Forest Department of the Government of Bangladesh, tigers killed 120 men in 2009 alone, or about one every three days. Some fisherwomen were also killed while fishing inside the forest. Some deaths go uncounted, however, because the documentation applies only to victims who are officially registered forestry workers. The government normally provides a lump sum of 100,000 BDT (1240 US$) per person to the families of victims but getting this compensation often involves bribery and suffers delays. More than 1,000 women are recorded who have lost their husbands in tiger attacks in the Sundarbans (Kazim 2011). Commonly referred to as "tiger widows", these women have become a symbol of misfortune in the village and in their in-law's houses. Sometime they are ill treated after the deaths of their husbands (LEDARS 2010). One tiger widow from Chandipur recalled her sad experiences:

After the death of my husband by a tiger attack, my miserable life started. I took shelter in my parents' home with my two kids. Working in a shrimp farm, sorting shrimps, only gives me 40 BDT (50 US cents) per day. The number of meals per day decreased; quite often I skip my meals to give some food to my children.

Misfortune also haunts the children of tiger widows. They may face harsh words from their classmates, for instance, that their fathers were killed because they were "bad" men. Because of such treatment and because of their poverty, many children leave school and try to eke out a living by engaging in labour work that earns them little income. Without education and other support, male children eventually turn to the forests, like their deceased fathers, putting themselves thus at the same risk (Kazim 2011; LEDARS 2010). Further, human activities also play role in intensifying certain risk activities in the forest. For instance; one key informant (an NGO official who is working with tiger widows) noted that:

Human activities largely influence the behavior of tigers. People are fishing and poaching in no-take-areas in the Sundarbans, thus the habitats and food sources of tigers are largely ransacked. Now tigers are roaming larger areas in the forest in search of food and attacking forest-goers. Day by day incidents of tiger attack and trespassing into nearby villages are increasing. Yet, the tiger is an integral part of resources management of the Sundarbans. If there were no tigers, the Sundarbans would perish within twenty years due to over-exploitation and illegal exploitation.

The socio-cultural setting of the communities also increases the impacts of their risk exposure. Although both poor and better off fishers are affected by dacoits, the poor suffer more and experience more profound shocks. Shocks are particularly biased towards women in the households or women-headed households in the fishing communities. Women and girls are usually involved in fishing practices that are time consuming, such as using drag nets for collecting shrimp and prawn postlarvae, for erratic and meager returns[f]. Women are usually assigned to the less strenuous parts of manual jobs and get seventy percent of the wage of their male counterparts, despite their ability to do more. Limited scope for income generation as well as wage differentiation put women-headed households at the lowest income level in the communities. Girls become a family liability due to the practice of dowry. Marriage of girls was thus a common shock for almost all households interviewed, even though it is not totally unanticipated when baby girls are born. Wedding-related expense may also push households into bankruptcy. In their study in rural Bangladesh, Baulch and Davis (2008) find that dowry represents the largest sum of yearly lump expenditure (35%) for households, and wedding expenses are higher in a bride's family (23%) than in a groom's (21%). Thus the number of girls in a family makes the family more vulnerable. Due to dowry and other reasons like childhood marriage, the rates of divorce and wife abandonment are increasing in fishing communities, some fishers indicated.

[f]Women and girls are reported to have gynecological problems after spending prolonged periods in water; risk of crocodile attack is also reported.

In sum, for most fishing households, shocks are recurrent, cumulative and transferable to subsequent generations. Fishing households may suffer several shocks within a short period rather than a single one. This exposure to consecutive shocks makes their livelihoods precarious: "a single blow can be endured by most people, but when several blows fall one after the other, then it becomes very hard for any individual to cope" (Krishna 2010: 18). Recurring shocks make them very vulnerable to further risks, which may push them into extreme poverty or diminish their opportunities to get out of poverty. Yet, as exposure to shocks and impacts of shocks are not uniform for all fishers, responses also vary accordingly. The next section focuses on different coping strategies of fishing households in response to different shock impacts.

Coping Strategies of the Fishing Households

For fishing households in the Sundarbans, reduced consumption is the first strategy to deal with crises of no or insufficient income. Usually the head of family and income earner gets the first priority in terms of access to limited food, with women having the last priority. The proportion of cheaper vegetables increases with the reduction of rice in daily consumption during periods when prices increase. Taking rice and other daily necessities on loan from next door neighbours is also a common strategy to smooth consumption. Diversified economic portfolios are another strategy of coping. For instance, women collect shrimp and prawn postlarvae as their main gainful activity, but also work in shrimp farms, weed grass from agriculture fields, collect paddy, mend and prepare nets, collect mangrove leaves for fuel, prepare traditional quilts, work as housemaids, and prepare and sell charcoal from mangrove wood. Another dominant strategy is to remove children from school; boys are put to work in fishing jobs, even though they receive lower wages than adults. Similarly, girls join in collecting shrimp and prawn postlarvae. The reasons for child labour are explained by one fisherwoman from Mothurapur:

There are always income opportunities in the forest, if they can catch a big crab and sell it at BDT 80 (1 US$), then I can buy two kilograms of rice. Rather than starving with children, better to earn with them.

The multi-species fisheries of the Sundarbans also offer job flexibility in terms of target species. During our study period, we observed that most interviewed fishers converted from catching fish species to harvesting crab because fish catches had declined, while the price of crabs rose. Crab collection also requires less labour power (only two persons) and it faces less risk of tiger attack. This coping strategy of changing target species was at first not taken up widely by lower caste fishers who, with their strong hereditary profession, consider fishing to mean catching fish not crabs. Times are changing, however, and crab collection is nowadays seen as rewarding. Thus fishers adopt diversification as way to manage risks associated with their biological and economic environments (Minnegal and Dwyer 2008).

Trust, reciprocity and kinship together constitute another coping strategy that draws on family ties and social networks. To meet immediate crises, such as dowry, fishers most commonly take loans from their relatives. When fishers go to the Sundarbans, they are usually accompanied by their next of kin (e.g. their son, brother or father), who will not leave them if there is any mishap. This trust and loyalty acts as their main security in their fishing operation (Kazim 2011). One fisher from Chandipur underscored the issue:

During fishing in the forest if a tiger attacks me, my brother will not leave me, and he will fight back to rescue me, and I will do the same in his case. If dacoits kidnap me and one of kin is with me that will give me a feeling that I am not abandoned in the risky forest.

We heard of a number of cases where fellow fishers fought in the forest with a tiger when it attacked one of their fishing mates.

Belief and rituals together make up another strategy to cope with the risk of a tiger attack in the forest. Before going to the forest, traditional Hindu fishers perform various rituals and worship the goddess *Bon Bibi* (Forest Lady) in a way that is different from mainstream Hindu beliefs. There are several statues of the forest goddess *Bon Bibi* scattered throughout the forest for worship by forest-goers. They believe that *Bon Bibi* is always vigilant in the forest to protect them from evil forces and it is she who can offer protection from tigers. This ritual practice and associated beliefs, they feel, provide them with the mental strength to engage in risky fishing practices in the wilderness of the forest.

Coping with income loss by increasing pressure on the fisheries resources is a widespread practice for fishers. Shrimp and prawn postlarvae collection, which is widely practiced by fisherwomen, is considered environmentally destructive, due to loss of large number of juvenile fish and crustaceans as by-catch. Along with other resource users, some fishers are involved in illegal logging, poaching of wildlife as well as in banned and destructive fishing practices, such as use of poison and catching of undersized and berried species.

For traditional fishers, outmigration was rarely mentioned as a coping strategy, because some fishers feared that it may lead to loss of entitlement to the *khas* land where they are living, even if they do not formally own it. Most fishers think that they have limited capacity to survive if they migrate to other areas. Citing the benefits of common pool resources, one fisherman from Mothurapur said:

"Here we can stay on *khas* land; if I have no food my child can at least collect some fish. If I go to any city, where I will stay, who will give me food, if I don't have a job for one day?

Finally, outside intervention sometime shapes the coping mechanisms of fishers. After cyclone Aila, there was an influx of governmental, donor and NGOs activities into the areas that brought changes in the livelihoods of fishing communities. Sanitation and drinking water facilities have been improved and rehabilitation activities (like building houses, maintenance of roads and ponds) created temporary job opportunities for many fishers. After encountering relief activities and participating in different awareness programs, most interviewed fishers are now interested in education and concerned to ensure a better future for their children. Some fishers in Chandipur and Dumuria take out micro-credit loans offered by different NGOs to meet immediate needs. Being largely illiterate, they only obtain short-term benefits from these loans, and often become heavily indebted in the long run when they are unable to repay them. Few fishers have savings or insurance schemes as a part of loan arrangements. Cases of fraudulent activities by insurance companies, however, make poor or landless fishers reluctant to be involved in any NGO lending scheme. Instead, they prefer to buy food and other necessities from grocery shops on loan, which they pay off during the peak fishing periods when income is better.

Although the majority of fishers are similarly exposed to shocks, coping heterogeneity exists across poor and better off fishing households (Table 2). The better off fishers are able to elevate their incomes by switching target species by using of different fishing gears (to ward off seasonality and low catch). This adaptive strategy requires, however, financial capital to buy different gears and to cover other ancillary costs, as well as skills that most poor fishers cannot afford or do not possess. Through land ownership, better off fishers could collect a number of material benefits (e.g. bank loans) and non-material benefits (e.g. access to social networks). Hence, a local proverb says "*Kheter kuna, durer sona,*" which translates to "a small portion of land is more valuable than gold". It is thus not surprising that the majority of the better off fishers were seen to convert their fishing income into land through direct purchase or mortgage. One key informant from Chandipur explained:

Incomes from forest fishing are diverse and attractive but tend to disappear like a bubble due to the extravagant behavior of fishers. Those who are able to lock their fishing income into land are successful.

Table 2: Key characteristics of poor and better off fishing households in the Sundarbans (Based on interviews with fishers and participant observation)

Poor households	Better off households
i.Fishers work as labour or on profit share schemes without ownership of fishing gears and craft and land.	i.Fishers who have at least homestead land, or if living on *khas* land, have other entitlements to land
ii.Houses are small with thatched roofs	ii.Houses have corrugated GI (galvanised iron) roof sheet
iii.Frequently take loans (*dadon*) for buying food or for other daily expenses	iii.To some extent, have diversified livelihoods outside of fishing
iv.Higher dependency ratios with small children, especially girls	iv.Usually don't take loans or *dadon* for daily expenses
v.Widow headed households without any other active income earners of the family	v.Possess small capital to lend to others on interest
vi.Fishers using inexpensive drag and pull nets for collection of shrimp and prawn postlarvae without any other income source	vi.Have ownership of fishing gears and a boat or involved in the fish trade
vii.Suffer food insecurity on daily or weekly basis; sometime go without one or two meals	vii.Enjoy food security all year round
viii.Youngsters do not go to school but are forced to work by the family out of necessity	viii.Children usually go to school, but if they work, it is for adding income to the family rather than due to dire need
ix.Reciprocal relations mainly exist within own community and relatives but not beyond	ix.Usually have reciprocal relations with people beyond their own communities and with powerful locals

Islam and Chuenpagdee

Islam and Chuenpagdee *Maritime Studies* 2013 12:7, doi: 10.1186/2212-9790-12-7

Type of gears and target species are significant in terms of degree of risk during fishing in the forest. Better off fishers usually use more efficient fishing gears and safer fishing methods than poor fishers. Further, in Bangladesh, the local power structure controls the ways the resources and help from the government reach the poor (Lewis and Hossain 2008). Thus, connection to locally powerful elites provides a cushion for the better off during period of crisis. Those who are locally powerful can negotiate by bribing forest officials or giving protection money to dacoits in advance to continue fishing in the forest.

To sum up, fishing households employ a number of coping strategies that include reduction and adjustment of consumption, income diversification through pooling labour and changing gear, illegal fishing, and drawing from mutual insurance and social networks, to mention some (Table 1). Yet, the capacity of a household to cope with the effects of shock exposure depends on the household's productive capacity (e.g. assets, endowments and labour), and family characteristics (dependency ratios), access to social networks, power, and other factors. Unfortunately, as for the poor elsewhere in the world, poor fishing households in the Sundarbans have less of these attributes what means that negative shocks trap them in poverty (cf. Takasaki et al. 2004). This will be discussed further in the next section.

DISCUSSION

Poor people globally are preoccupied with dealing with risks and uncertainty, and their failure to adequately deal with shocks often acts as main cause of their poverty (World Bank 2001). For the poor with lower per capita income, unmitigated shocks can have devastating impacts on their livelihoods (Fafchamps and Lund 2003). This proposition is highly relevant to small-scale fishing households around the world, which are enmeshed within risk and uncertainty (Béné and Friend2009). The livelihoods of the small-scale fishers of the Sundarbans are similarly highly prone to shock, which emanates from both risky and non-risky events (Figure 2). This shock exposure is a major cause of poverty (cf. Dercon 2010) and in the Sundarbans it reduces the well-being of the fishers in several ways. For instance, seasonality directly results in low income through loss of fishing days. This manifestation of shock exposes them to further risk (cf. Fafchamps 1999). In the absence of formal health insurance for poor rural fishers, another example of risk exposure is that the death of the main income earner, or his or her chronic illness creates both physiological and economic shocks, which can lead even better off households to bankruptcy and perpetuation of poverty. These observations confirm the findings of Hulme (2004). In the face of income loss, the poor need surplus accumulation to compensate for possible losses, but making savings requires "room to maneuver" (Jentoft and Midré 2011; Clay and Schaffer 1984) that the poor fishers of the Sundarbans simply do not have. The high risk forest environment and certain changes in land usage patterns, such as the expansion of coastal aquaculture activities in their area, put limits on the fishing and living space of poor fishers. Their "room to maneuver" is also restricted due to specific social relationships, such as caste structure and gender relations (cf. Cleaver 2005; Borooah 2005). Women are vulnerable to poverty not only because of their social status, but also because of their role as "shock absorbers" (Mendoza 2009).

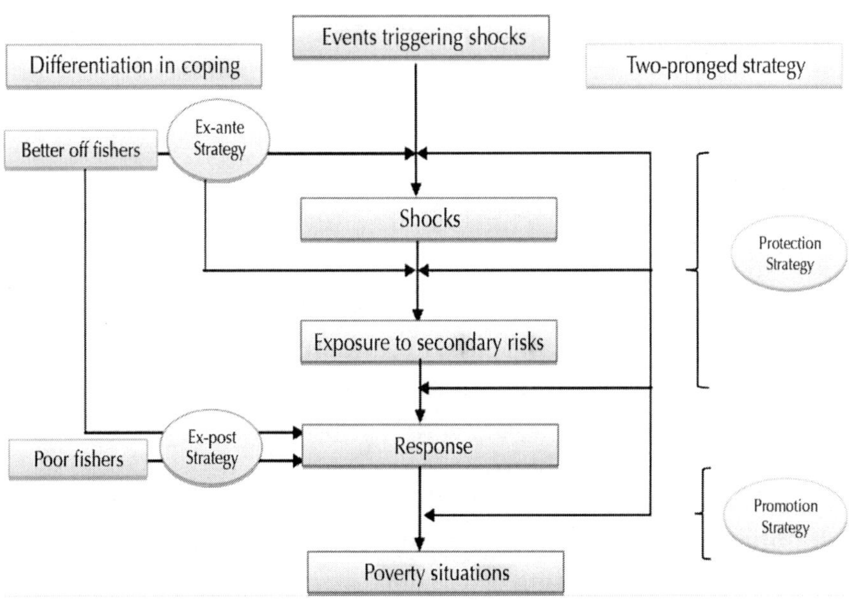

Figure 2: Impacts of risks and shocks on poverty situation and coping and response strategies.

In particular, shocks also lead to the exposure to secondary risk as illustrated in Figure 2. These secondary risks are evident in the case of "tiger widows", who after facing the shocking experience of the tragic death of their husband further face the secondary risk of social exclusion and risk of abject poverty. In response to shocks and risks the poor often adopt *ex-post* risk-coping strategies, which only enable them to continue to survive (Figure 2). Yet, a number of coping strategies to reduce shock exposure deepen their precarious conditions. As found in this study, poor fishing households mostly choose to invest in low return peripheral fishing in the Sundarbans and forego higher return on similar investments in deep forest fishing, in order to avoid serious hardship and destitution induced by the possible loss of investment (cf. Dercon 2010) by the assault of criminal gangs or the tragic situation created by tiger attack. Taking children out of school, poor nutrition due to reduction in the number of meals and reduction of the quality of meals are some other erosive coping strategies that affect current and future capacity to avert poverty. Better off fishers, on the other hand, employ a different set of strategies, many of which are ex-*ante*, which might not lead to complete eradication of the impacts of shock, but that largely offset them and protect fishers from the exposure to secondary risks (Figure 2). Wealthier fishers are found to develop risk management strategies that are more resilient because they have more diversified and efficient fishing gears and are able to provide bribes and pay extortion where needed. Greater mobility and greater "room to maneuver" in the forest provides them with an income edge over the poor members of the communities, and thus further widens the existing income inequality within the communities.

Recognizing these different responses from better off and poor fishers, we argue for a two pronged approach to interventions, as shown in Figure 2. A protection-oriented component is required to reduce vulnerability to risk exposure, while a promotional component aims to increase income, productivity, or employment prospects (Matin and Hulme 2003; Krishna 2010). Both of these policies are intertwined and reinforce each other. For instance, access to formal bank credit schemes will not only protect households from exploitation by money lenders, but will also promote income generation through investments in productive assets.

Given that seasonality and shocks affect their income and restrict their upward mobility (cf. Krishna 2010), fishers need to be protected from events that erode their income. Some key informants perceive that although complete elimination of the sources of risk may not be possible, some risk events are manipulated by human activities and are negotiable. Ironically, most fishers said that criminal gangs of dacoits are more harmful than tigers. Most fishers complain they are tired of having to meet the extortion and ransom demands to get access to fishing. So it is imperative to provide them "protective security" (Sen 1999), through, among other things, better governance. The national law of Bangladesh formally favors landless people to get access to government owned *khas*land, but acquisition is largely discriminatory and the processes bear potential for conflicts with local landlord elites. Secure ownership of *khas* land in a suitable setting should be a priority for livelihood strengthening of poor fishing households. Considering the limited feasibility of insurance schemes by private enterprises, public micro-insurance of all legal fishing practices can be an effective strategy. A small premium could be taken when fishing permits are issued. This will also encourage fishers to practice legal fishing, which will reduce illegal and over exploitation of resources as well as serve as a buffer against sudden shocks. Having buffers and protective security will reverse risk averse behaviour of poor fishers to a certain extent and that, in turn, will boost their capacity to take on more risky but higher-return fishing activities in the forest. However, such changes of attitude need to be promoted by endowing fishers with socio-economical capitals.

In terms of promotion, raising income is not all that is required for risk management and reduction of poverty for small-scale fishers, it is also urgent to enhance the set of livelihood choices for risk spreading. Considering the diverse sources of risks women face and their history of job multiplication, land based job opportunities for women need to be promoted. Shifting the occupation of fisherwomen from forest fishing (particularly environmentally destructive shrimp and prawn postlarvae collection activities) would help to take pressure off the forest and also to reduce high dependency of entire households on vulnerable fisheries and uncertain incomes (cf. Takasaki et al. 2004). More importantly, to prevent intergenerational continuities of poverty, more effective *ex-ante* and *ex-post*mechanisms are required (Santos 2010). Our study identified some promising outside interventions after cyclone Aila. Now (2011) in Chandipur, about eighty percent of children (5 years of age or older) go to school whereas only 5 percent of adult fishers (+30 years) have five years of schooling. The government now gives monthly allowances to students in primary school. Particularly, the present study observed that school feeding programs, that provide nutritious biscuits to students, have positive impacts on school attendance. Given limited means and resources, targeting support is probably the most efficient solution (Dercon 2005). Following this policy, vulnerable fishing households need to be brought into the social safety net through, for example, enrolling them in the existing Vulnerable Group Feeding program which is targeted to vulnerable people in society. Most lower caste poor fishers suffer from a lack of interaction and diversity both in terms of their fishing group as well as in mixing with other communities. As a result they suffer social exclusion. This kind of segregation bars them from participation in the social and economic growth opportunities in the area (cf. Crona and Bodin 2006) and inhibits them from exploring new opportunities. Again, in the longer term, eradication of rural poverty is only possible by economic development (Fafchamps1999). Hence, it is important to bring fishers into mainstream development processes, recognizing their different coping mechanisms, and including them in delineating risk management options. This implies that it is crucial to provide them access to education, skills, healthcare, information, and credit, which will increase their opportunity to share in societal wealth creation (Dercon 2010; Takasaki et al. 2004).

CONCLUSIONS

In this paper, we examine the risks and shocks faced by the fishers of the Sundarbans, how they cope with risk exposure and shocks, what factors differentiate them in their adaptive capacity, and what implications differential capacity may have on their poverty situations. Our study shows that small-scale fishers in the Sundarbans face disruptive shocks that are numerous, severe, and widespread and that this shock exposure is a major driver that pushes or entraps them in poverty. In responding to shock exposure, fishing households in the Sundarbans have developed a number of strategies which are diverse and vary according to asset ownership. Yet, in absence of any effective buffer, frequent shocks create deprivation among poor fishers who are thus not able to employ sound coping strategies. On the other hand, the adaptive strategies of better off fishers are more effective. This finding suggests that holding socio-economic assets is a key tool to guard against shocks and differentiates among the capacities of fishers to cope with or negotiate risk and shock impacts. Under such conditions, our study submits that reducing risk and shock exposure should be at the core of poverty reduction efforts for Sundarbans fishing communities. For instance, better off households in the Sundarbans may not be poor today, but recurrent exposure to shock can push them rapidly into poverty, because they might survive one shock but not recurrent shocks. Thus poverty alleviation strategies should aim at not only lifting the shock-ridden poor out of poverty, but also to protect risk-vulnerable (better off) fishers from getting into poverty. Hence, our study argues for a two-pronged strategy of protection and promotion to contain the risk factors in the household's environment, to mitigate the household's exposure to shock and to strengthen its capacity to cope with and manage risk exposure.

AUTHORS' CONTRIBUTIONS

MMI and RC shared responsibility in conceptualization of research questions. MMI was responsible for fieldwork, data analysis and preparation of manuscript. RC provided input to the structure of the manuscript and helped read and revise it. All authors read and approved the final manuscript.

ACKNOWLEDGEMENTS

Funding for this research of the first author including his empirical research was provided by the Bremen International Graduate School for Marine Sciences (GLOMAR). The idea for the paper was developed during the visit of the first author to International Coastal Network, Memorial University, Canada, where the second author is located. The manuscript has benefited from comments of Michael Flitner from the University of Bremen, Germany and Maritime Studies Editor Derek Johnson. We are grateful to two anonymous reviewers for their very helpful comments.

REFERENCES

1. Allison, EH, AL Perry, M-C Badjeck, WN Adger, K Brown, D Conway, AS Halls, GM Pilling, JD Reynolds, NL Andrew, and NK Dulvy. 2009. Vulnerability of National Economies to the Impacts of Climate Change on Fisheries. Fish Fish 10: 173–196.
2. Andrade, H, and G Midré. 2011. The Merits of Consensus: Small-Scale Fisheries as a Livelihood Buffer in Livingston, Guatemala. In Poverty Mosaics: Realities and prospects in Small-scale Fisheries, ed. Jentoft S, Eide A, 427–448. Dordrecht Springer.
3. Asian Development Bank. 1998. Summary of Initial Environmental Examination for Sundarbans Biodiversity Conservation Project in Bangladesh. Asian Development Bank.http://www.adb.org/documents/environment/ban/ban-sundarbans.pdf *webcite*, Accessed August 23, 2011
4. Baulch, B, and P Davis. 2008. Poverty Dynamics and Livelihood Trajectories in Rural Bangladesh. International Journal of Multiple Research Approaches 2 (2): 176–190.
5. Béné, C, and RM Friend. 2009. Water, Poverty and Inland Fisheries: Lessons from Africa and Asia. Water International 34 (1): 47–61. Publisher Full Text
6. Borooah, VK. 2005. Caste, Inequality and Poverty in India. Rev Dev Econ 9: 399–414.
7. Cashdan, EA. 1985. Coping with Risk: Reciprocity among the Basarwa of Northern Botswana. Man New Series 20 (3): 454–474.
8. Chambers, R. 2006. Editorial Introduction: Vulnerability, Coping, and Policy. IDS Bull 37 (4): 33–40.
9. Chaudhuri, S, J Jalan, and A Suryahadi. 2002. Assessing Household Vulnerability to Poverty from Cross-Sectional Data: A Methodology and Estimates from Indonesia. Department of Economics, Columbia University, New York. Discussion Papers 0102–52
10. Chuenpagdee, R, and K Juntarashote. 2011. Learning from the Experts: Attaining Sufficiency in Small-Scale Fishing Communities in Thailand. In Poverty Mosaics: Realities and prospects in

Small-scale Fisheries, ed. Jentoft S, Eide A, 309–331. Dordrecht Springer.

11. Clay, EJ, and B Schaffer. 1984. Conclusion: Self Awareness in Policy Practice. In Room for Manoeuvre: An Explorafion of Public Policy in Agricuhural and Rural Development, ed. Clay EJ, Schaffer B, 191–193. Cranbury, New Jersey: Heinemann.
12. Cleaver, F. 2005. The Inequality of Social Capital and the Reproduction of Chronic Poverty. World Dev 33 (6): 893–906.
13. Crona, B, and Ö Bodin. 2006. What You Know is Who You Know? Communication Patterns among Resource Users as a Prerequisite for Co-management. Ecol Soc 11 (2): 1–7.
14. Dercon, S. 2002. Income Risk, Coping Strategies, and Safety nets. World Bank Research Observer 17 (2): 141–166.
15. Dercon, S. 2005. Risk, Poverty and Vulnerability in Africa. Journal of African Economics 14 (4): 483–488.
16. Dercon, S. 2006. Vulnerability: A Micro-perspective. In Annual World Bank Conference on Development Economics-Europe: Securing development in a unstable world, ed. Bourguignon F, Pleskovic B, van der Gaag J, 117–145. The World Bank, Washington, D.C.
17. Dercon, S. 2010. Risk, Vulnerability and Human Development: What We Know and What We Need to Know? In Risk, Shocks, and Human development: On the brink, ed. Fuentes-Nieva R, Seck P, 13–35. Basingstoke: Palgrave Macmillan.
18. Dercon, S, J Hoddinott, and T Woldehanna. 2005. Shocks and Consumption in 15 Ethiopian villages, 1999–2004. J Afr Econ 14 (4): 559–585.
19. Edvardsson, IR, D Tingley, AJ Conides, B Drakeford, and D Holm. 2011. Fishermen's risk perception in four European countries. Maritime Studies 10 (1): 139–159.
20. Fafchamps, M. 1999. Rural Poverty, Risk, and Development. Center for the Study of African Economies. Oxford: University of Oxford.
21. Fafchamps, M, and S Lund. 2003. Risk-Sharing Networks in Rural Philippines. J Dev Econ 71 (2): 261–287.
22. Hoddinott, J, and A Quisumbing. 2010. Methods for Microeconometric Risk and Vulnerability Assessment. In Risk,

shocks, and human development: On the brink, ed. Fuentes-Nieva R, Seck P, 62–94. Basingstoke: Palgrave Macmillan.

23. Hoogeveen, J, E Tesliuc, R Vakis, and S Dercon. 2004. A Guide to the Analysis of Risk, Vulnerability and Vulnerable Groups. Social Protection Unit, Human Development Network, The World Bank. http://siteresources.worldbank.org/INTSRM/Publications/20316319/RVA.pdf *webcite*, Accessed November 1, 2009

24. Hoq, ME. 2007. An analysis of Fisheries Exploitation and Management Practices in Sundarbans Mangrove Ecosystem. Bangladesh. Ocean & Coastal Management 50: 411–427.

25. Hossain, N. 2009. Accounts of Crisis: Poor People's Experiences of the Food, Fuel and Financial Crises in Five Countries. Report on a pilot study in Bangladesh, Indonesia, Jamaica, Kenya and Zambia. London: Institute of Development Studies.

26. Hulme, D. 2004. Thinking 'Small' and the Understanding of Poverty: Maymana and Mofizul's story. J Hum Dev 5 (2): 161–176.

27. Islam, MS, and MA Wahab. 2005. A Review on the Present Status and Management of Mangrove Wetland Habitat Resources in Bangladesh with Emphasis on Mangrove Fisheries and Aquaculture. Hydrobiologia 542 (1): 165–190.

28. Jentoft, S, and G Midré. 2011. The Meaning of Poverty: Conceptual Issues in Small-scale Fisheries Research. In Poverty Mosaics: Realities and Prospects in Small-scale Fisheries, ed. Jentoft S, Eide A, 43–68. Dordrecht: Springer.

29. Kazim, H. 2011. The Outcasts: Bangladesh's Tiger Widows Fight Exclusion. Spiegel Online.http://www.spiegel.de/international/world/0 *webcite*,1518,744594,00.html, Accessed October 2, 2011

30. Khuda, ME. 2008. Transparency and Accountability in Forest Conservation and Management: Problems and Way Out. Executive Summary. Dhaka: Transparency International Bangladesh.

31. Kissling, E, EH Allison, JA Seeley, S Russell, M Bechmann, SD Musgrave, and S Heck. 2005. Fisherfolk are Among Those Most at Risk to HIV: A Cross-country Comparison of Estimated

Prevalence and Numbers Infected among Groups at Risk. AIDS 19: 1939–1945.

32. Krishna, A. 2010. One Illness Away. Why People Become Poor and How they Escape Poverty. Oxford: Oxford University Press.
33. LEDARS. 2010. Tiger Widows-A Hidden Issue in the Sundarbans. Tiger Widow Newsletter. http://www.ledars.org/livelihood_security_program.php *webcite*, Accessed October 2, 2011
34. Lewis, D, and AA Hossain. 2008. Tale of Three Villages: Power, Difference and Locality in Rural Bangladesh. Journal of South Asian Development 3 (1): 33–51.
35. 2002. Proceedings of the International Fishing Industry Safety and Health Conference,Lincoln JM, Hudson DS, Conway GA, Pescatore R Woods Hole, Massachusetts: Department of Health and Human Services.
36. Matin, I, and D Hulme. 2003. Programs for the Poorest: Learning from the IGVGD Program in Bangladesh. World Dev 31 (3): 649–667.
37. Mendoza, RU. 2009. Aggregate Shocks, Poor Households and Children: Transmission Channels and Policy Responses. Global Social Policy 9: 55–78.
38. Minnegal, M, and PD Dwyer. 2008. Managing risk, resisting management: stability and diversity in a southern Australian fishing fleet. Hum Organ 67: 97–108.
39. Mitra, M. 2000. The Sundarbans: A Riparian Commons in Search of Management. Eighth Conference of the International Association for the Study of Common Property. IN, USA: Bloomingdale.
40. Morduch, J. 1995. Income and Consumption Smoothing. J Econ Perspect 9 (3): 103–114.
41. Morduch, J. 1999. Between the state and the market: Can informal insurance patch the safety net? The World Bank Research Observer 14 (2): 187–207.
42. Mosley, P, and A Verschoor. 2005. Risk attitudes and the 'Vicious Circle of Poverty'. Eur J Dev Res 17 (1): 59–88.
43. Quisumbing, A, R Meinzen-Dick, and L Bassett. 2008. Helping Women Respond to the Global Food Price Crisis. IFPRI Policy Brief 7. Washington, DC: IFPRI.

44. Rosenzweig, M, and H Binswanger. 1993. Wealth, Weather Risk and the Composition and Profitability of Agricultural Investments. Econ J 103: 56–80.

45. Rouf, MA, and KR Jensen. 2001. Coastal Fisheries Management and Community Livelihood: Possible Strategy for the Sundarbans, Bangladesh. Thailand: ITCZM Monograph No. 04.

46. Salas, S, M Bjørkan, F Bobadilla, and MA Cabrera. 2011. Addressing Vulnerability: Coping Strategies of Fishing Communities in Yucatan, Mexico. In Poverty Mosaics: Realities and Prospects in Small-scale Fisheries, ed. Jentoft S, Eide A, 195–220. Dordrecht: Springer.

47. Santos, VI. 2010. The Effects of Earthquakes on Children and Human Development in Rural El Salvador. In Risk, shocks, and human development: On the brink, ed. Fuentes-Nieva R, Seck P, 1128–1144. Basingstoke: Palgrave Macmillan.

48. Sen, A. 1999. Development as Freedom. Oxford: Oxford University Press.

49. Sinha, S, M Lipton, and S Yaqub. 2002. Poverty and "Damaging Fluctuations": How do they relate? Journal of Asian and African Studies 37 (2): 186–243.

50. Smith, ME. 1998. Fisheries Risk in Modern Context. Maritime Anthropological Studies 1: 29–48.

51. Tai, X, S Li, MW Feldman, GC Daily, and J Li. 2010. Rural Households' Risks Management Strategies and Vulnerability to Poverty in Western Rural China. Montpellier:ISDA. http://www.isda2010.net/var/isda2010/storage/original/application/aeb7d95cb639bb08a017c5d311fc0085.pdf *webcite*, Accessed November 1, 2009

52. Takasaki, Y, BL Barham, and OT Coomes. 2004. Risk Coping Strategies in Tropical Forests: Floods, Illnesses, and Resource Extraction. Environ Dev Econ 9: 203–224.

53. The Royal Society. 1992. Risk: Analysis, Perception and Management. London: The Report of a Royal Society Study Group.

54. Tingley, D, J Asmunsson, E Borodzicz, A Aonides, B Drakeford, IR Eovarosson, D Holm, K Kapiris, S Kuikka, and B Mortensen. 2010. Risk Identification and Perception in the Fisheries Sector:

Comparisons between the Faroes, Greece, Iceland, and UK. Marine Policy 34 (6): 1249–1260.

55. UNDP. 2007. Fighting Climate Change: Human Solidarity in a Divided World, Human Development Report. http://hdr.undp.org/en/media/HDR_20072008_EN_Complete.pdf *webcite*, Accessed November 1, 2009

56. Webb, P, and A Harinarayan. 1999. A Measure of Uncertainty: The Nature of Vulnerability and its Relationship to Malnutrition. Disasters 23 (4): 292–305.

57. WFP (World Food Programme). 2009. Pilot Monitoring of High Food Price Impact at Household Level in Selected Vulnerable Areas. Indonesia: Mimeo.

58. World Bank. 2001. World Development Report 2000/2001: Attacking Poverty. Oxford and New York: Oxford University Press.

chapter 7

The Presence of Microcystins in Fish Cyprinus Carpio Tissues: A Histopathological Study

Amalia Mitsoura[1], Ifigenia Kagalou[13], Nikolaos Papaioannou[2], Panagiotis Berillis[1], Eleni Mente[1], and Theodoti Papadimitriou[12]

[1]Department of Ichthyology and Aquatic Environment, School of Agricultural Sciences, University of Thessaly, Fytoko, Volos, 38446, Greece

[2]Faculty of Veterinary Medicine, Aristotle University of Thessaloniki, Thessaloniki, 54124, Greece

[3]Management Body of Ecodevelopment Area of Karla, Mavrovouni, Kefalovriso, Velestino, 37500, Greece

ABSTRACT

The occurrence of heavy cyanobacterial blooms has become a worldwide problem, as a consequence of eutrophication of the aquatic ecosystems; furthermore, 60% to 75% of these blooms have been found to be toxic. Microcystins (MCYSTs), the predominant toxins of cyanobacterial blooms, are associated with mortality and illness in both animals and humans. Laboratory-controlled experiments studying the effects of different microcystins on the common carp (*Cyprinus carpio*) have revealed various histopathological alterations. The aim of the present study is to investigate the effect of chronic or subchronic exposure of fish to microcystins under natural environmental conditions by examining the possible histopathological changes associated with a dense cyanobacterial bloom and determining the microcystin contents of fish tissues. Common carps (*C. carpio*) were caught from Lake Karla (Greece), during a dense cyanobacterial bloom. The concentration of MCYSTs in the fish liver, kidney and muscle tissues was measured by enzyme-linked immunosorbent assay. The pseudogaster contents were analysed, and a histopathological examination was performed using light and electron microscopy. Severe alterations were detected in the liver and the kidney, suggesting that the toxic effects were caused by various pollutants that were particularly associated with microcystins. The histopathological findings are also discussed, taking into consideration the health conditions of the common carp as a commercial fish species. The mechanisms of expansion of the microcystins and the poisoning of aquatic organisms (e.g. fish) are not yet known in the Lake Karla ecosystem. Future research may focus on identifying the changes caused by microcystins and other factors that exert similar effects on fish tissues, as well as on establishing the overall combined effect of all these factors on fish health.

BACKGROUND

The frequent occurrence of cyanobacterial blooms has been regarded as a serious global public health problem and a major environmental issue. Cyanobacteria can produce several toxic metabolites known as cyanotoxins (Ressom et al. 1994; Blaha et al. 2009). Many species of cyanobacteria produce toxic metabolites, peptides and alkaloids that are a serious threat to the various uses of freshwater lakes and reservoirs. Toxin-producing cyanobacteria that are widely distributed in freshwaters include the planktonic N_2-fixing genera of *Anabaena, Aphanizomenon, Nostoc, Cylindrospermopsis* and the non N_2-fixing genera, such as *Microcystis, Planktothrix* and*Oscillatoria* (Welker et al. 2004). Among these cyanobacteria, microcystins (MCYSTs) are the most abundant group. Exposure to MCYSTs imposes a health risk on aquatic organisms, wild life, domestic animals and humans through ingesting the cyanobacteria present in the water or the food (Duy et al. 2000; Malbrouck and Kestemont 2006).

Fish, a group of organisms that represents one of the main inhabitants of the aquatic systems, are frequently exposed to MCYSTS both directly and passively, leading to their poisoning and/or their subsequent mortality (Carbis et al. 1996; Ernst 2008).

Fish typically either ingest cyanobacteria or prey that has already fed on cyanobacteria (Tencalla et al. 1994; Fisher and Dietrich 2000). To a lesser extent, they can also absorb the toxins directly from the water (Phillips et al. 1985; Smith et al. 2008). Currently, there is a large body of literature describing experimental studies of cyanobacterial toxins in aquatic systems and their acute toxicity effects; however, there are gaps about the toxicological effects of these toxins under field conditions in environmentally relevant concentrations. Although acute toxicity experiments are useful in the study of toxicokinetics and histopathological changes, such experiments do not represent the mode of exposure in a natural environment (Ferrão-Filho and Kozlowsky-Suzuki2011). Because the chronic and subchronic effects in aquatic organisms might be more relevant than the acute lethal effects, studies addressing the exposure of biota in cyanobacteria-rich lakes have attracted substantial attention (Ibelings and Chorus 2007; Ibelings and Havens 2008).

It is well known that one cyano-toxigenic mechanism is the potent inhibition of the protein phosphatases 1 and 2A; this inhibition results in the abrogation of the protein phosphorylation status, which is directly associated with the cytotoxic effects and tumour-promoting activity of cyanotoxins (Carmichael 1994; Hooser 2000). In addition, studies of fish pathology have shown that MCYST exposure can produce histopathological effects in the gills, intestine and heart (Atencio et al. 2008; Jiang et al. 2011). Hepatic tumours and severe hepatic haemorrhages, as well as the disruption of the hepatic cytoskeleton and the subsequent, progressive liver necrosis and apoptosis, have been widely reported in fish (Tencalla et al. 1994; Fischer et al. 2000). The degree of these MCYST-induced effects depends on the exposure route. However, most of the studies on MCYSTs have been performed using an IP injection or an oral uptake as the exposure route.

Cyprinus carpio (common carp) is a widespread species found in various freshwater habitats, including almost all freshwater Greek lakes. The cyano-toxicological effects on the common carp are thought to be quite important given its commercial importance as a product of inland fisheries and aquaculture. Planktivorous fish, such as the carp, intentionally ingest cyanobacteria and, in the process, are also exposed to cyanobacterial metabolites through the aquatic food web (Malbrouck and Kestemont 2006).

Although these species are frequently exposed to cyanotoxins in their natural environment, they are also considered to be among the most tolerant in terms of survival. No evidence exists regarding the sublethal effects of cyanotoxins, including pathological alterations. Studies on endemic fish species in Europe, Australia and USA have shown that fish liver histopathology is a useful biomarker of exposure to various contaminants (Au 2004; Feist et al. 2004).

The primary aim of each of these studies was to identify histological changes in selected target organs of bio-indicator fish species with regard to one or more specific contaminants. Regarding cyanotoxins, in most cases, the liver and renal histological alterations were highly important (Fisher and Dietrich 2000; Molina et al. 2005; Lang et al. 2006 Li et al. 2007a; Gutierrez-Praena et al. 2011).

In this context, the purpose of the present study is to assess the occurrence and distribution of MCYST in the tissues of the fish species *C. carpio*, as well as to evaluate the histopathological alterations under cyanobacteria-rich conditions. The histopathological findings were revealed by light and electron microscopy. To our knowledge, this is the first study evaluating the histopathology of a freshwater biomarker under natural conditions to provide information about the public health issue arising from human consumption.

Lake Karla (Central Greece) is a unique example (in Europe) of a shallow lake ecosystem that was dried in the 1960s and has been reconstructed, establishing a 'new' ecosystem. During the past 2 years of the lake's rehabilitation (2009 to 2011), frequent and extensive cyanobacterial blooms have occurred that were dominated by toxin-producing species (Oikonomou et al. 2012). During the same period, many episodes of fish mortality were also reported. These events have received intense media coverage due to the lake's importance as a major water reservoir in Greece. Fishing is also among the traditional economic activities in the area, and the common carp is considered to be the main commercial fish species.

METHODS

Lake Karla: Limnological Features of the Study Area

Lake Karla occupied the lowest part of the Thessaly plain and was considered to be one of the most important wetlands in Greece until 1962. Surface runoff from the watershed and the floodwaters of the Pinios River (discharging via a constructed ditch) supplied the lake with large quantities of freshwater. In 1962, the lake was completely drained to create more land for agriculture. The reconstructed Lake Karla is located on the lower depression of the Thessaly plain, a region of Central Greece (Figure 1). The lake lies between latitude 39°26′49″ and 39°32′03″ N and longitude 22°46′47″ and 23°51′50″ E and has a surface area of 38 km^2 with a perimeter of 228 km. The hydrological regime of the lake is determined by the inputs (the rainfall on the lake and the tributary inflows) and the outputs (evaporation). The lake has no natural outflow because the constructed tunnel draining into the Pagasitikos bay is currently closed. Considering the present environmental conditions, Papadimitriou et al. (2011) reported on the water chemistry, and an in-depth analysis of the water column and sediment interactions in Lake Karla has also been published by Jouni (2011). Both studies reported on the highly eutrophic conditions of the lake and highlighted its nutrient-rich content and high chlorophyll-a values. Moreover, there was also an evidence of phosphorous mobilisation from the sediment to the water column. In the same period, Oikonomou et al. (2012) confirmed the occurrence and dominance of toxic cyanobacteria species of *Anabaenopsis* and *Planktothrix*, as well as a diverse microbial community indicative of a hypertrophic status.

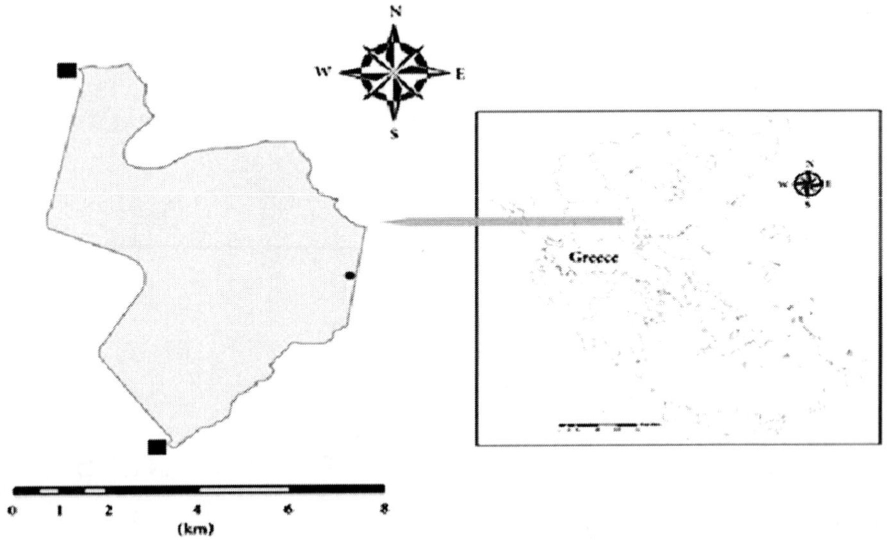

Figure 1: Map of the re-constructed Lake Karla located in the Thessaly region of Central Greece (Oikonomou et al.2012).

Fish Collection and MCYST Detection

Thirty specimens of *C. carpio* with a mean body weight and a mean body length of 1,032 ± 121 g and 30 ± 4.2 cm, respectively, were collected from Lake Karla via two surveys during a period of dense cyanobacterial bloom (May and June 2011) using a trammel net that has a 60-mm inner and 300-mm outer mesh size. Ten *C. carpio* fish were also obtained from a fish farm (Hatchery station of river Louros-Ioannina, Hellenic Ministry of Agriculture) and were used as controls. To extract the toxins from the fish organs, the fish were sacrificed, and the liver, kidney and muscle tissues were excised, weighed and immediately frozen. Subsequently, all of the tissues were homogenised separately, extracted in 100% methanol (Magalhães et al. 2001), stirred overnight at room temperature and then centrifuged at 1,300 g for 15 min using a Universal 32 centrifuge (DJB Labcare Ltd., Buckinghamshire, England, UK). The supernatants were collected and stored overnight at 4°C. A 5-ml aliquot of each supernatant was concentrated under nitrogen stream to 350 µl to remove the organic solvent. A 100-µl aliquot of the concentrated sample extract was diluted with 900 µl of distilled water according to Sipia et al. (2002). The final sample was clarified using membrane filters (pore size of 0.45 μm and diameter of 4 mm). The sample solutions were immediately analysed by enzyme-linked immunosorbent assay (ELISA). For each ELISA assay, the negative control and the four standards were assayed at least in duplicate. The results are expressed in nanogrammes of MCYST-LR equivalents per gramme of fish tissue.

MCYSTs were also measured in the water of Lake Karla. Two forms of MCYSTs were investigated: dissolved in water (extracellular) and cell-bound in seston (intracellular). For the latter, 1,000 mL of water was filtered on a Whatman GF/C filter (Sigma Aldrich, St. Louis, MO, USA) which was immediately frozen at −20°C. MCYSTs were extracted from the filter after placement in 100% methanol and stirring overnight at room temperature followed by centrifugation at 1,300×g for 15 min. This extraction procedure was repeated three times, and the three supernatants were pooled. The organic solvent was removed by placing the extract under nitrogen stream. The remaining concentrated sample was subjected to ELISA. The results are expressed as microgrammes of cellular MCYST-LR equivalents per litre. For analysis of dissolved MCYSTs, the filtered water was applied directly to ELISA. A commercial Abraxis Microcystin ELISA kit was used (Warminster, PA, USA) following the instructions of the manufacturer.

The recovery of the method was determined by analysing the samples before and after the addition of the pure MCYST and then subtracting the concentration of the MCYSTs present in the sample prior to spiking. The matrix effect (i.e. the effect of animal tissue) was checked by spiking the control tissues with the MCYST-LR standard (2 μg/g). The response was compared to that of the 100% methanol spiked with the same amount of the standard.

Microscopic Analyses

Histological samples from the excised tissues, including the liver and the kidney, were subjected to light and electron microscopy. For light microscopy, the samples were initially fixed in a 10% formalin buffer for 24 h at 4°C and were then immediately dehydrated in a graded series of ethanol, immersed in xylene and embedded in paraffin wax using an automatic processor. Sections of 5 to 7 μm were then mounted. After deparaffinisation, the sections were rehydrated, stained with hematoxylin and eosin (Humason 1972) and mounted with Cristal/Mount (Sigma Aldrich, St. Louis, MO, USA). Subsequently, all of the tissues were examined microscopically, and their histological abnormalities were recorded.

For electron microscopy, tissue specimens were prefixed in 2.5% glutaraldehyde diluted in a 0.1-M sodium cacodylate solution for 24 h at 4°C. The specimens were washed in the same buffer before and after fixation. Post-fixation was performed with 1% osmium tetroxide in 0.1-M sodium cacodylate for 2 h at 4°C. The specimens were washed in the same buffer before and after post-fixation and then rinsed in distilled water. Then, the specimens were dehydrated in a graded ethanol series and were subsequently immersed and left overnight in a 1:1 mixture of propylene oxide and the embedding resin. The final step of the embedding took place in capsules containing agar resin. Polymerisation of the resin was completed after 48 h at 60°C. Ultrathin sections (60 to 80 nm) were cut with a Reichert Supernova ultramicrotome (DeKalb, IL, USA). The sections were mounted on a copper grid and stained with uranyl acetate and lead citrate. The tissue sections were examined in a Philips CM10 electron microscope (Amsterdam, The Netherlands).

The common carps are stomachless fish. The short oesophagus connects the posterior pharynx to the anterior part of the intestine, the pseudogaster. Microscopic analysis of the pseudogaster contents was also performed on the examined fish specimens. The pseudogaster was removed from fresh carps, and samples of its contents were collected and kept at 1°C to 5°C until further analysis. Two aliquots of each sample were taken, and one of the aliquots was diluted in distilled water. Dilution was performed in a glass test tube by mixing 330 μl of the sample with 330 μl of distilled water. The non-diluted pseudogaster contents (330 μl) were placed on one end of the slide. The cover slip was placed at a 45° angle on top of the sample to avoid creating air bubbles. Similarly, 330 μl of the diluted pseudogaster contents was placed on the other end of the slide, and optical microscopy images were obtained from both sides of the slides.

Statistics

The data are expressed as the means ± SD. A two-way analysis of variance (ANOVA) was used to compare the means of the MCYSTs contents between the tissues and the sampling periods. The results were considered statistically significant when $P < 0.05$. When the ANOVA results indicated a significant effect, Tukey's multiple comparison test was used to compare the differences between the means. All statistical analyses were performed with SPSS vers. 20.0 for Windows (Chicago, IL, USA).

RESULTS

MCYST in the Fish Tissues and Lake Water

All fish samples of *C. carpio* examined during the present study contained MCYSTs (Table 1). According to the statistical analysis, there were significant differences between the tissues ($n = 20$, $F = 12.53$, $P < 0.05$). However, there were no significant differences in MCYST concentration between the sampling periods ($n = 20$, $F = 0.05$, $P > 0.05$). The highest MCYST concentration was found in the liver (732 ± 350 ng/g), followed by the kidney (362 ± 207 ng/g), while the lowest concentrations were detected in the muscle tissues (114 ± 25 ng/g) (Table 1). During the second survey, in June, the kidney had a higher concentration of MCYST than the liver tissues (696 ± 258 and 346 ± 156 ng/g, respectively); again, the lowest MCYST values were found in the muscle tissues (108 ± 33 ng/l) (Table 1). The examined tissues of the control *C. carpio* individuals contained no MCYSTs when examined by ELISA.

Table 1: MCYST concentrations in *C. carpio* tissues (ng/g), extracellular MCYST(μg/l) and intracellular MCYST (μg/l) in May and June 2011

	May 2011	June 2011
C. carpio liver	732 ± 350	346 ± 156
C. carpio kidney	362 ± 207	696 ± 258
C. carpio muscle	114 ± 25	108 ± 33
Extracellular	2.03 ± 0.32	3.01 ± 0.41
Intracellular	4.19 ± 0.33	5.5 ± 0.29

Values are given as mean ± SD. In all of the control *C. carpio* individuals' examined tissues, there were zero levels of MCYST.

Mitsoura *et al.*

Mitsoura *et al. International Aquatic Research* 2013 5:8 doi:10.1186/2008-6970-5-8

The extracellular MCYST values were 2.03 ± 0.32 μg/l and 3.01 ± 0.41 μg/l for May and June, respectively. The respective intracellular MCYST values were 4.19 ± 0.33 μg/l and 5.5 ± 0.29 μg/l (Table 1) for the same time periods as above.

The recovery of MCYST that we obtained from the spiked samples was 77 ± 2.5% for liver, 73 ± 3.2% for kidney and 72.6 ± 2.12% for muscle. The matrix effect was negligible (from 0.08% to 5.2% of the differences between the matrix and the methanol results, with an average of 1.9 ± 0.7%).

Mortality and Macroscopic Observations

No fish mortalities were observed during the studied period, and the appearance of the examined organisms was macroscopically normal. All of the examined samples (100%) of the fish pseudogaster contents contained various cyanobacterial species, with the dominant species being *Microcystis aeruginosa* and *Planktothrix agarrdii* (Figure 2). While examining the test organs, macroscopic lesions were observed in the liver and the kidney. Morphological changes included liver discoloration and brittleness, as well as ecchymoses and petechiae (Figure 3). The kidney appeared brittle and normal in colour. Neither the organ displayed appeared enlarged. No pathological changes were observed in the control samples.

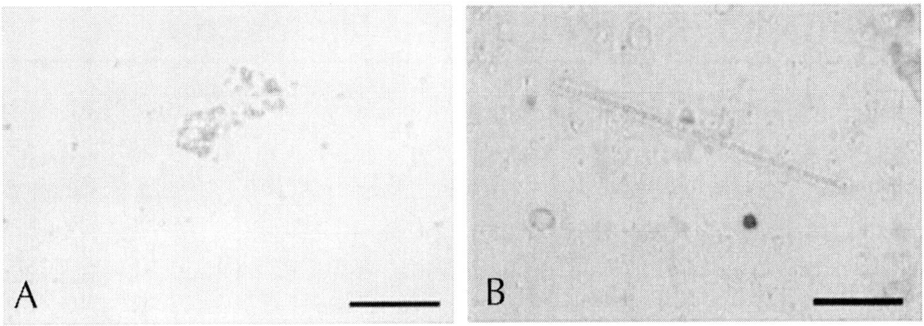

Figure 2: Microscopic examination of *Cyprinus carpio* stomachic contents. (A) *Microcystis aeruginosa* and (B) *Planktothrix agarrdii*. Bar = 25 μm.

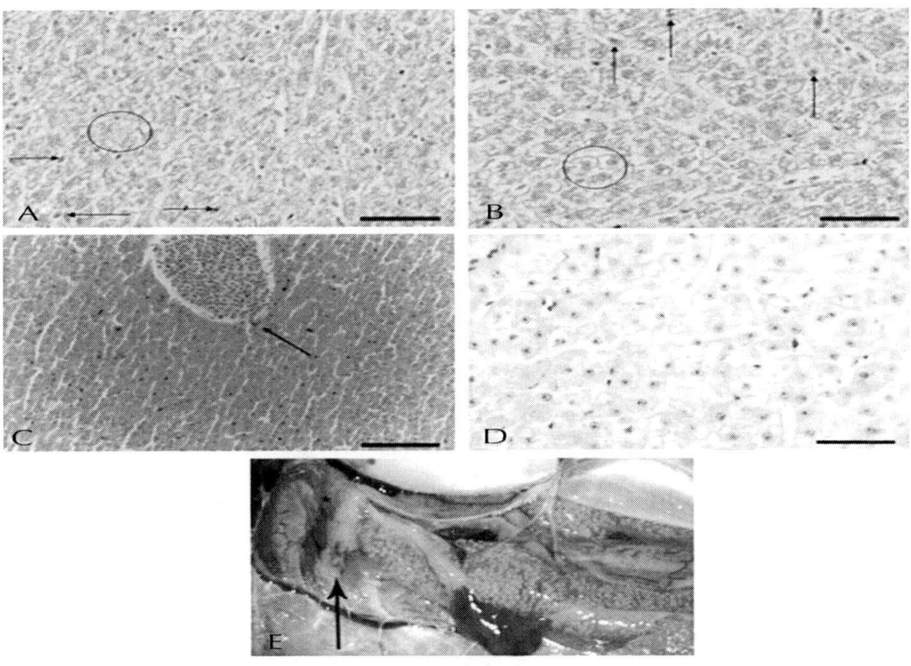

Figure 3: *Cyprinus caprio* liver. (A) Hydropic degeneration, granular glycogen (circle) and sporadic haemorrhagic symptoms (arrows). (B) Onion-like cells (circle) and sporadic haemorrhagic symptoms (arrows). (C) Capillary fracture (arrow). (D) Control, there are no histopathological degenerations. Bar=62.5 μm. (E) Macroscopic degenerations of the liver. Discoloration (arrow) and petechiaes (star) were observed.

Histopathology under Light Microscopy

Histopathological changes were observed in the liver and the kidney of the fish specimens in comparison with the control ones. However, no differences were observed among the sampling surveys. Histopathological lesions were detected in the liver and the kidney and were characterised by hydropic degeneration and necrosis. Pathological changes in the fish liver included loss of the architecture structure, onion-like cells, focal necrosis, granular glycogen, nuclei pyknosis (Figure 3) and sporadic haemorrhagic symptoms. The kidney pathology was characterised by the degeneration of the renal tubule, glomerulopathy, glomerular atrophy and a dilated Bowman's capsule (Figure 4). No pathological changes were observed in the muscles.

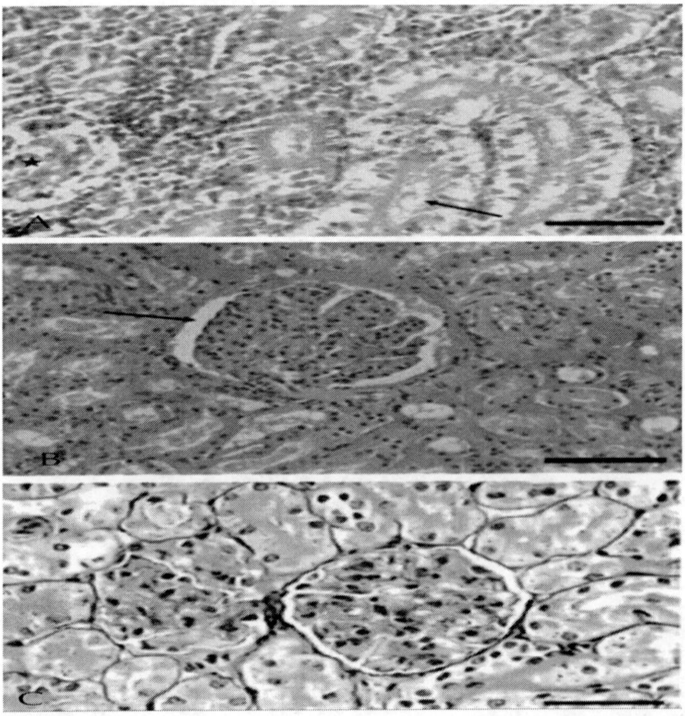

Figure 4: *Cyprinus carpio* kidney. (A) Degeneration of the renal tubular (arrow) and glomerular atrophy (star). Bar = 62.5 μm. (B) Glomerulopathy and dilation of Bowman›s capsule (arrow). (C) Control, there are no histopathological degenerations. Bar = 43.48 μm.

Ultrastructural Histopathological Observations

Histopathological alterations were observed in the liver and the kidney of all fish samples except for the control ones. Both organs appeared swollen, with a loss of the parenchymal architecture. An apparent lysis of the membranes of the hepatic cells resulting in necrotic cells was observed, along with vacuolisation and the presence of lipid droplets. The fragmentation of the nuclear envelope, the swelling of mitochondria, the fragmentation and vesicularisation of the endomembrane system, the pyknosis of nuclei and karyorrhexis were also observed in the liver (Figure 5). Nuclei pyknosis, nuclear envelope fragmentation and proliferation of the lysosomes were observed in the kidney (Figure 6).

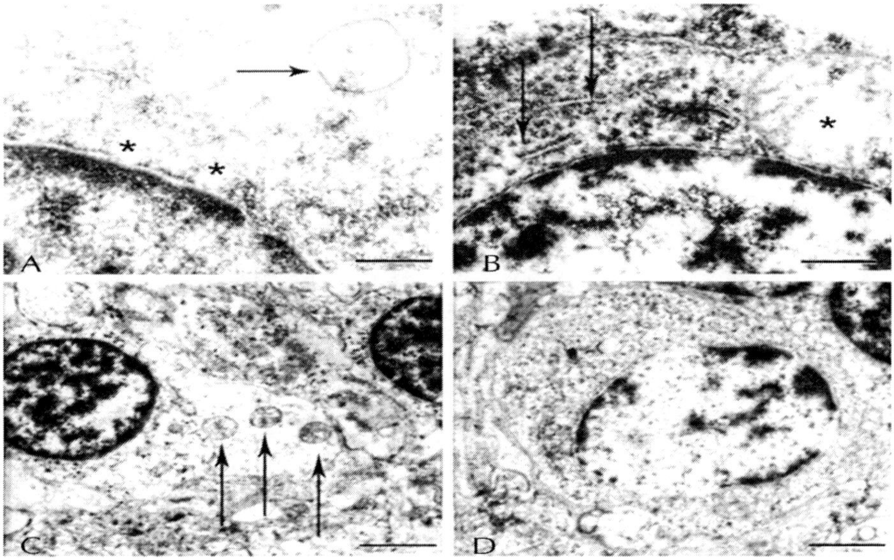

Figure 5: Ultrastructural observation of *Cyprinus carpio*'s liver tissue. (A) Nuclear envelop fragmentation (stars) and a swelling mitochondrion (arrow). Bar = 0.37 µm. (B) Fragmentation of endoplasmic reticulum (arrows) and mitochondria internal membrane system (star). Bar = 0.60 µm. (C) Lysis of the hepatic cell›s plasma membrane. Mitochondria (arrows) in the extracellular space. Bar = 1.74 µm. (D) Karyorrhexis. Bar = 1.74 µm.

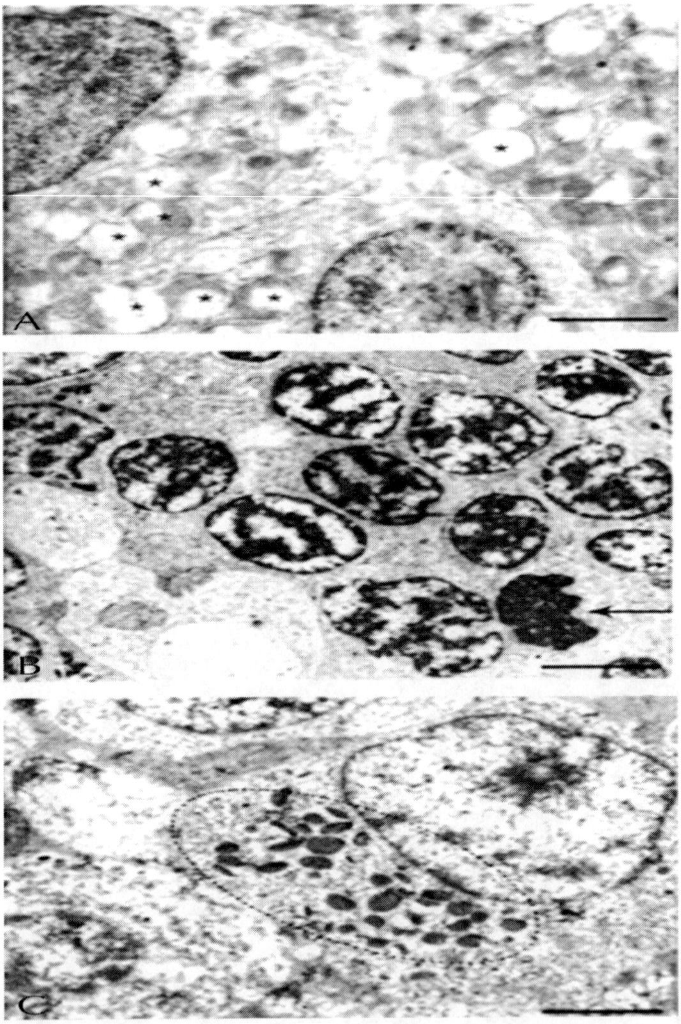

Figure 6: Ultrastructural observation of *Cyprinus carpio*'s kidney tissue. (A) Lipid droplets (stars) are present. Bar = 1.74 μm. (B) Pyknotic nuclei (arrow). Bar = 3.33 μm. (C) Proliferation of lysosomes in the cell (circle). Bar = 1.74 μm.

DISCUSSION

The only study before Lake Karla dried out was by Ananiadis (1956). He reported signs of eutrophication and occurrence of few cyanobacterial species. Our data concerning lake water, suggest that the reconstructed Lake Karla is experiencing the occurrence of significant MCYST concentrations. Papadimitriou et al. (2011) previously reported the presence of MCYST concentrations in Lake Karla ranging between 0.75 and 3.90 μg/l, while Oikonomou et al. (2012) and Papadimitriou et al. (2013) confirmed the occurrence of the toxic cyanobacterial species of*Anabaenopsis, Planktothrix and Microcystis* in Lake Karla. The above cyanobacterial species found in Lake Karla have been shown to produce a variety of toxins and alkaloids with toxic activity in many lakes worldwide (Sivonen and Jones 1999; Sabour et al. 2005; Kurmayer et al. 2005; Hisem2008). MCYST concentrations (intracellular and extracellular) found in Lake Karla are similar to those reported for other Mediterranean lakes in Turkey (Albay et al. 2003) and in Portugal (Vasconcelos et al. 1996), but generally, lower to those of the temperate lakes in Canada (Kotak et al. 1996) or in Finnish lakes (Lindholm et al. 2003) and also lower than those reported for Brazil lagoons (Magalhães et al. 2001). Extracellular and intracellular MCYST concentrations found in Lake Karla are comparable to those found in another shallow lake in Greece, Lake Pamvotis (Papadimitriou et al. 2012a). It is worth noting that the comparable MCYST concentrations found in Lake Pamvotis, were associated with the bioaccumulation of MCYST in tissues of aquatic organisms (Papadimitriou et al. 2012a).

Studies addressing the chronic effects resulting from the exposure of cyprinids to sublethal concentrations of MCYSTs are quite limited. Our study focuses on the histopathological alterations observed in the *C. carpio* species found in the eutrophic Lake Karla, thus addressing the effects of the environmentally relevant MCYST concentrations. This study revealed that tissues from all fish samples caught during the sampling surveys contained MCYSTs. This result suggests that the MCYST content in the aquatic environment was adequate to promote MCYST accumulation in the exposed fish. It is well documented that the primary target organ for MCYST accumulation is the liver (Ernst et al. 2006; Papadimitriou et al. 2012a; Moutou et al. 2012), whereas muscle usually presents the lowest MCYST content. The preferential accumulation in the liver may be attributable to the high density of the organic anionic transporters on the surface of hepatocytes, while the process known as presystematic hepatic elimination could prevent or at least minimise the distribution of MCYSTs to other parts of the body (Fischer et al. 2005). However, there is also an evidence that the carp's kidney is the first organ to be affected by MCYST in terms of pathological changes (Fisher and Dietrich 2000). MCYSTs produced by cyanobacteria in an aquatic environment have been shown to exert adverse effects on fish. Fish are exposed to MCYSTs directly during feeding and/or passively through their continuous contact with their aquatic environment; cyanobacterial metabolites are known to be transported by the aquatic food web (Xie et al. 2004; Smith et al. 2008). Cyanotoxicity can result in two types of structural changes. One is the direct toxic effect of the pollutant, which leads to tissue degeneration and necrosis, and the other is the development of compensatory mechanisms, such as cellular hyperplasia, to address the stressor (Li et al. 2007b). The histopathological changes observed in tissues are the result of histological-level reactions of the fish; thus, histopathology represents a useful tool to assess the degree of toxicity.

According to Palikova et al. (2011), cyanobacteria are regular components of the cyprinid diet, and it appears that *M. aeruginosa* comprises a significant portion of the carp diet when a bloom formation occurs (Carbis et al. 1997). Nevertheless, carps are not able to avoid the ingestion of toxic cyanobacteria and their toxins in eutrophicated lakes (Tencalla et al. 1994). *M. aeruginosa*and *P. agarrdii* found in the pseudogasters of the examined fish were also found in the water of Lake Karla according to the studies of Papadimitriou et al. (2013). This confirms the direct exposure of fish originated from Lake Karla to cyanobacteria and to MCYSTs through feeding. Many previous studies have demonstrated the acute toxicological effects induced by MCYSTs in fish using carps as bioassay models. Laboratory-controlled experiments using different MCYSTs, doses and routes of administration in the common carp (*C. carpio*) have shown severe histopathological effects (Rabergh et al. 1991; Fisher and Dietrich 2000; Jiang et al. 2011). Jiang et al. (2011) exposed *C. carpio* individuals to 10 µg/l MC-LR for 14 days, and the results included some liver histopathological changes, such as slight swelling of hepatic cells and partially dissolved parenchymal architecture characterised by vacuolar degeneration with damage of the nuclei (pyknosis, karyolysis). Although the dose of 10 µg/l MC-LR is higher than the MCYST concentrations found in Lake Karla, the histopathological observation found in common carps from Lake Karla are similar. This may be explained by the effect of chronic or subchronic exposure of fish to cyanobacterial blooms containing MCYSTs. Our histopathological observations seem to be in agreement with previous reports concerning cyanobacterial toxicity (Carbis et al.

1996; Fisher and Dietrich 2000; Malbrouck and Kestemont2006; Qui et al. 2007; Jiang et al. 2011). Concerning the liver histopathology, the fish exhibited hydropic degeneration and necrosis, in agreement with the findings reported by Rabergh et al. (1991), Snyder et al. (2002), Sugaya et al. (1990), Tencalla et al. (1994), Fisher and Dietrich (2000) and Liu et al. (2002). In contrast to mammals, only a few studies have demonstrated haemorrhagic effects due to cyanobacteria and MCYSTs in fish (Tencala and Dietrich 1997; Tencalla et al. 1994; Jiang et al. 2011). Kidney alterations included degeneration of the renal tubule, glomerulopathy and dilation of Bowman›s capsule. According to Carbis et al. (1996), Fischer and Dietrich (2000) and Kotak et al. (1996), the MCYST-induced renal pathology appears to be generally restricted to the proxima in the posterior part of the kidney. Our results seem to confirm these previously published findings.

Very few *in vivo* studies have been performed regarding the toxic effects of MCYSTs on the ultrastructures of the hepatocytes in the fish, and very little knowledge is available about the kidney's ultrastucture histopathology (Li et al. 2001; Atencio et al. 2008; Trinchet et al. 2011). Our main histological findings were loss of the parenchymal architecture, hepatocyte necrosis with vacuolisation of the cytoplasm and the presence of lipid droplets. Vacuolisation has been reported in isolated hepatocytes from the common carp (Li et al. 2001) after oral exposure to MCYSTs. According to Atencio et al. (2008) and Molina et al. (2005), vacuolisation might indicate an imbalance between the rate of synthesis of substances in the parenchymal cells and the rate of release of these substances into the systemic circulation. Atencio et al. (2008) have observed glomerulopathy with thickening of the basal membrane, an increased number of lysosomes in the proxima tubules and generalised vacuolisation. We also found degenerations that were mainly associated with the irregularity of the endomembrane system, the swelling of mitochondria and the fragmentation of the mitochondria internal membrane system; these findings are more or less consistent with the observations made by Carbis et al. (1996) after exposing common carps to the MCYST.

It is important to note that the cyanobacterial bloom usually contains many different toxins that have been found to be more toxic than the individually purified component toxin(s) (Ibelings and Chorus 2007). Thus, our histopathological observations provide information on a natural model of disease based on the synergies between the toxicity of the various toxins and the other factors, rather than on the quantities of the individual compounds. Moutou et al. (2012) studied the response of the oxidative system in the same fish species under MCYST-rich conditions. They reported that under natural conditions, the response of the GSH/GSSH system and the catalase activity may also depend on other factors besides continuous exposure.

Lang et al. (2006) suggested a categorisation system for the diagnosis of liver histological alterations in terms of the toxicological relevance of these alterations based on the findings in flatfish species. Recently, van Dyk et al. (2011) have applied this system to evaluate pollution-related histopathological changes in the catfish. These categories include non-specific lesions, early toxicopathic non-neoplastic lesions, pre-neoplastic lesions and neoplasms. The alterations listed within each of these categories are widely accepted as useful indicators for monitoring the biological effects of contaminants on fish (Feist et al. 2004). Using the proposed categories as guidelines, it is clear that many of these alterations were also observed in *C. carpio* during the present study, such as early toxicopathic, non-neoplastic lesions, including hepatocellular necrosis, nuclei pyknosis, vacuolisation and steatosis.

In conclusion, common carps from Lake Karla that were exposed to a cyanobacterial bloom contained high amounts of MCYSTs in the examined tissues. Regarding the risk that MCYST toxicity poses to public health, the World Health Organization (World Health Organization 1998) proposes 0.04 μg MC-LR equivalent/kg per day as the tolerable daily intake for MCYSTs. The estimated daily intake for *C. carpio* samples from Lake Karla exhibited MCYST amounts above the WHO guideline (World Health Organization 1998); thus, there might be potential harmful effects on human health from the lifelong consumption of contaminated fish that cannot be overlooked.

In general, our results confirmed the hypothesis that chronic exposure to a cyanobacteria-rich environment and, thus, to MCYST can lead to pathological changes in the exposed carps. The potential ecological risk for the species *C. carpio*, which always dominates eutrophic, hypertrophic lakes and reservoirs, is also demonstrated. However, because MCYSTs almost never occur in nature as single species but rather occur as a mixture of toxins, the present toxicological profile could obviously be the result of multiple cyanotoxins that were present in the lake water and exerted a synergistic effect on the health of *C.*

carpio. In our study, fish were collected during the spring and the early summer; therefore, it is unlikely that the histopathological differences identified would be related to the seasonal variations. Furthermore, we did not estimate the fish age, but all fish samples were of similar body size; thus, it is likely that all fish were of the same age class. However, taking into consideration the different accumulation rates in the different age classes (Papadimitriou et al. 2012b), there is a need for further research regarding the factors, such as seasonal variation and fish age, when histopathological observations are evaluated. Given the number of contradictory results regarding the effects of cyanotoxins in various biomarker studies, histopathological observations could be quite sensitive biomarkers that reflect the cyanotoxicity effects at the cellular level. The results of the current study may contribute to supporting the cause-effect relationship between fish pathology and the pollution levels in the freshwater environment.

Finally, studies about the effects of cyanobacteria and the accumulation of their toxins in the Mediterranean region are of great importance, as the incidence and persistence of toxic blooms in this region are greater than those observed in temperate regions. Monitoring programmes, specifically at environmentally sensitive sites such as the protected Lake Karla, should include the establishment of baseline histopathological data for the endemic and bio-indicator fish species of the region.

CONCLUSIONS

The results of the present study contribute to our knowledge on the accumulation of microcystins in fish tissues under algal bloom rich conditions. Carps from Lake Karla that were exposed to a cyanobacterial bloom contained high amounts of MCYSTs in the examined tissues appearing also histopathological changes.

Our results also confirmed that the liver accumulated the highest MCYST concentrations, while the lowest concentrations were detected in the muscle tissues. Histopathological findings could serve as sensitive signals concerning cyanotoxicity. In terms of public health the consumption of carps as lifelong dietary items might cause harmful effects on human health.

AUTHORS' CONTRIBUTIONS

AM was responsible for the sampling, analysis and laboratory handling. IK deployed the research protocol, contributed to the analysis of the data, discussion, writing, and reviewing. NP was responsible for the histopathological observations with the optical microscope and contributed in results evaluation. PB was responsible for electron microscopy and ultrastructural histopathological diagnosis, contributed to the data analysis, discussion, writing, and reviewing. EM was responsible for the fish sampling, contributed in analysing the data, discussion of the results, writing and editing. TP made the MCYST detection, contributed to sampling, statistical analysis, discussion, writing and reviewing. All authors read and approved the final manuscript.

ACKNOWLEDGEMENTS

Laboratory work was partially financed by the postgraduate taught degree programme 'Sustainable Management of Aquatic Environment' by the Department of Ichthyology and Aquatic Environment, University of Thessaly.

REFERENCES

1. Albay M, Akcaalan R, Tufekci H, Metcalf J, Beattie K, Codd G (2003) Depth profiles of cyanobacterial hepatotoxins (microcystins) in three Turkish freshwater lakes. Hydrobiologia 505:89–95
2. Ananiadis CI (1956) Limnological study of Lake Karla. Bull Inst Oceanogr 1083:1–19
3. Atencio L, Moreno I, Jos A, Pichardo S, Moyano R, Blanco A, Camean A (2008) Dose-dependent antioxidant responses and pathological changes in tenca (*Tinca tinca*) after acute oral exposure to Microcystis under laboratory conditions. Toxicon. 52:1–12
4. Au D (2004) The application of histo-cytopathological biomarkers in marine pollution monitoring: a review. Mar Pollut Bull. 48:817–834

5. Blaha L, Babica P, Maršálek B (2009) Toxins produced in cyanobacterial water blooms – toxicity and risks. Interdiscip Toxicol. 2(2):36–41

6. Carbis CR, Mitchell GF, Anderson JW, McCauley I (1996) The effects of microcystins on the serum biochemistry of carp, *Cyprinus carpio* L, when the toxins are administered by gavage, immersion and intraperitoneal routes. J Fish Dis. 19:151–159

7. Carbis CR, Rawlin GT, Grant P, Mitchell GF, Anderson JW, McCauley I (1997) A study of feral carp,*Cyprinus carpio* L., exposed to Microcystis aeruginosa at Lake Mokoan, Australia, and possible implications for fish health. J Fish Dis. 20:81–91

8. Carmichael WW (1994) The toxins of cyanobacteria. Sci Am. 270:78–86

9. Duy TN, Lam PK, Shaw GR, Connell DW (2000) Toxicology and risk assessment of freshwater cyanobacterial (blue-green algal) toxins in water. Rev Environ Contam Toxicol. 163:113–186

10. Ernst B (2008) Investigations of the impact of toxic cyanobacteria on fish Dissertation, University of Kostanz

11. Ernst B, Hoeger SJ, O'Brien E, Dietrich DR (2006) Oral toxicity of the microcystin containing cyanobacterium *Planktothrix rubescens* in European whitefish (*Coregonus lavaretus*). Aquat Toxicol. 79:31–40

12. Feist SW, Lang T, Stentiford GD, Kohler A (2004) Biological effects of contaminants: use of liver pathology of the European flatfish dab (*Limanda limanda* L.) and flounder (*Platichthys flesus* L.) for monitoring. 38: Copenhagen: ICES, p 42

13. Ferra˜o-Filho AS, Kozlowsky-Suzuki B (2011) Cyanotoxins: bioaccumulation and effects on aquatic animals. Mar Drugs. 9:2729–2772

14. Fischer WJ, Hitzfeld BC, Tencalla F, Eriksson JE, Mikhailov A, Dietrich DR (2000) Microcystin-LR toxicodynamics, induced pathology, and immunohistochemical localization in livers of blue-green algae exposed rainbow trout (*Oncorhynchus mykiss*). Toxicol Sci. 54:365–373

15. Fischer WJ, Altheimer S, Cattori V, Meier PJ, Dietrich DR, Hagenbuch B (2005) Organic anion transporting polypeptides

expressed in liver and brain mediate uptake of microcystin. Toxicol Appl Pharmacol. 203:257–263

16. Fisher W, Dietrich D (2000) Pathological and biochemical characterization of 4 MC-induced hepatopancreas and kidney damage in carp (*Cyprinus carpio*). Toxicol Appl Pharmacol. 164:73–81
17. Gutierrez-Praena D, Pichardo S, Jos A, Camean AM (2011) Toxicity and glutathione implication in the effects observed by exposure of the liver fish cell line PLHC- 1 to pure cylindrospermopsin. Ecotoxicol Environ Saf. 74:1567–1572
18. Hisem D (2008) Toxicity of Heterocytous Cyanobacteria to Model Invertebrate Artemia salina. Is the toxicity to invertebrate specific and environmentally depended? Bachelor Thesis, Faculty of Science, The University of South Bohemia
19. Hooser SB (2000) Fulminant hepatocyte apoptosis in vivo following microcystin LR administration to rats. Toxicol Pathol. 28:726–733
20. Humason GL (1972) Animal tissue techniques San Francisco: W.H. Freeman and Company
21. Ibelings B, Chorus I (2007) Accumulation of cyanobacterial toxins in freshwater "seafood" and its consequences for public health: a review. Environ Pollut. 150:177–192
22. Ibelings B, Havens KE (2008) Cyanobacterial toxins: a qualitative meta-analysis of concentrations, dosage and effects in freshwater, estuarine and marine biota. Adv Exp Med Biol. 619:675–732
23. Jiang JL, Gu XY, Song R, Zhang Q, Geng JJ, Wang XY, Yang LY (2011) Time- dependent oxidative stress and histopathological alterations in *Cyprinus carpio* L. exposed to microcystin-LR. Ecotoxicology. 20:1000–1009
24. Jouni S (2011) Current trophic status of Lake Karla, Greece, and proposal for remediations Dissertation, University of Edinburgh
25. Kotak BJ, Semalulu S, Friytz DL, Prepas EE, Hrudey SE, Coppock RW (1996) Hepatic and renal pathology of intraperitoneally administered microcystin-LR in rainbow trout (*Oncorhynchus mykiss*). Toxicon. 34:517–525
26. Kurmayer R, Christiansen G, Gumpenberger M, Fastner J (2005) Genetic identification of microcystin ecotypes in

toxic cyanobacteria of the genus Planktothrix. Microbiology 2005(151):1525–1533

27. Lang T, Wosniok W, Barsiene J, Broeg K, Kopecka J, Parkoonen J (2006) Liver histopathology in Baltic flounder (*Platichthys flesus*) as indicator of biological effects of contaminants. Mar Pollut Bull. 53:488–496
28. Li X, Liu YD, Song LR (2001) Cytological alterations in isolated hepatocytes from common carp (*Cyprinus carpio* L.) exposed to microcystin-LR. Environ Toxicol. 16:517–522
29. Li L, Xie P, Li S, Qiu T, Guo L (2007) Sequential ultrastructural and biochemical changes induced in vivo by the hepatotoxic microcystins in liver of the phytoplanktivorous silver carp*Hypophthalmichthys molitrix*. Comp Biochem Phys C. 146:357–367
30. Li S, Xie P, Li L, Liang G, Zheng L (2007) Tissue distribution of microcystins in bighead carp via interaperitoneal injection. Bull Environ Contamin Toxicol. 79:297–300
31. Lindholm T, Vesterkvist P, Spoof L, Lundbergniinisto C, Meriluoto J (2003) Microcystin occurrence in lakes in Åland, SW Finland. Hydrobiologia 505:129–138
32. Liu Y, Song L, Li X (2002) The toxic effects of microcystin LR on embryo-larval and juvenile development of Loach, *Misgurnus mizolopis*. Toxicon. 40:395–399
33. Magalhães VF, Soares R, Azevedo S (2001) Microcystin contamination in fish from the Jacarepagua Â Lagoon (Rio de Janeiro, Brazil): ecological implication and human health risk. Toxicon. 39:1077–1085
34. Malbrouck C, Kestemont P (2006) Effects of microcystins on fish. Environ Toxicol Chem. 25:72–86
35. Molina R, Moreno I, Pichardo S, Jos A, Moyano R, Monterde JG, Camean A (2005) Acid and alkaline phosphatase activities and pathological changes induced in Tilapia fish (*Oreochromis* sp.) exposed subchronically to microcystins from toxic cyanobacterial blooms under laboratory conditions. Toxicon. 46:725–735
36. Moutou K, Tsikogias S, Papadimitriou T, Kagalou I (2012) Oxidative stress in *Cyprinus carpio* to analyze microcystin impact

in eutrophic shallow lakes: a preliminary study. J Environ Monit. 14(8):2195–2203

37. Oikonomou A, Katsiapi M, Karayanni H, Moustaka-Gouni M, Kormas K (2012) Plankton microorganisms coinciding with two consecutive mass fish kills in a newly reconstructed lake. Sci World J. 504135:
38. Palikova M, Mares J, Kopp R, Hlavkova J, Navratil S, Adamovsky O, Chmelar L, Blaha L (2011) Accumulation of microcystins in Nile Tilapia, *Orechromis niloticus* L., and effects of a complex cyanobacterial bloom on the dietetic quality of muscles. Bull Environ Contamin Toxicol. 87:26–30
39. Papadimitriou T, Stampouli Z, Kagalou I (2011) Preliminary results on the cyanotoxicity in the "new" Lake Karla (Thessaly-Greece). In: Proceedings of the 12th international conference on environmental science and technology. Rhodes Island. pp 1416–1423 8-10 Sept
40. Papadimitriou T, Kagalou I, Stalikas C, Pilidis G, Leonardos I (2012) Assessment of microcystins distribution and biomagnification in tissues of the aquatic food web compartments from a shallow lake and potential risks for public health. Ecotoxicology. 21(4):1155–1166
41. Papadimitriou T, Kagalou I, Leonardos I (2012) Seasonally accumulation of microcystins in the various tissues of an endemic and protected fish species (*Rutilus panosi*) with different sizes. Clean-Soil Air Water. 40(4):402–407
42. Papadimitriou T, Katsiapi M, Kormas KA, Moustaka-Gouni M, I K (2013) Artificially-born "killer" lake: phytoplankton based water quality and microcystin affected fish in a reconstructed lake. Sci Total Environ. 452–453:116–124
43. Phillips MJ, Roberts RJ, Stewart JA, Codd GA (1985) The toxicity of the cyanobacterium *Microcystis aeruginosa* to rainbow trout, *Salmo gairdneri* Richardson. J Fish Dis. 8:339–344
44. Qui T, Xie P, Ke Z, Li L, Guo L (2007) In situ studies on physiological and biochemical responses of four fishes with different trophic levels to toxic cyanobacterial blooms in a large Chinese lake. Toxicon. 50:365–376

45. Rabergh CM, Bylund G, Eriksson JE (1991) Histopathological effects of microcystin- LR, a cyclic peptide toxin from the cyanobacterium (blue-green alga) *Microcystis aeruginosa*, on common carp (*Cyprinus carpio* L.). Aquat Toxicol. 20(3):131–146
46. Ressom R, Soong FS, Fitzgerald J, Turczynowicz L, El Saadi O, Roder D, Maynard T, Falconer IR (1994) Health effects of toxic cyanobacteria (blue-green algae) Canberra: National Health and Medical Council, Australian Government Publishing Service
47. Sabour B, Loudiki M, Oudra B, Vasconcelos V, Oubraim S, Fawzi B (2005) Dynamics and toxicity of*Anabaena aphanizomenoides* (cyanobacteria) waterblooms in the shallow brackish Oued Mellah (Morocco). Aquat Ecosyst Health Manage. 8:95–104
48. Sipia V, Lahti K, Kankaanpaa H, Vuorinen P, Meriluoto J (2002) Screening for cyanobacterial hepatotoxins in herring and salmon from the Baltic Sea. Aquat Ecosyst Health Manage. 5(4):451–456 Sivonen K, Jones G (1999) Cyanobacterial toxins. In: Chorus I, Bartram J (ed) Toxic Cyanobacteria in Water, London: E & FN Spon, WHO
49. Smith JL, Boyer GL, Zimba PV (2008) A review of cyanobacterial odours and bioactive metabolites: impacts and management alternatives in aquaculture. Aquaculture. 280:5–20
50. Snyder GS, Goodwin AE, Freeman DW (2002) Evidence that channel catfish, *Ictalurus punctatus*(Rafinesque), mortality is not linked to ingestion of the hepatotoxin microcystin-LR. J Fish Dis. 25:275–285
51. Sugaya Y, Yasuno M, Yanai T (1990) Effects of toxic *Microcystis viridis* and isolated toxins on goldfish. Jpn J Limnology. 51:149–153
52. Tencala F, Dietrich D (1997) Biochemical characterization of microcystin toxicity in rainbow trout (*Oncorhynchus mykiss*). Toxicon. 35(4):583–595
53. Tencalla F, Dietrich D, Schlatter C (1994) Toxicity of *Microcystis aeruginosa* peptide toxin to yearling rainbow trout (*Oncorhynchus mykiss*). Aquat Toxicol. 30:215–224
54. Trinchet I, Djediat C, Huet H, Dao S, Edery M (2011) Pathological modifications following sub-chronic exposure of medaka fish (*Oryzias latipes*) to microcystin-LR. Reprod Toxicol. 32:329–340

55. van Dyk J, Cochrane M, Wagenaar G (2011) Liver histopathology of the sharptooth catfish *Clarias gariepinus* as a biomarker of aquatic pollution. Chemosphere. 87(4):304–311
56. VasconcelosV, Sivonen K, EvansWR, CarmichaelWW, Namikoshi M (1996) Hepatotoxic microcystin diversity in cyanobacterial blooms collected in Portuguese freshwaters. Water Res. 30:2377–2384
57. Welker M, Brunke M, Preussel K, Lippert I, von D¨ohren H (2004) Diversity and distribution of*Microcystis* (Cyanobacteria) oligopeptide chemotypes from natural communities studied by single colony mass spectrometry. Microbiology. 150:1785–1796
58. World Health Organization (WHO) (1998) Cyanobacterial toxins: microcystin-LR. In: Guidelines for drinking water quality 2: Geneva: World Health Organization. pp 95–110 Addendum to
59. Xie LQ, Xie P, Ozawa K, Honma T, Yokoyama A, Park HD (2004) Dynamics of microcystins-LR and -RR in the phytoplanktivorous silver carp in a sub-chronic toxicity experiment. Environ Pollut. 127:431–439

Chapter 8

Cultural and Health Implications of Fish Advisories in a Native American Community

Elizabeth Hoover

American Studies and Ethnic Studies, Brown University, Box 1886, Providence, RI 02860, USA

ABSTRACT

Introduction

Fish advisories are issued in an effort to protect human health from exposure to contaminants, but Native American communities may suffer unintended health, social, and cultural consequences as a result of warnings against eating local fish. This paper focuses on the Mohawk community of Akwesasne, which lies downstream from a Superfund site, and explores how fish advisories have impacted fish consumption and health.

Methods

65 Akwesasne community members were interviewed between March 2008 and April 2009. Interviews were semi-structured, lasted from 30–90 minutes and consisted of open-ended questions about the impacts of environmental contamination on the community. Detailed field notes were also maintained during extensive visits between 2007–2011. Interviews were transcribed, and these transcripts as well as the field notes were analyzed in NVivo 8.0. This research received approval from the Akwesasne Task Force on the Environment Research Advisory Committee, as well as the Brown University Institutional Review Board.

Results

Three-quarters of the 50 Akwesasne Mohawks interviewed have ceased or significantly curtailed their local fish consumption due to the issuance of fish advisories or witnessing or hearing about deformities on fish. Many of these respondents have turned to outside sources of fish, from other communities or from grocery stores. This change in fish consumption concerns many residents because cultural and social connections developed around fishing are being lost and because fish has been replaced with high-fat high-carb processed foods, which has led to other health complications. One-quarter of the 50 interviewees still eat local fish, but these are generally middle-aged or older residents; fish consumption no longer occurs in the multi-generational social context it once did.

Conclusions

Human health in Native American communities such as Akwesasne is intimately tied to the health of the environment. Fish advisories should not be used as an institutional control to protect humans from exposure to contaminants; if Akwesasne are to achieve optimal health, the contaminated environment has to be remediated to a level that supports clean, edible fish.

INTRODUCTION

We turn our minds to all the Fish life in the water. They were instructed to cleanse and purify the water. They also give themselves to us as food. We are grateful that we can still find pure water. So, we turn now to the Fish and send our greetings and thanks.

Now our minds are one.

--Haudenosaunee Thanksgiving Address (Patterson 1999)

For traditional Haudenosaunee (also known as Iroquois) people, the *Ohenton Kariwatehkwen* or "Thanksgiving Address" is recited at the opening and closing of important events, as a reminder of essential elements to be collectively thankful for. The translated excerpt above highlights the importance of fish, which historically were an important source of food for many Haudenosaunee nations, including the Mohawk.[a] In communities such as Akwesasne, the relationship between fish—whose duty it is to cleanse the water and offer themselves as food—and humans—whose role it is to respectfully harvest these fish—has been interrupted by environmental contamination. Because concepts of health for Mohawk people extend beyond the individual to the community and the environment (Arquette et al. 2002), this interrupted relationship with the fish has resulted in altered diets with resulting health impacts, and the fear that language and culture related to fish will be lost.

[a]The Haudenosaunee, also known as the Iroquois or Six Nations, are a confederacy of nations traditionally from the region that is now New York State, but now spread across New York, eastern Canada, Wisconsin, and Oklahoma. The six nations of the confederacy include the Mohawk, Oneida, Onondaga, Cayuga, Tuscarora, and Seneca. Akwesasne is one of five Mohawk reservations, which also includes Kahnawake and Kanesatake in Quebec and Wahta and Tyendinaga in Ontario. The Six Nations reservation in Ontario is home to Mohawk people as well as Haudenosaunee people of the other five nations as well.

Much of the literature on fish advisories has focused on concerns about whether these advisories properly inform minority subsistence fishermen and their families about the risks of consuming contaminated fish (Chess et al. 2005; Beehler et al. 2003; Tan et al. 2011; Imm et al. 2005). Following a conventional human health risk model in which prevention of exposure protects health, the goal of much of this scholarship is ensuring that the fish avoidance message reaches all audiences. Less focus has been given to the impact on communities who follow these advisories, and the feasibility of ever reversing the impact of these advisories even after site cleanup.

Through interviews with Akwesasne Mohawk community members and environmental officials, I explore the impact fish advisories have had on this community, the extent to which the community decreased or ceased their fish consumption, and the unintended health and cultural consequences of fish advisories. I also explore the motivations of people who have decided to continue to eat fish despite the advisories, and conclude with a discussion of future research and outreach needed in the community. The overarching message conveyed by community members and scholars who are pushing for more holistic forms of risk assessment (Arquette et al. 2002; Ranco et al. 2011; Harper et al. 2012; Donatuto and Harper 2008) is that optimum human health cannot be achieved in Native American communities such as Akwesasne until ecological health is achieved as well.

BACKGROUND

Akwesasne is a Mohawk community of about 13–15,000 people[b] that shares borders with New York, Ontario, and Quebec. Located at the confluence of four rivers—the St. Regis River, the Raquette River, the Grasse River, and the St. Lawrence River—the community relied for generations on the abundance of fish and wildlife, as well as the rich alluvial soils for farms (see Figure 1).

[b]An estimate of Akwesasne's population is given because residents in this community are notoriously difficult to enumerate. Akwesasro:non have been suspicious of, and resistant to, national censuses, and some residents are enrolled with both the St. Regis Mohawk Tribe and the Mohawk Council of Akwesasne. This estimate was used in establishing the demographics of the community for the extensive health studies conducted by SUNY Albany (see for example Fitzgerald et al. 1998 and Schell et al. 2009).

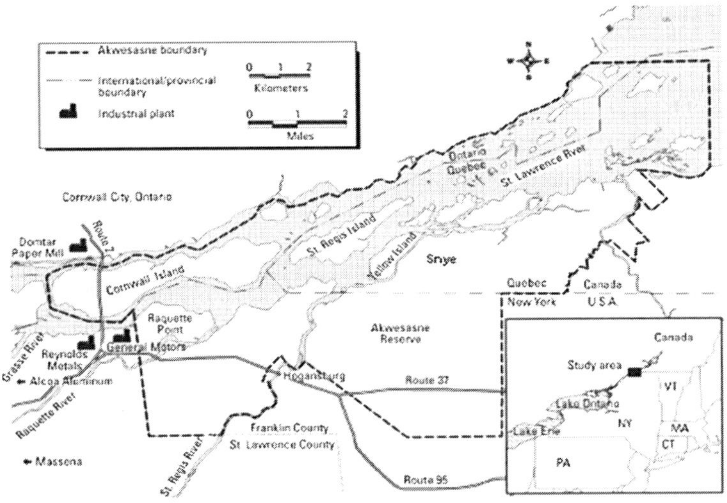

Figure 1: Map of Akwesasne.

The St. Lawrence Seaway project, begun in 1954, widened and deepened the river, and created a series of canals and locks that opened the region to ocean-going vessels. In 1957 the Moses-Saunders Power Dam was constructed on the St. Lawrence River and attracted industry with its low-cost hydroelectricity. The Aluminum Company of America (ALCOA) had already established a factory a few miles west of Akwesasne in 1903 on the Grasse River and was joined by the General Motors (GM) aluminum plant in 1958 and Reynolds Metals in 1959, both just west of the reservation, upstream and upwind. On the Canadian side of the river, a paper mill was built in 1881, which was acquired by Dominion Tar & Chemical in 1961 and rebranded as Domtar in 1965.

In 1976 Health and Welfare Canada approached the Mohawk Council of Akwesasne (MCA), the tribal government for the northern half of the community, to determine if there were elevated mercury levels in the people of Akwesasne, since mercury had been identified as a problem in Native communities across Canada. The presence of paper companies such as Domtar adjacent to, and upstream from, Akwesasne led to the concern that mercury could be a threat to this community as well. In 1978 MCA took samples of fish and found PCBs, mercury, and Mirex, which led them to recommend that women of childbearing age, children under 15, and pregnant women cease consumption of fish from the St. Lawrence (Hauptmann 1988:64).

In 1981, two dormant sludge pits filled with polychlorinated biphenyls (PCBs) were discovered behind GM, adjacent to the Raquette Point region of the reservation, and by 1984 the entire 270 acre General Motors site was declared a Superfund site. Following tests done by a NY State wildlife epidemiologist that found high levels of PCBs in fish and aquatic wildlife, an official three-part health risk assessment was developed that examined contaminant levels in fish (Sloan and Jock1990), wildlife (Skinner 1992) and breast milk (Fitzgerald et al. 1992). Sloan and Jock (1990:26) found that "PCB, dioxin, and mercury throughout the study area exceeded criteria for the protection of piscivorous wildlife." Tests done on 343 fish collected from 12 locations on the St. Lawrence River near the GM site showed total PCB levels ranging between 3 ppm and 8,000 ppm (lipid basis), which exceeded the tolerance limits established by the federal government of 2 ppm (wet weight) (Kinney et al. 1997:314).

Following tests done around the GM Superfund site, the Health Service for the St. Regis Mohawk Tribe (SRMT), the tribal government for the southern half of the community, issued an advisory in July of 1986 recommending that women of childbearing age, pregnant and nursing women, and children under 15 should entirely avoid the consumption of contaminated fish. They also gave a list of species for everyone to avoid, and a separate list from which residents should only eat one half pound per week.[c] This news further destroyed the local fishing economy, which had previously supported a number of Mohawk families and had already begun to diminish after the MCA fish advisory.

[c]Lactating women and women of childbearing age are to avoid all contaminated fish (carp, catfish and suckers). Adults should only eat one half pound per week of yellow perch, pumpkinseed, rock bass, whitefish, bowfin. Everyone should avoid carp, channel catfish, walleye, pike, red horse suckers, white suckers, and brown bullhead.

The results of the breast milk section of the health risk assessment (Fitzgerald et al. 1992), as well as continued studies that resulted from a partnership between the Akwesasne community and the State University of New York (SUNY) at Albany, demonstrated that fish consumption led to higher levels of PCBs in Akwesasne residents. Fingerprinting analyses established that fish caught in the St. Lawrence River offshore from the GM site were contaminated with the same lightly chlorinated PCB congeners as the sediment collected offshore from the GM plant. This contamination was primarily Aroclor 1248, the PCB mixture used in GM's die casting machinery (Hwang et al. 1993; Fitzgerald et al. 1995). This contamination was then traced from fish to humans: breast milk samples from women who ate local fish had a congener pattern that was much closer to perch, the preferred species of fish, than that found in women who ate little or no fish (Fitzgerald et al. 1998; Hwang et al. 2001). Similarly, Mohawk men who ate the most fish had a congener pattern similar to the fish studied (although their serum was more likely to contain more chlorinated PCB mixtures such as Aroclor 1254 and 1260, which have been traced to the Great Lakes, than the local mixture, Aroclor 1248) (Fitzgerald et al. 2007). This series of studies was significant because it demonstrated how PCBs could be fingerprinted as they migrated offsite from an industrial source, and traced into fish and then humans. Many Mohawks I spoke with referred to the St. Lawrence as the "lifeblood" of the community. By the contamination of the river, and hence the fish, Mohawk bodies were subsequently contaminated as well. Therefore cessation of fish consumption, which distanced Mohawks from this river, was lauded by the public health community as a means for preventing further exposure to contamination.

Environmental health studies conducted by the SUNY Albany research team and the Akwesasne community extended into a second Superfund Basic Research Project grant from 1995–2000. Papers published based on this project demonstrated that higher PCB levels in Mohawk participants were potentially connected to abnormal thyroid functioning in adolescents (Schell et al. 2004,2008, 2009; Schell and Gallo 2010); diabetes (Codru et al. 2007); higher levels of total serum lipids that contribute to heart disease (Goncharov et al. 2008); altered cognitive function in adolescents (Newman et al. 2006, 2009) as well as altered cognitive function in older adults (Haase et al. 2009); earlier onset of menarche in girls (Denham et al. 2005); and reduced testosterone levels in men (Goncharov et al. 2009).

The General Motors Superfund site has been undergoing remediation for decades but may finally be nearing completion. The Environmental Protection Agency (EPA) issued a Record of Decision in 1990 for GM's wastewater lagoons and the contaminated adjacent river sediment and in 1992 for GM's industrial landfill. The dredging of the St. Lawrence River sediments, along with a cap in areas where the cleanup goals were not met, was completed in 1995. From 2000–2004, GM remediated the inactive lagoons at the facility, excavating contaminated sludge and soils, stabilizing them and shipping to an offsite facility. The Raquette River bank soils and sediments were also remediated, and contaminated soils were removed at the toe of the slope of the Industrial Landfill, which reached out to the Raquette Point portion of the reservation. In 2004–2005 GM remediated Turtle Cove, which had been renamed "Contaminant Cove" by NY State Department of Environmental Conservation (NYSDEC) workers. The GM plant closed in May 2009, was bulldozed, and the remains shipped to an offsite landfill in 2011 (USEPA 2011). In 2013–2015 another four lagoons and two sludge pits will be cleaned up, and the edge of the landfill will be pulled back 150 ft from the shore of the St. Lawrence River and reservation boundary. The last of the general site cleanup and restoration activities will occur in 2016 (Arquette 2012). According to the EPA, current human exposures at this site are under control but contaminated groundwater migration is not (USEPA 2012).

METHODS

In order to explore how a Native American community located downstream from a Superfund site has been impacted by contamination and the ensuing environmental health studies, from March 2008 through April 2009 I interviewed 65 Akwesasne Mohawk community members, ranging in age from 25 to 90, with a majority ($n = 41$, 63%) in their 40s and 50s.[d] Eight participants were in their 20s to 30s, and 16 participants were older than 60. Those in their 40s and 50s were targeted, as they were the most likely to have taken part in the environmental health studies during the 1980s–1990s. Slightly over half of the interviewees (57%, $n = 37$) were women.

[d]Participants were not asked their exact age. Some participants offered their precise age, others indicated a general age range (e.g., 50s) during the interview.

All interviews were semi-structured, lasted from 30–90 min and consisted of open-ended questions about the impacts of the environmental contamination on the community, fish consumption, and current health concerns. During these interviews, I asked 50 interviewees (18 men and 32 women, 68% in their 40s and 50s) directly about their fish consumption, as well as that of their families, and how this may have changed as a result of the fish advisories. It is from this sub-sample that the data for this paper are drawn. Questions included: Do you still eat fish? As much as you used to? If you stopped, or reduced your fish eating, at what point did you do so, and why? Were your changes due to advisories or because you noticed changes in the fish? Do members of your family all eat the same amount of fish?

I made contact with most interviewees through snowball sampling, and in addition approached two members of the SRMT Environment Division, two members of the MCA Department of Environment, and six individuals who were at some time affiliated with the grassroots organization Akwesasne Task Force on the Environment (ATFE). All interviews were recorded and transcribed with all identifying information removed to protect confidentiality if the interviewee chose this option. For those who did not choose to remain confidential, I received permission to use their names. In addition to interviews, detailed field notes were maintained during extensive visits to Akwesasne from 2007 to 2011. Transcripts and notes were then analyzed in NVivo 8.0, a program for qualitative data entry, coding, sorting, and retrieval. Data coding was done in an iterative fashion, with additional readings of the transcripts leading to additional codes as more was learned from the materials. Prior to conducting this research, I received approval from the Akwesasne Task Force on the Environment Research Advisory Committee, as well as the Brown University Institutional Review Board.

RESULTS AND DISCUSSION

Fishing Tradition

Prior to the fish advisories issued in the 1980s, fishing had been a central part of the diet, economy, and social culture of Akwesasne for centuries. More than just a means of acquiring a dietary mainstay, fishing was described by community members as a livelihood, a lifestyle, and a culture. Almost everyone I spoke to in the community had a connection in some way to fish or fishing. The process of catching and cooking fish out of the river was at the root of many of the interviewees' childhoods and something that connected them to their ancestors. People in their 50s on up through their 90s recalled with youthful excitement their childhood experiences of going to the fish boxes that each family kept on the shore of the river to pull out the evening's supper. People fondly reminisced about fishing with their fathers on the river, helping their fathers prepare fishing equipment, or helping their mothers clean and cook the fish. Species such as sturgeon, perch, and bullhead were mentioned most frequently, and they were eaten smoked or fried. Fish was eaten several times a week for an ordinary dinner, and in large quantities at "fish fries" to celebrate special occasions and family gatherings.

When fish advisories were issued that called for people to diminish or eliminate fish from their diet, many residents felt that they had lost more than just omega-3 fatty acids from their diet; another part of their culture was being eroded by outside influences. A cessation in fishing gradually diminished Mohawk culture in several ways. As Henry Lickers describes, the language and culture around tying knots in nets as well as the social interactions that occurred around the process of creating these nets are lost when there is no longer a use for those nets:

People forget, in their own culture, what you call the knot that you tie in a net. And so, a whole section of your language and culture is lost because no one is tying those nets anymore. The interrelation between men and women, when they tied nets, the relationship between adults or elders and young people, as they tied nets together, the stories... that whole social infrastructure that was around the fabrication of that net disappeared (interview 10).

Similarly, the language around the names and descriptions of certain fish is lost. As one older man described to me, "A lot of that has been forgotten, the fish names in our language. Because a lot of the fishermen when they go fishing they talk about their Indian names to them, there is no English part of it, but that has been sort of forgotten now" (interview 39). One young mother, Randi, described how even though the youth were learning the Mohawk language, words related to activities no longer widely practiced, like fishing, "are never going to be spoke again because those things are now in the past... so only very elderly people are going to know those words, so that's a loss" (interview 54).

Changes in Community Fish Consumption

Data gathered during the health studies demonstrated a decrease in fish consumption among pregnant women (Fitzgerald et al. 1995, 2004) and Mohawk men (Fitzgerald et al. 1999). These papers cite fish advisories as the reason for the decline in fish consumption. Many of the Akwesasne community members I interviewed also described a decline in fish consumption, attributed to the fish advisories, but also to visual changes in the fish and a diminished fish population. On the other hand, some have maintained fish consumption based on a cultural connection that ties them to fish or because they felt their age precluded them from the more pressing reproductive and developmental concerns associated with the main target demographic of the fish advisories.

When asked whether they still ate local fish, three-quarters of the interviewees I spoke with (37 out of 50) replied that they had either dramatically decreased or entirely ceased their local fish consumption, even though for most of them it was previously an important part of their diet. Of those who had decreased fish consumption, eight interviewees described fish meals as a rare, special occasion treat. As Howard, an elder in his 80s explained, "I eat fish once or twice a year, not like every day" (interview 13). Another woman remarked that when she does have a little bit of fish on these occasions, she worries, "You know in the back of your mind that you're going to be glowing (laughs). You know what I mean? You know it is there, the fear is still there" (interview 27). Others have sworn off fish entirely and express aversion even to the idea. As Gina described, the only circumstance under which she would eat local fish would be, "Maybe if somebody raised them and then threw them in the river and you caught them that same day" (interview 4). Even though the fish advisories targeted mainly women of childbearing age and children, three of the men I spoke with shared what they saw as a common sentiment among men: if it was bad for the women, they should not eat it either. Nineteen (19) of the interviewees specified that not only had they given up eating fish, but so had the rest of their families.

Even prior to the announcement of fish advisories, which 29 interviewees indicated to me was what drove them from eating fish, some residents began noticing or hearing about visual clues that fish were not safe. One Raquette Point resident, Mark, described to me catching "fish with humongous tumors on them," or "funny color eyes" (interview 34). Others ($n = 6$) recalled how the fishermen were catching fish with black spots on them, with bugs inside, or with sores. Another man, Robert (interview 32), remembered cutting open fish with black spines, which he described as resulting from heavy metals contamination. Gina recollected, "We'd see like a big black spot on them or a glob of green and they would tell us that's what the PCBs are doing" (interview 4). Whether or not all of these physical changes witnessed in the fish can be attributed to PCBs is debatable, but more importantly, seeing or hearing about these physical deformities discouraged Mohawks from eating local fish.

Problematically, not all contaminated fish showed such visual cues. In 1985, NY State wildlife epidemiologist Ward Stone took samples of a sturgeon caught by Mohawk fishermen in order to test it for PCBs. When he came back with his results, which showed the fish to contain levels of PCBs above what the USDA considered safe for consumption, he was aghast to learn that the fishermen had already eaten the sturgeon.

The fact that fish could be contaminated without showing visible evidence led many community members for whom it was financially feasible (including 11 of these interviewees) to rely solely on outside sources of fish. For three related interviewees, this fish was coming from as far away as British Columbia. For three others it was from other communities nearby, such as Tyendinaga.[e] Robert explained how he gets his perch "out of upper Canada where they're not polluted yet" (interview 32). Some realized the irony in that they were probably still consuming contamination, just from another place they were less familiar with. Chris, an iron worker who had spent most of his life in Akwesasne but had also traveled extensively, exclaimed how "people think that if the fish comes from someplace else rather than right here, then it is ok. They don't realize every Great Lake dumps into the next Great Lake, which dumps into the St. Lawrence River. It is one big sewer" (interview 29). To avoid even the concern, four interviewees reported that they would only eat fish from the supermarket. As Alice, a lab technician for the health clinic described, "So we end up being supermarket Indians, buying tilapia from Hannaford's, not so much perch or walleye" (interview 62). For those who can afford to buy fish from outside the community this helped to satisfy the nutritional void created by the fish advisories, but not some of the social and cultural roles described earlier.

[e]A Mohawk community about 150 miles west of Akwesasne in Deseronto, Ontario.

Henry Lickers, who works for the MCA Department of Environment, described the rapid decline in fish consumption since moving to the community 30 years ago. When he first arrived in the community, he reports that 90% of the people he visited were eating fish. Then as the fish advisories became more prominent, people began changing their behavior. When he would stop by their house at dinnertime:

Suddenly, the old man or whoever it is was cooking the fish would put it in the cupboard and shut the door. And then they would be cooking something else, you know. "Well, you know, Henry has been talking about this. And you don't want to show him that you don't believe what he's talking about, because I really like fish, you know. And besides, I'm over 60, and it's not going to hurt me. And I don't want to have any more kids, so I'm okay." But you got funny things like that occurring (interview 10).

Henry no longer eats fish because he feels that he has a responsibility to set an example: "I don't eat fish from the St. Lawrence. I believe the same way, if people saw me eating, then they would say 'oh, then we can go back.' And I don't think that that's responsible. If I'm going to tell them not to, well then I better not as well." At the same time, he recognized that some people do still eat fish, even if they do not openly admit it. It is possible that for the earlier cited studies in which Fitzgerald was documenting a decline in fish consumption, as well as in the interviews I was conducting, that people under-reported their fish consumption because they recognize that according to the fish advisories they are not supposed to be eating fish, and they do not want to be judged for their choices.

One-quarter of the interviewees (13 out of 50) I asked about fish consumption expressed that they continued to eat local fish because they felt a cultural obligation to do so ($n = 4$), were not concerned about the warnings based on personal experiences ($n = 4$), or have decided to resume fish consumption now that they are no longer in their child-bearing years ($n = 5$). Richard described to me the traditional connection and responsibility that Mohawks and the fish have to each other, and for this reason, he continues to eat the fish. As he described, the Creator put the food in the water:

We give thanks for that food and we have to use it… I mean it doesn't make sense scientifically, but it makes sense spiritually and mentally that you should eat that, you know. You can't just put it aside and say, "well your work is not good enough," or something, you know? They're still given out what their original instructions were, and it's us that are at fault, it's our fault that they're like that, you know (interview 20).

Even though as a Mohawk he is not responsible for the contamination that has affected the fish, as a human being he is implicated in the problem, and therefore it is even more important that he works to maintain this relationship with the fish. Because the job given by the Creator to fish is to offer themselves as food, and the job given to humans is to respectfully harvest these fish, people like Richard who are working to maintain tradition feel obligated to maintain these roles. I heard similar narratives around the preservation of heritage seed varieties: the duty of these seeds is to sprout every spring, and the duty of humans is to plant them. If Mohawks fail to plant these seeds, "the plants will go back to the Sky World because they volunteered to come to the earth to help man to survive" (Brenda, interview 21). The concerns around the disuse of fish and heritage seed varieties stem back to cultural stories about ungrateful humans who have their food sources taken from them and who only regain them after learning lessons about maintaining ceremonies and traditional roles.

For some community members, an impression that the site remediation has led to lower levels of contamination in the fish or a nuanced understanding of more and less contaminated species and methods of preparation has contributed to their choice to eat local fish. One woman, who worked on the environmental health studies as a field assistant and was part of ATFE, described how her family continued to eat fish, and her kids "love it. They eat it whenever they can get it. I know that the area has been remediated and the fish isn't that bad anymore. So I hadn't told them not to eat it. So we just continue" (interview 26). Another ATFE member, Joyce, described how "the levels with the fish going down, the PCB levels going down…I feel more comfortable eating fish now. So I don't think I'm going to pick up that much contamination with PCBs anymore" (interview 16).

Another woman, Randi, who had relatives who worked on the health studies and with ATFE, noted that many people in the community have vilified the consumption of all fish. She noted that if caught eating local fish, pregnant women could expect a similar reaction as though they were smoking or drinking. She expressed disappointment that the only lesson that people seemed to take away from the health studies is not to eat fish:

I feel like sometimes I could try to educate people about what fish is good for you and what is bad for you, but sometimes it is just, why bother? You know my 30-second conversation is not going to undo 12 years of ingrained messages—"don't eat any more fish"... So I don't fight it too much, I just eat my fish in private (interview 54).

She laughed that people could eat fast food and then criticize her for eating fish. Similarly, an individual employed by the Environment Division stated that he felt the nutritional benefits of fish outweighed the potential contamination in fish since the beginning of the remediation of the industrial sites.

For other community members, personal and family experience with fish that have not led to ill health has encouraged them to continue to eat local fish. Agnes, who also worked on the environmental health studies, described how "we were brought up by the river and on the river. We were brought up to fish, we were brought up to swim in the river, and we were brought up on a boat. I don't have no fear of contamination. It was just a part of my life" (interview 59). She still eats fish as well. Nelson, a farmer and construction worker from the Snye region of the reservation, expressed skepticism towards all of the fish advisories because "we've been fishing all of our lives and we're still here. And my aunt, we just buried her last week. My great aunt was 102" (interview 40).

To a great extent, fish consumption in the community is divided along generational lines. In several families, members described to me that younger women who were planning to have children would not eat fish, but older women would go back to eating fish. For example, as Brenda, who is in her 50s, expressed, "I'm not young anymore so it doesn't matter. I eat the fish" (interview 21). Elizabeth, who is also in her 50s, also described how she went ten years without eating fish and would not let her kids have any. But she has gone back to it recently: "Let's just say I'm getting older now. I don't care, I love fish" (interview

22). However, even though this more advanced generation has returned to fish consumption, many interviewees were not convinced that the younger generation, even if given the chance, would eat fish. Middle-aged and older community members who had gone back to eating fish noted that they had not raised their kids to do so because of the warnings, and now they "didn't develop a taste for it" as Joyce describes. Seven interviewees described how their children and grandchildren currently had no desire to eat fish and are unlikely to show an interest in it even if it were determined to be clean at some point. As Agnes described, "They weren't brought up with the fish so they're not going to turn around and change their ways" (interview 59).

Even aside from the issue of contamination, ten of the community members I spoke with expressed the opinion that the fish population is too low to support the community. As Joyce, whose father was a fisherman, noted, "There isn't enough of a fish population to make a living off of anymore." She and others referred to the cormorant, a voracious bird that is new to the area and has been decimating fish stocks, especially the perch populations. Others pointed to the dams and locks now in place on the St. Lawrence River that prevent the fish from getting upstream and spawning as they once did. Ernie, a 90-year-old elder who witnessed the transformation of the St. Lawrence from a river to a seaway, described how, in the process of dredging channels and blasting through rock ledges in the river, the fish spawning grounds were destroyed.

[The blasting of rocks] affected the spawning grounds of fish, not only by the blasting but also because of when the blasting was done, they had to clean out all the broken bottom soil and then deposit it somewhere. And of course the easiest place to do it were the inlets and the bays where there were spawning areas and so for a long time fish couldn't make a living out there and so a lot of their work was not done. The fish as you know, have sort of a cleaning action there in swimming – absorbing the water and taking in contaminants, deposit it down in the bottom of the river, so getting it out of the way. And so now we had to do without the fish for years.

As mentioned in the Thanksgiving Address, part of the instruction given to fish is to cleanse and purify the water. As Ernie has noted, this job has been hampered by changes made to the river. As Richard remarked above, the other instruction given to the fish is to offer themselves as food. Contamination released into the river and some residents' concerns about taking this contamination into their own bodies have dramatically altered the feasibility for this job to be carried out as well.

Costs and Benefits of Fish Consumption

For some, current rates of diabetes, heart disease, and obesity among Mohawks have led them to wonder if trading local fish for inexpensive processed foods was the healthiest decision. Currently about 25% of the community suffers from diabetes (Rourke 2009, director of "Let's Get Healthy" program, personal communication). Of the 38 interviewees who expressed opinions about the causes of diabetes in the community, half of them ($n = 19$) pointed to a change in diet brought about as a result of the contamination of the environment. One man, Richard D., who works for the MCA Department of Environment, wants someone to do a study to see who currently has better health: the individuals who ignored the fish warnings and continued to eat a traditional diet or those who heeded the warnings to avoid fish and instead substituted a high carbohydrate, high fat diet, "like me, and developed obesity and blood pressure and diabetes and stuff like that. Like who's better off? I'd like to see a study of that" (interview 45). He attributes the high rates of diabetes to the community's collectively changed diet. "There's a lack of healthy food here. I mean, used to be we'd get bullheads out of here for consumption. I wouldn't touch them now." So while the fish advisories were intended to protect Mohawk health, the shift in diet away from fish to other affordable sources of nutrition also caused health problems.

Jim, who worked for the SRMT Environment Division at the time the contamination was discovered, expressed mixed feelings for the fish advisories that strongly encouraged people to change their diets: "The problem we didn't anticipate though was the change in the diet and the change in lifestyle we feel has contributed to the diabetes in the community and to the other illnesses in the community that has occurred since then. So that concerns me" (interview 36). In criticizing the conventional risk assessment model, Akwesasne community members Tarbell and Arquette (2000) noted that sometimes the greatest health effects are seen outside of chemical exposures and are thus not included in risk assessments. At Akwesasne, health was impacted by the environmental contamination even without the ingestion of fish: fear of exposure led to the replacement of this low-fat source of protein and other important nutrients with high-fat and high-carbohydrate sources of food. Tarbell and Arquette (2000:102) posit, "Diabetes is on the rise because more people no longer eat traditional foods and no longer participate in cultural activities that once provided healthy forms of exercise." SUNY Albany researchers conducting environmental health studies with Mohawk adolescents also noted that while the community might have decreased their exposure to fish-borne contamination, they have lost a primary source of protein and other important nutrients such as calcium, iron, zinc, and omega-3 fatty acids (Fitzgerald et al. 2004). The replacement of fish with cheap foods has had the effect of "further exacerbating chronic, diet-related health problems in the community, such as diabetes and cardiovascular disease" (Schell et al. 2003:961).

Despite these concerns, these researchers have expressed that reducing fish consumption has been more beneficial to health than continued fish consumption because of the risks of contaminant exposure. In a recent paper, Schell et al. (2012) assessed the benefits of consuming less local fish (lower PCB levels in the youth they tested) versus the costs (cultural loss and higher rates of diabetes and obesity). They concluded that the more holistic risk-based environmental decision-making proposed by ATFE members Arquette et al. (2002) should be better considered by regulatory agencies, and human biologists should give more focus to the non-nutritional components of many foods, such as persistent organic pollutants (POPs). David Carpenter (personal communication, 2008) has argued that, especially since some studies done at Akwesasne have connected PCB levels with potential health effects, the cessation of fish consumption was the best option for Mohawks, although more should have been done to help people find healthier food substitutes. Carpenter also questioned whether the touted benefits of fish consumption are enough to counterbalance the potential impacts of the contaminants (Bushkin-Bedient and Carpenter 2010). Turyk et al. (2012) argued that most of our knowledge about the nutritional benefits of fish consumption is based on marine fish, which generally have higher concentrations of omega-3 fatty acids than freshwater fish. They pointed to studies by Philibert et al. (2006) and Godin et al. (2003) that found no association between local fish intake and serum omega-3 fatty acids in Great Lakes fishermen. Since omega-3 fatty acids are one of the most highly cited health-promoting compounds in fish, this has led Turyk et al. (2012) to conclude that we do not have enough data to quantitatively analyze the costs and benefits of the consumption of fish from the Great Lakes and the St. Lawrence River.

At a recent community meeting (1/11/12) questions arose around whether the fish advisory had been the best course of action, considering the unintended health consequences such as obesity and diabetes that have been linked to a more modern diet. The researchers hosting the meeting acknowledged that their data demonstrated that youth born before the fish advisory (1985) had higher PCB levels than those born after, demonstrating the effectiveness of the advisory in lowering PCB body burdens (see Schell et al. 2003, 2012; Gallo et al. 2011). One participant pushed further—what about now, after the remediation work that has been done? In the discussion that followed, the general consensus was that more testing needed to be done on local fish populations to determine current contaminant levels. An Environment Division employee present at the meeting announced that there were plans in the coming year to collaborate with the NYSDEC to repeat a fish study done in 1988, and efforts were being made to convince EPA to do fish monitoring at the remedial sites. When I interviewed an Environment Division employee and asked if the fish will ever be considered safe to eat again, he replied, "I think so. I think that'll be as clean as the fish upstream." He remarked that the farther you go from GM, the cleaner the river gets, and the cleaner the fish get.

So, when you go down into Snye (a region of Akwesasne east of GM), we've taken the samples of fish and the fish are pretty clean. I think they are – we are still being cautious; we still don't want to say yes, you can eat the fish, because we are still not sure what the proper level is that's safe. Is it going to be 0.05 parts per million, is it going to be 0.5 parts per million you know, 0.005... you know there is still science that's going on. So, we want to be very sure of what we're doing before we say it's okay. I think it's going to happen eventually you know" (interview 15).

In order for the tribal government to be able to properly advise residents about the risks and benefits of eating local fish, more testing needs to be done, and the results conveyed in a manner that the community can understand and apply.

Risk Avoidance and Reduction

The case of Akwesasne is illustrative of unintended health and cultural consequences of relying on risk avoidance rather than risk reduction methods of preventing human exposure to contamination (O'Neill 2003NEJAC 2002). *Risk reduction strategies* look to risk-producers to prevent or eliminate environmental contamination in order to avoid human exposure. In the case of Akwesasne, risk reduction strategies would have entailed greater monitoring of General Motor's operations to prevent decades' worth of PCB contamination to the surrounding area. A greater enforcement of risk reduction would also have led to the immediate and complete removal of PCB-contaminated waste from the GM site, rather than a decades-long cleanup that resulted in a 12 acre landfill, and a reliance on continued fish advisories to prevent Mohawks from being exposed to contamination.*Risk avoidance strategies* call upon the risk-bearers to alter their practices so as to avoid the harms of exposure to contamination. Fish advisories are an example of this strategy: the onus is on the risk-bearers, in this case the fish consumers, rather than those who caused the risk.

O'Neill (2003) points out that reducing human health risks by targeting the first link in the chain that connects environmental contamination to human health—in this case removing the source of the PCB contamination—means that ecological health benefits as well. Intervening late in the chain and breaking the link at the point of human exposure, in this case by preventing fish consumption, leaves a greater amount of contamination unabated, has greater negative environmental effects, and is a form of cultural discrimination.

Risk-avoidance strategies also rely implicitly on the assumption that there are readily available substitutes for local fish and the customs that accompany their gathering (NEJAC 2002). As we have seen from the case in Akwesasne, these substitutes were not available to all residents, and there are no substitutes for the cultural activities and knowledge exchange that once happened around fishing. Fish was not just a source of protein for Mohawks, but a cultural object of importance that could not easily be factored into the assessment of mortality and morbidity risks that currently comprise health risk assessments (Donatuto et al. 2011). In order to properly calculate whether risk-reduction strategies are an acceptable solution to environmental contamination, it is necessary to look beyond the risk to a population of cancer deaths, and consider the threats to a healthy, culturally specific lifestyle as defined by the Mohawks themselves. This more complete assessment would include cultural indicators such as access to a traditional diet and the passing down of traditional knowledge (Johnson and Ranco 2011).

While fish advisories were necessary in the 1980s to protect Mohawk health when GM's contamination was first discovered, EPA has not made any concerted attempts to ensure that advisories will only be necessary in the short term (O'Neill 2003). While fish advisories are often necessary to protect human health in the short term, there is a need to emphasize more permanent and judicious fixes to problems of contamination. The EPA's most recent Five Year Report about the GM site states that "remedial actions have been completed in the St. Lawrence River, Raquette River, and Turtle Cove, and, *when combined with the existing fish advisories*, these measures address unacceptable exposure pathways in these areas" (USEPA 2010: ES1;*italics* mine). This report takes for granted that fish advisories are an acceptable tool for preventing human exposure to contaminants, similar to a cap on the river bottom that isolates contaminated sediment. Acceptance of the ongoing fish advisories allows GM and the EPA to avoid a more thorough and permanent cleanup.

CONCLUSIONS

Human health in Native American communities is intimately tied to the health of the environment. Akwesasne Mohawks (Arquette et al. 2002:262) have defined health as "based on peaceful, sustainable relationships with other peoples including family, community, Nation, the natural world, and spiritual beings. Health is supported by the solid foundation of a healthy natural world." Human health in a community such as Akwesasne cannot be understood independent of the health of the natural environment, and especially in this case, the health of the fish.

When Mohawk mothers who participated in the breast milk study demonstrated that removing local fish from their diets decreased the PCB contamination in their breast milk, they showed that exposure to PCBs was avoidable, and thus according to conventional risk assessment the problem was eliminated. What was not predicted, and the reason why indigenous scholars such as Arquette et al. (2002) and Ranco et al. (2011) are calling for more holistic risk assessment, was that avoiding fish consumption had other health implications, both physical and cultural. For community members who continue to consume fish, this consumption is often socially fractured rather than part of a broader social context. As described above, fish is consumed along generational divides by Mohawks who see themselves as beyond their childbearing years, or "in private" as one woman described, in order to avoid judgment.

If the Akwesasne community is going to achieve optimal health, the contaminated environment has to be remediated to a level that supports clean, edible fish. This will not happen as long as fish advisories are considered an acceptable institutional control to protect humans from exposure to contaminants. The accepted culture around environmental cleanup must shift away from one of risk avoidance, a distributive justice situation where those who did not benefit from industry are forced to pay the price in order to protect their health. At the General Motors Superfund site in Massena, economic considerations were given priority over the health and culture of Mohawk people, in an attempt to secure a source of employment for the residents of Massena. Despite these efforts, and $49.5 billion in bailout money, General Motors filed for bankruptcy in June 2009 and spun off a holding company to handle its idle properties, Motors Liquidation Corp. When it emerged from bankruptcy, GM was freed of responsibility for rehabilitating dozens of toxic waste sites in 13 states where it had manufacturing plants. Revitalizing Auto Communities Environmental Response, or the RACER Trust, is an environmental trust that assumed ownership of 89 former General Motors properties and is tasked with completing remediation and selling off dozens of former GM properties, including the one adjacent to Akwesasne. The new General Motors, freed of its old liabilities, is struggling back towards success in the auto market, while the Massena town residents who fought to shelter the company from high cleanup expenses are left without jobs, and the Mohawk are left living adjacent to an industrial landfill that they suspect will continue to pollute their environment.

Researchers and environmental officials working in Akwesasne have stated that a new round of studies determining current contamination levels in the fish is necessary to determine the safety of local fish consumption. Researchers have additionally called for studies of the nutritional content of the fish in order to properly conduct a cost-benefit analysis as to whether the nutritional benefits of the fish outweigh the risks posed by contamination.

Once information about local fish is obtained, it could be disseminated via a model illustrated by DeWeese et al. (2009), who produced advisory maps for Anishnaabe communities that provided lake-specific, risk-based, culturally sensitive consumption advice on color-coded maps for two groups: children under age 15 years and females of childbearing age, and males 15 years and older and females beyond childbearing age. Because the maps were easy to read and developed in conjunction with community members, DeWeese et al. (2009) found they significantly increased the percentage of survey participants who indicated awareness of advisory information and increased preference for smaller walleye, which contain lower levels of contamination than larger fish. After future testing of Akwesasne's local fish population, similar maps could be produced and distributed as a way of making this information accessible to the community. At Brown University,[f] we are currently developing a project with the Narragansett Tribe in which local fish will be tested, and based on the results, cards will be developed and distributed to fishermen to keep in their tackle boxes to help them determine which species of fish to keep and which to toss back based on contaminant levels. We are also developing fish puzzles for families that help illustrate which parts of the fish are more or less contaminated in order to facilitate the consumption of the less contaminated portions. Each of these small projects described above can help a community to maintain some level of fish consumption rather than cutting it entirely from their diet, as most people at Akwesasne have even though environmental specialists in the community point to some alternatives. What should be highlighted though is that these alternate species and methods of preparation should not be considered as a solution, but rather a step along the process towards remediating environmental contamination to a level in which culturally preferred fish species and methods of preparation can be safely utilized again.

[f]The Community Engagement Core of the Brown Superfund Research Project, consisting of the author, Marcella Thompson, and Robert Vanderslice, working in conjunction with Dinalyn Spears, head of the Natural Resources Department of the Narragansett Indian Tribe.

Akwesasne is a case where measures taken to protect community health—adherence to fish advisories to prevent exposure to contamination—have inadvertently led to diet-related health consequences as well as concerns around the loss of language, culture, and social connections attached to fishing. While Akwesasne community members, environmental specialists, and their allies in the scientific community are continuing to push for additional cleanup and fish sampling, this case should also serve as an example of why risk avoidance methods such as fish advisories should not be considered a viable long-term solution to preventing human exposure to contamination.

ACKNOWLEDGEMENTS

The author would like to acknowledge the Akwesasne Task Force on the Environment (ATFE) and members of the Akwesasne community who offered their time for these interviews. I would also like to acknowledge members of Brown University's Contested Illness Research Group for providing feedback on an earlier draft, and Dr. Nicholas Reo for guest editing this special issue. This research was funded by a National Science Foundation Cultural Anthropology Dissertation Improvement Grant, a Switzer Environmental Fellowship, a Lynn Reyer Tribal Community Development Grant and a Ford Foundation Dissertation Fellowship.

REFERENCES

1. Arquette C (2012) GM remediation update. http://www.srmtenv.org/index.php?spec=sf_generalmotors_ru. Accessed 4 Dec 2012
2. Arquette M, Cole M, Cook K, LaFrance B, Peters M, Ransom J, Sargent E, Smoke V, Stairs A (2002) Holistic risk-based environmental decision making: a native perspective. Environ Health Perspect 110(supplement 2):259-264
3. Beehler GP, Vena JE, McGuiness BM (2003) Characterizing Latino anglers' environmental risk perceptions, sport fish consumption, and advisory awareness. Med Anthropol Q 17:99-116

4. Bushkin-Bedient S, Carpenter DO (2010) Benefits versus risks associated with consumption of fish and other seafood. Rev Environ Health 25:161-191
5. Chess C, Burger J, McDermott MH (2005) Speaking like a state: environmental justice and fish consumption advisories. Soc Nat Resou 18:267-278
6. Codru N, Schymura M, Negoita S, Rej R, Carpenter DO, Akwesasne Task Force on the Environment (2007) Diabetes in relation to serum levels of polychlorinated biphenyls and chlorinated pesticides in adult native Americans. Environ Health Perspect 115:1442-1447
7. Denham M, Schell L, Deane G, Gallo MV, Ravenscroft J, DeCaprio A, Akwesasne Task Force on the Environment (2005) Relationship of lead, mercury, mirex, dichlorodphenyldichloroethylene, hexachlorobenzene and polychlorinated biphenyls to timing of menarche among Akwesasne Mohawk girls. Pediatrics 115:e127-e134
8. DeWeese AD, Emiecik NE, Chiriboga ED, Foran JA (2009) Efficacy of risk-based, culturally sensitive Ogaa (Walleye) consumption advice for Anishnaabe tribal members in the Great Lakes region. Risk Anal 29:729-742 | Publisher Full Text
9. Donatuto J, Harper BL (2008) Issues in evaluating fish consumption rates for native American tribes. Risk Anal 28:1497-1506
10. Donatuto J, Satterfield TA, Gregory R (2011) Poisoning the body to nourish the soul: prioritizing health risks and impacts in a Native American community. Health Risk Soc 13:103-127
11. Fitzgerald EF, Hwang S, Brix KA, Bush B, Quinn J, Cook K (1992) Chemical contaminants in the milk of Mohawk women from Akwesasne. Report for the Health Risk Assessment of the General Motors Central Foundry Division Superfund Waste. Albany: New York State Department of Health.
12. Fitzgerald E, Hwang S, Brix K, Cook K, Worsick P (1995) Fish PCB concentrations and consumption patterns among Mohawk women at Akwesasne. J Expo Anal Env Epid 5:1-19
13. Fitzgerald E, Hwang S, Bush B, CookKWP (1998) Fish consumption and breast milk PCB concentrations among Mohawk women at Akwesasne. Am J Epidemiol 148:164-172 |

14. Fitzgerald E, Deres D, Hwang S, Bush B, Yang B, Tarbell A, Jacobs A (1999) Local fish consumption and serume PCB concentrations among Mohawk men at Akwesasne. Environ Res 80:S97-S103 0013-9351/99
15. Fitzgerald E, Hwang S, Langguth K, Cayo M, Yang B, Bush B, Worswick P, Lauzon T (2004) Fish consumption and other environmental exposures and their associations with serum PCB concentrations among Mohawk women at Akwesasne. Environ Res 94:160-170 |
16. Fitzgerald E, Hwang S, Gomez M, Bush B, Yang B, Tarbell A (2007) Environmental and occupational exposures and serum PCB concentrations and patterns among Mohawk men at Akwesasne. J Expo Sci Env Epid 17:269-278
17. Gallo MV, Schell LM, DeCaprio AP, Jacobs A (2011) Levels of persistent organic pollutant and their predictors among young adults. Chemosphere 83:1374-1382 |
18. Godin C, Shatenstein B, Paradis G, Kosatsky T (2003) Absence of cardiovascular benefits and sportfish consumption among St. Lawrence river anglers. Environ Res 93:241-247
19. Goncharov A, Haase R, Santiago-Rivera A, Morse G, McCaffrey RJ, Rej R, Carpenter DO, Akwesasne Task Force on the Environment (2008) High serum PCBs are associates with elevation of serum lipids and cardiovascular disease in a Native American population. Environ Res 106:226-239 |
20. Goncharov A, Rej R, Negoita S, Schymura M, Santiago-Rivera A, Morse G, Carpenter DO (2009) Lower serum testosterone associated with elevated polychlorinated biphenyl concentrations in Native American men. Environ Health Perspect 117:1454-1460 |
21. Haase R, McCaffrey RJ, Santiago-Rivera AL, Morse GS, Tarbell A (2009) Evidence of an age-related threshold effect of polychlorinated biphenyls (PCBs) on neuropsychological functioning in a Native American population. Environ Res 109:73-85 |
22. Harper B, Harding A, Harris S, Berger P (2012) Subsistence exposure scenarios for tribal application. Hum Ecol Risk Assess 18:810-831

23. Hauptmann L (1988) Formulating American indian policy in New York state, 1970–1986. State University of New York. Albany: Press.
24. Hwang S, Gensburg L, Fitzgerald E, Herzfeld P, Bush B (1993) Fingerprinting sources of contamination: statistical techniques for identifying point sources of PCBs. J Occup Med Toxicol 4:365-382
25. Hwang S, Yang B, Fitzgerald E, Bush B, Cook K (2001) Fingerprinting PCB patterns among Mohawk women. J Expo Anal Env Epid 11:184-192
26. Imm P, Knobeloch L, Anderson HA, Great Lakes Sport Fish Consortium (2005) Fish consumption and advisory awareness in the great lakes Basin. Environ Health Perspect 113:1325-1329 |
27. Johnson J, Ranco DJ (2011) Risk assessment and Native Americans at the cultural crossroads: making better science or redefining health? In: Ottinger G, Cohen B (eds) Technoscience and environmental justice: transforming expert cultures through grassroots engagement, Cambridge: MIT Press.
28. Kinney A, Fitzgerald E, Hwang S, Bush B, Tarbell A (1997) Human exposure to PCBs: modeling and assessment of environmental concentrations on the Akwesasne reservation. Drug Chem Toxicol 20:313-328 |
29. NEJAC (National Environmental Justice Advisory Council) (2002) Fish consumption and environmental justice. US Environmental Protection Agency. Washington DC.http://www.epa.gov/environmentaljustice/resources/publications/nejac/fish-consump-report_1102.pdf. Accessed 1 February 2013
30. Newman J, Aucompaugh A, Schell L, Denham M, DeCaprio AP, Gallo MV, Ravenscroft J, Kao C, Hanover MR, David D, Jacobs A, Tarbell A, Worswick P, Akwesasne Task Force on the Environment (2006) PCBs and cognitive functioning of Mohawk adolescents. Neurotoxicol Teratol 28:429-
31. Newman J, Gallo MV, Schell LM, DeCaprio AP, Denham M, Deane GD, Akwesasne Task Force on the Environment (2009) Analysis of PCB congeners related to cognitive functioning in adolescents. Neurotoxicology 30:686-696 |

32. O'Neill CA (2003) Risk avoidance, cultural discrimination, and environmental justice for indigenous peoples. Ecol Law Quart 30:1-57
33. Patterson N (1999) The fish. In: Force HET (ed) The words that come before all else, Akwesasne: Native North American Traveling College.
34. Philibert A, Vanier C, Abdelouahab N, Chan HM, Mergler D (2006) Fish intake and serum fatty acid profiles from freshwater fish. Am J Clin Nutr 84:1299-1307 |
35. Ranco DK, O'Neill CA, Donatuto J, Harper BL (2011) Environmental justice, American Indians and the cultural dilemma: developing environmental management for tribal health and well-being. Environ Just 4:221-230
36. Schell LM, Gallo MV (2010) Relationships of putative endocrine disruptors to human sexual maturation and thyroid activity in youth. Physiol Behav 99:246-253
37. Schell LM, Hubicki LA, DeCaprio AP, Gallo MV, Ravenscroft J, Tarbell A, Jacobs A, David D, Worswick P (2003) Organochlorines, lead, and mercury in Akwesasne Mohawk youth. Environ Health Perspect 111:954-961 |
38. Schell L, Gallo MV, DeCaprio AP, Hubicki LA, Denham M, Ravenscroft J, The Akwesasne Task Force on the Environment (2004) Thyroid function in relation to burden of PCBs, p,p'-DDE, HCB, mirex and lead among Akwesasne Mohawk youth: a preliminary study. Environ Toxicol Pharm 18:91-
39. Schell LM, Gallo MV, Denham M, Ravenscroft J, DeCaprio AP, Carpenter DO (2008) Relationship of thyroid hormone levels to levels of polychlorinated biphenyls, lead, p, p0- DDE, and other toxicants in Akwesasne Mohawk youth. Environ Health Perspect 116:806-813 |
40. Schell LM, Gallo MV, Ravenscroft J, DeCaprio AP (2009) Persistent organic pollutants and anti-thyroid peroxidase levels in Akwesasne Mohawk young adults. Environ Res 109:86-92 | Publisher Full Text | PubMed Central Full Text
41. Schell L, Gallo MV, Cook K (2012) What's NOT to eat—food adulteration in the context of human biology. Am J Hum Bio 24:139-148

42. Skinner L (1992) Chemical contaminants in wildlife from the Mohawk Nation at Akwesasne and the vicinity of the General Motors Corporation/Central Foundry Division, Massena, NY Plant. Albany, NY: New York State Department of Environmental Conservation.
43. Sloan R, Jock K (1990) Chemical contaminants in the fish from the Mohawk Nation at Akwesasne and the vicinity of the General Motors Corporation/Central Foundry Division. Albany, NY: Massena NY Plant. New York State Department of Environmental Conservation.
44. Tan M, Ujihara A, Kent L, Hendrickson I (2011) Communicating fish consumption advisories in California: what works, what doesn't. Risk Anal 31:1095-1105
45. Tarbell A, Arquette M (2000) Akwesasne: a Native American community's resistance to cultural and environmental damage. In: Hofrichter R (ed) Reclaiming the environmental debate: the politics of health in a toxic culture, Cambridge: MIT Press.
46. Turyk M, Bhavasar S, Bowerman W, Boysen E, Clark M, Diamond M, Mergler D, Pantazopoulos P, Schantz S, Carpenter DO (2012) Risks and benefits of consumption of Great Lakes fish. Environ Health Perspect 120:11-18 http://dx.doi.org/10.1289/ehp.1003396
47. USEPA (2010) Second five-year review report General Motors (Central Foundry Division) Superfund site. St Lawrence County, Town of Massena, New York. http://cfpub.epa.gov/supercpad/SiteProfiles/index.cfm?fuseaction=second.additional&id=0201644. Accessed 4 Dec 2012
48. USEPA (2011) General Motors (Central Foundry Division). More in-depth site details. http://cfpub.epa.gov/supercpad/cursites/csitinfo.cfm?id=0201644. Accessed 4 Dec 2012
49. USEPA (2012) Superfund information systems. Superfund site progress profile General Motors (Central Foundry Division) EPA ID: NYD091972554. http://cfpub.epa.gov/supercpad/cursites/csitinfo.cfm?id=0201644 e. Accessed 4 Dec 2012

Chapter 9

Contamination of Water Resources by Pathogenic Bacteria

Pramod K Pandey[1], Philip H Kass[1], Michelle L Soupir[2], Sagor Biswas[1], and Vijay P Singh[3]

[1]Department of Population Health and Reproduction, University of California, Davis, California, USA

[2]Department of Agricultural and Biosystems Engineering, Iowa State University, Ames, Iowa, USA

[3]Department of Biological and Agricultural Engineering & Zachry Department of Civil Engineering, Texas A & M University, College Station, Texas, USA

ABSTRACT

Water-borne pathogen contamination in water resources and related diseases are a major water quality concern throughout the world. Increasing interest in controlling water-borne pathogens in water resources evidenced by a large number of recent publications clearly attests to the need for studies that synthesize knowledge from multiple fields covering comparative aspects of pathogen contamination, and unify them in a single place in order to present and address the problem as a whole. Providing a broader perceptive of pathogen contamination in freshwater (rivers, lakes, reservoirs, groundwater) and saline water (estuaries and coastal waters) resources, this review paper attempts to develop the first comprehensive single source of existing information on pathogen contamination in multiple types of water resources. In addition, a comprehensive discussion describes the challenges associated with using indicator organisms. Potential impacts of water resources development on pathogen contamination as well as challenges that lie ahead for addressing pathogen contamination are also discussed.

INTRODUCTION

Water-borne pathogen contamination in ambient water bodies and related diseases are a major water quality concern throughout the world. Pathogen contamination is a serious issue for almost all types of ambient water bodies, making its recognition and understanding essential (U.S. EPA [2012a]). The United Nations identified improving water quality as one of the eight Millennium Development Goals (MDGs). Its target is to reduce the number of people without access to safe water by 50% by 2015 (WHO [2011]). Because of the overwhelming scientific evidence for climate change (IPCC [2007]), it is also important to understand how perturbations in weather patterns can potentially impact pathogen levels in water resources. To meet future demands of water for food, energy, and ecosystems, increasing water storage structures (i.e., dams) must be a component of long-range planning (World Bank [2010]). However, such new structures can potentially degrade water quality and exacerbate public health risk.

While several review papers are currently available (Bradford et al. [2013]; Pachepsky and Shelton [2011]; Pang [2009]; Jin and Flury [2002]; John and Rose [2005]; Jamieson et al. [2004]; Jamieson et al. [2002]; Arnone and Walling [2007]; Kay et al. [2007]), there is a manifest need for additional transdisciplinary studies that assimilate knowledge gained from multi-research endeavors studying pathogen contamination, and provide a comprehensive synopsis in order to comprehend the entirety of the problem. Therefore, the goal of this review is to present a broad research scope assessment of pathogen contamination of water resources and the associated challenges it presents. We synthesize the potential health risks imposed by pathogens in water resources by providing existing knowledge that covers surface water, groundwater, fresh water, and saline water. Further, the impact of water resources development on pathogen contamination, future challenges, and recommendations are summarized. In addition, we provide a brief discussion describing water-borne pathogen footprints and potential challenges associated with the use of indicator organisms for assessing water quality.

Health Risk

Water-borne diseases (i.e., diarrhea, gastrointestinal illness) caused by various bacteria, viruses, and protozoa have been the causes of many outbreaks (Craun et al. [2006]). In developing countries, such as those in Africa, water-borne diseases infect millions (Fenwick [2006]). According to World Health Organization (WHO), each year 3.4 million people, mostly children, die from water-related diseases (WHO [2014]). According to United Nations Children's Fund (UNICEF) assessment, 4000 children die each day as a result of contaminated water (UNICEF [2014]). WHO ([2010]) reports that over 2.6 billion people lack access to clean water, which is responsible for about 2.2 million deaths annually, of which 1.4 million are in children. Improving water quality can reduce the global disease burden by approximately 4% (WHO [2010]).

Although water-associated diseases in developing countries are prevalent, they are also a serious challenge in developed countries. A study by Arnone and Walling ([2007]), who compiled data of outbreaks in the U.S. (1986 – 2000), reported 5,905 cases and 95 outbreaks associated with recreational water. Gastrointestinal Illness (GI) caused by variety of different microbes and germs, which causes symptoms, such as diarrhea, nausea, vomiting, fever, abdominal pain, was responsible for about 29.53% cases. More than 27% of cases were caused by Shigella spp. In addition, 10.99%, 10.08%, and 6.59% of the cases were caused by Cryptosporidium parvum, Adenovirus 3, and Leptospira, respectively. Nearly 23% and 21% of the outbreaks were caused by GI and Shigella spp, respectively. In addition, 16.84%, 12.63%, and 7.37% of the outbreaks were caused by Naegleria fowleri, E. coli 0157:H7, and Schistosoma spp., respectively. Besides acute gastroenteritis, major etiological agents such as Giarida, Cryptosporadium, E. coli 0157:H7, V. cholera, and Salmonella were the agents responsible for many outbreaks (Craun et al. [2006]). During the same period 437,082 cases and 48 outbreaks were caused by contaminated drinking water, of which about 95.89% of the cases were caused by Cryptosporidium parvum. Nearly 42% and 31% of the outbreaks were caused by Giardia lamblia and GI, respectively. Reporting statistics on water-borne outbreaks in the U.S., Craun et al. ([2006]) found that at least 1870 outbreaks (23 per year) occurred between 1920 and 2002. These reported outbreaks and their reported incidence of illnesses are likely to be an underestimation of actual numbers because of nonreported cases and missing exposure information. To protect public health, the U.S. EPA's National Primary Drinking Water Regulations (NPDWRs) contain standards describing the Maximum Contaminant Level (MCL) – the highest level of a contaminate allowable in drinking water. The U.S. EPA has defined the MCL of various microorganisms, such as Cryptosporidium, Giardia lamblia,Legionella, and Total Coliforms (including fecal coliform and E. coli), and viruses (U.S. EPA[2012b]). The Maximum Contaminant Level Goal (MCLG) – the level of a contaminant in drinking water below which there is no known risk to public health, has also been proposed by the U.S. EPA. The MCLC levels for Cryptosporidium, Giardia lamblia, Legionella, and Total Coliforms are zero. The EPA requires 99% removal of Cryptosporidium in drinking water, and the removal percentages of Giardia lamblia and viruses are 99.9 and 99.99%, respectively. Although there is no limit for Legionella, EPA believes that if Giardia lamblia and viruses are removed/inactivated, then drinking water likely to be free of Legionella. The U.S. EPA requires routine sampling of drinking water for testing total coliform and E. coli, and if a routine sample is positive, then repeat samples are required. If, in any repeat sample, total coliform or E. coli is detected then the drinking water has an acute MCL violation. For a drinking water system that collects fewer than 40 routine samples per month, no more than one sample can be total coliform-positive per month. For a system that collects more than 40 routine samples, no more than 5% of samples total coliform-positive in a month is allowed (U.S. EPA [2012b]).

Each year approximately 42,000 cases of salmonellosis are reported in the U.S. (CDC [2014]). Schistosomiasis is not reported in the U.S.

because it is not endemic; however, 200 million people are infected worldwide. In 2011, about 1,060 cases of Guinea worm disease, caused by the parasite Dracunculus medinensis, were reported in many remote parts of Africa that do not have safe drinking water. Malaria, a protozoal disease of the Genus Plasmodium transmitted by mosquitos breeding in contaminated water, affects 300–500 million people, and causes over one million deaths each year (more than 90% of deaths in Africa). Overall the morbidity and mortality caused by contaminated water are enormous and need to be controlled by improving the security of safe water (i.e., recreational as well as drinking water) in both developing and developed countries.

Historical Perspective of Water-Borne Diseases

Water contamination has a long presence in human history, with descriptions in the Sushruta Samshita about water-borne diseases resembling cholera in an Indian text written in Sanskrit as early as 500–400 B.C. (Colwell [1996]). Although cholera infections have not been reported in recent years in developed countries mainly due to improved sanitation, millions of people each year continue to get infected by Vibrio cholera in developing countries (Nelson et al. [2009]). The World Health Organization reports about 3–5 million cholera cases and 10,000 – 120,000 deaths, mainly in developing countries, due to cholera every year. Over time, cholera has caused millions of deaths in developing as well as developed countries (Colwell [1996]; Okun [1996]). For instance, a major outbreak of cholera was reported in London in 1849. Dr. John Snow, a physician to Queen Victoria, showed a relationship between people infected by cholera and contaminated water (Snow [1854]; Colwell [1996]). Jordan et al. ([1904]), Ruediger ([1911]), Simons et al. ([1922]), and Rudolfs et al. ([1950]) provide excellent reviews on incidents during the early 19th century. Colwell ([1996]) reported that in the mid and late 18th century, cholera infected millions of people all over the world. The worst outbreak in recent memory occurred in Haiti following the devastating earthquake affecting the capital and surrounding regions, with almost a half a million cases, killing thousands of people (CDC [2011]).

Water-Borne Pathogen Footprints and Challenges

Indicator organisms are commonly used to assess the levels of pathogens in water resources; i.e., water-borne pathogen footprints of water resources. Monitoring the levels of indicator organisms (such as fecal coliforms, E. coli) (Figure 1) is a common approach for quantifying the potential pathogen loads in ambient water bodies. For decades, public health officials/scientists have evaluated water quality by enumerating fecal coliforms and E. coli levels in rivers, lakes, estuaries, and coastal waters (Malakoff [2002]; Pandey et al. [2012a]; Pandey et al. [2012b]; Pandey and Soupir [2013]). There is, however, much debate regarding current indicator organisms and their ability to represent the potential presence of pathogenic bacteria. In addition, identifying the source of pathogens (e.g., human waste, animal waste, wildlife excreta, and waterfowl droppings) (Figure 2) is challenging (Malakoff [2002]; Dickerson et al. [2007]). There is potential to use a relatively new approach such as microbial source tracking (MST) to trace the origin of fecal coliform (Scott et al. [2002]; Grave et al. [2007]; Dickerson et al. [2007]; Ibekwe et al. [2011]; Ma et al. [2014]). In the past, the MST method was exploited by antibiotic resistance analysis to assess the impact of cattle on water quality on a watershed scale (Grave et al. [2007]). The authors suggested that host-origin libraries, based on a phenotypic method, are useful for tracking the pathogen sources. Many MST methods, however, rely on the assumption that some strains of bacteria are found only within a single kind or group of animals. This assumption can be debatable when it comes to the common fecal bacteria E. coli (Malakoff [2002]). Therefore, caution is needed while using E. coli for source tracking (Gordon [2001]). Further, the cost to develop libraries, implement extensive sampling programs needed for verifying the MST method, and calculate uncertainties associated with the method are legitimate issues, which requires attention before exploiting the MST method at watershed scale.

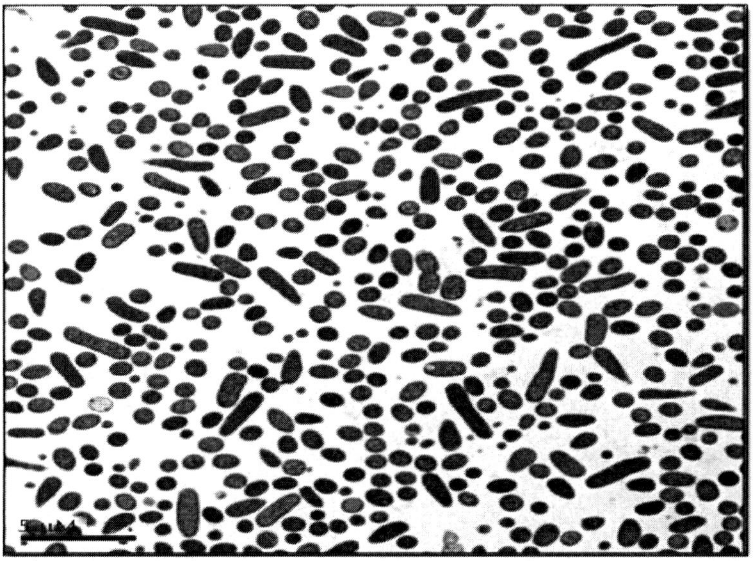

Figure 1: Transmission electron micrograph ofE. coli(0157:H7; ATCC: 35150).

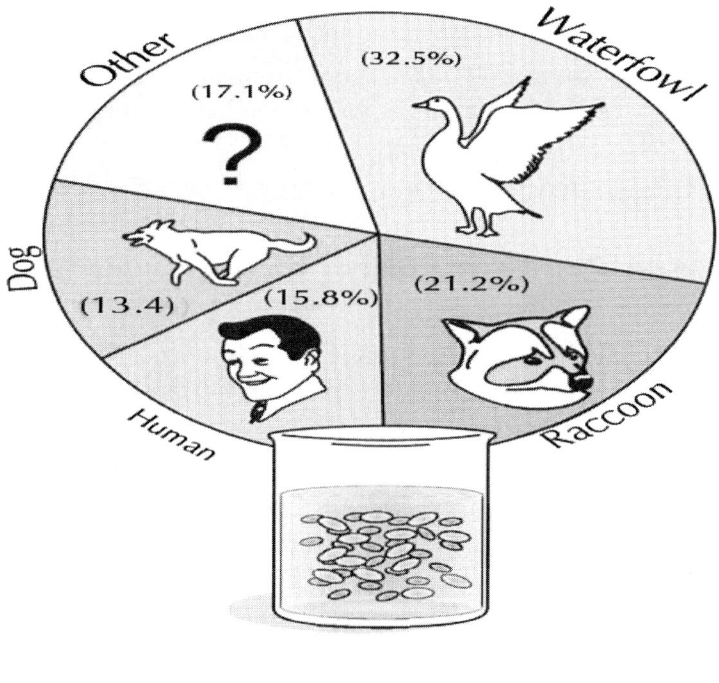

Figure 2: Challenges in identifying enteric pathogen sources (source: Malakoff, [2002]).

Currently, public health officials/scientists rely on exposure limits for assessing pathogen levels in water resources, which have been established to protect human health. The EPA defines acceptable recreational limits as those that will result in eight or fewer swimming-related gastrointestinal (GI) illnesses out of every 1,000 swimmers (U.S. EPA [1986]). The current U.S. EPA fresh water quality criteria for E. coli is a geometric mean not exceeding 126 CFU/100 ml, or no samples exceeding a single sample maximum of 235 CFU/100 ml (U.S. EPA [2001]). Criteria were developed based on the U.S. EPA measurements of total and Highly Credible Gastrointestinal Illnesses (HCGI), which correlated with E. coli densities (r=0.804) in fresh recreational waters (Dufour [1984]). Multiple studies have identified trends between indicator organisms in water and GI illness in humans, including vomiting, diarrhea, and fever (Cabelli [1983]; Wade et al. [2006]). Recent work by Edge et al. ([2010]) detected water-borne E. coli in 80% of water samples with E. coli levels of less than 100 CFU/100 ml. Another study by Wade et al. ([2006]) reported significant positive trends between increased GI illness and indicator organisms at the Lake Michigan beach, and a positive trend with indicators such as E. coli at a Lake Erie beach. Recently, the use of indicator organisms (e.g., fecal coliforms, E. coli) for assessing pathogen levels has been debated more often than ever; however, the use of indicator organisms is likely to continue for assessing pathogen levels in water resources potentially because of the lack of an alternative reliable solution.

Pathogen Contamination in Water Resources

The U.S. EPA, which monitors water quality of various ambient water bodies, estimated that pathogens impair more than 480,000 km of rivers and shorelines and 2 million ha of lakes in the U.S. (U.S. Environmental Protection Agency [2010a]). According to EPA estimates, pathogens are the leading cause of impairment for 303 (d) listed waters (i.e., list of impaired and threatened waters that the Clean Water Act requires all states to submit for EPA approval) (Figure 3) (U.S. EPA [2014a], [2014b], [2014c]). A total of 71,917 causes of impairment have been reported, and the top five causes of impairment are shown in Figure 3. Pathogen contamination clearly dominates the causes of impairment (U.S. EPA [2014a], [2014b], [2014c]).

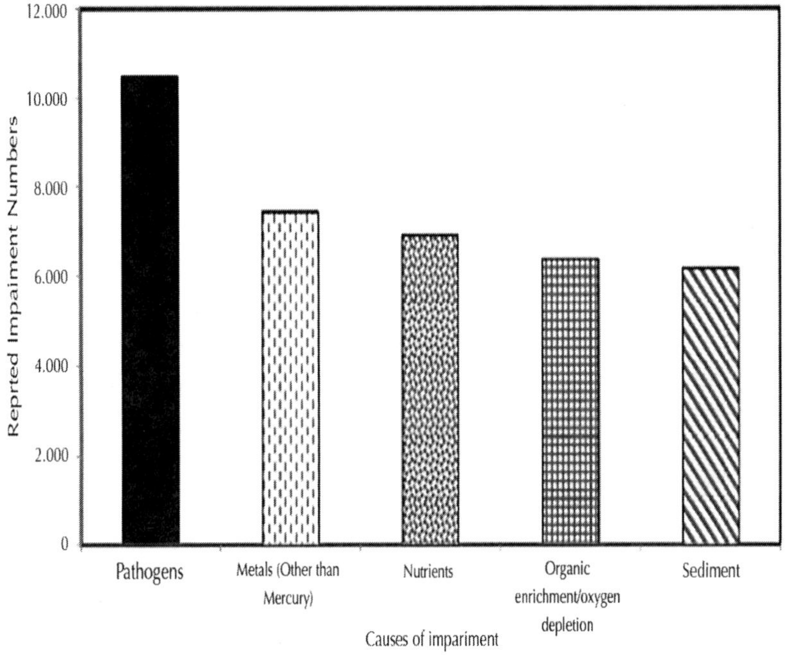

Figure 3: Causes of impairment in the U.S. (data source: U.S. EPA ([2014a],[2014b],[2014c])).

Studies by Diffey ([1991]), Brookes et al. ([2004]), Jamieson et al. ([2004]), Gerba and Smith ([2005]), Gerba and McLeod ([1976]), Hipsey et al. ([2008]), Pachepsky and Shelton ([2011]) reviewed the current studies of water-borne pathogen transport, with particular reference to freshwater and estuarine sediments. In addition, many current reviews focus on specific aspects of water resources, for instance, John and Rose ([2005]) focused on groundwater, Brookes et al. ([2004]) focused on reservoirs and lakes, Jamieson et al. ([2004]) focused on agricultural watersheds, and Kay et al. ([2007]) reviewed catchment microbial dynamics. The review study presented here uses a relatively broader approach for understanding how water-borne pathogens can potentially impact public health and various ambient water bodies. In addition, existing challenges, while assessing pathogen levels in water resources are discussed.

Coastal and Estuarine Environments

In the U.S., elevated pathogen levels are a leading cause of impairments of coastal environments (U.S. EPA [2014a], [2014b], [2014c]). Urban runoff and sewers have been identified as the primary source of coastal water impairments. Rippey ([1994]) reported about 400 outbreaks and 14,000 cases caused by pathogen contaminated coastal water since the late 1800s in the U.S. Impairments of coastal environments have major economic impacts on the U.S. For example, losses caused by pathogen contamination in Massachusetts are more than $75 million each year (Weiskel et al. [1996]). The studies, which elaborate various pathogens in coastal environment and their survival mechanism, are summarized in Table 1.

Table 1: Studies describing pathogen contamination in saline water (coastal and estuary environments)

Author(s) year	**Organisms**	**Results**	**Study remarks**
Coastal water			
Gerba and McLeod ([1976])	E. coli, fecal coliform	Longer survival in the sediment presence in seawater	Sediment influence on pathogen survival
Goyal et al. ([1977])	Total coliform, fecal coliform	Sediments of shallow canal can act as a reservoir	Pathogens distribution in water and sediment
Kapuscinski and Mitchell ([1983])	E. coli, bacteriophages	E. coli survives longer than bacteriophages	Survival of pathogens in sunlight
Rao et al. ([1984])	Enteroviruses (Polio and Rota)	Abundance viruses were attached with sediment	Viruses distribution in water and sediment
Weiskel et al. ([1996])	Fecal coliform	Waterfowl major source of fecal coliform inputs	Pathogen source and transport pathways
Sinton et al. ([1999])	Bacteria and Fecal bacteriophages	Somatic coliphages shown prolonged survival	Sunlight influence on sewage-polluted seawater
Solo-Gabriele et al. ([2000])	E. coli	Riverbanks as the primary pathogen source	Sources of pathogens on subtropical environment
Nasser et al. ([2003])	Cryptosporidium, viruses, E. coli	E. coli die-off was faster than other pathogens	Comparative survival of various pathogens

Schriewer et al. ([2010])	Bacteroidales, fecal indicator, protozoa, bacteria	Bacteroidales have shown higher predictive skill than fecal indicators	Bacteroidales as a predictor of pathogens in coastal water
Estuaries			
Ketchum et al. ([1952])	Coliform, zooplankton	Sactericidal and predation caused coliform die-off	Processes responsible for pathogens decrease
Smith et al. ([1978])	Echovirus 1, coxsackieviruses	Sediment prolonged viruses survival	Persistence of pathogen viruses
Rhodes and Kator ([1990])	E. coli	Mortality rises in sunlight	Indigenous microbiota and sunlight influence
White et al. ([1998])	Perkinsus marinus	Use of Kriging analysis for disease prevalence	Use of GIS in pathogen distribution analysis
Lipp et al. ([2001])	Vibrio vulnificus	Salinity controls the distribution of pathogens	Distribution of human pathogens
Desmarais et al. ([2002])	E. coli, C. perfringens	Pathogens re-grown with tides and sterile sediment	Influence of soil on fecal indicator in tidally influenced environment
Frias-Lopez et al. ([2002])	Clostridium, Campylobacter,Arobacter	Pathogen partitioning was found in surface and overlying water	Bacterial communities partitioning between sea water, dead coral surface
Chandran and Hatha ([2005])	E. coli, Salmonella	E. coli shows better survival capacity than Salmonella	Relative survival in microcosm studies
Baker-Austin et al. ([2009])	Vibrio vulnificus	Prevalence of antibiotic resistance in a human pathogen	Multi-site analysis shows widespread antibiotic resistance in pathogens

Pandey *et al.*

Pandey *et al. AMB Express* 2014 **4**:51, doi:10.1186/s13568-014-0051-x

The sources of coastal water contamination are: point discharges of treated and untreated sewage from shoreline outfalls, and non-point discharges. The non-point sources, such as runoff from naturally vegetated areas, discharge pathogens into coastal waters. Besides runoff from vegetated areas, the storm water runoff from urban, commercial, and industrial lands also discharges pathogens into coastal waters. In addition, other sources, such as malfunctioning or poorly sited septic systems, can also introduce significant amounts of pathogens (Sayler et al. [1975]; Howe et al. [2002]). Weiskel et al. ([1996]) reported that direct deposition of waterfowl feces was a considerable source of pathogens. Fayer and Trout ([2005]) summarized the transport of various pathogens, such as Giardia, Toxoplasma, and Cryptosporidium (zoonotic parasites) in the coastal environment. Moreover, the presence of sediment in seawater can also increase the survival chance of fecal coliforms, such as E. coli (Gerba nd McLeod [1976]; Goyal et al. [1977]). Solo-Gabriele et al. ([2000]) showed that the location and timing of storms of the coastal area in tropical and subtropical environments are also important factors that can potentially influence coastal water quality.

Previous studies have shown that the direct discharge of storm water runoff into coastal waters through storm drain systems can cause pathogen contamination, even where separate storm and sanitary sewer systems are in place. For instance, Weiskel et al. ([1996]) found that about 16% of the total fecal coliform inputs were caused by storm water entering Buttermilk Bay in Massachusetts. In addition, coastal rivers draining largely undeveloped watersheds with extensive riparian wetlands can be a natural source of fecal pathogens to coastal waters (Viau et al. [2011]; Staley et al. [2014]; Roberts et al. [2013]; Liang et al. [2013]; Wilkes et al. [2014]). On-site septic systems can also contribute significant amounts of fecal pathogens to coastal waters in low-lying fine-grained geological settings where saturated soils enhance pathogen growth. Weiskel et al. ([1996]) reported that shoreline wrack deposits could act as a reservoir of fecal bacteria, and the removal of wrack deposits from inter-tidal zones can improve the water quality of adjacent coastal waters.

Similar to the coastal environment, increasing water-borne pathogen levels in estuaries are a serious threat to public health. Human activities can impact estuary pathogen levels when they are adjacent to populated areas, and often provide a means of transportation and substantial recreation (Schriewer et al. [2010]; Pachepsky and Shelton [2011]). The most common pathogens, previously identified in estuaries by Rhodes and Kator ([1990]), were Vibrio cholerae,Giardia, Cryptosporidium, Salmonella, and Campylobacter spp. As shown in Table 1, the presence of various pathogens (e.g., E. coli, C. perfringens, Clostridium, Salmonella) has been reported in many previous studies. Municipal point sources are the primary cause of pathogen contamination in estuaries. Urban water disposed through combined sewer outflows is the cause of approximately 12% of estuary impairments in the U.S. (Arnone and Walling [2007]). Pathogens, including Vibrio vulnificus which carries the highest fatality rate of any food-borne pathogen in the U.S., were detected in the Gulf of Mexico Estuary (Lipp et al. [2001]; Baker-Austin et al. [2009]). Several studies discovered that bed sediment plays a vital role (i.e., with the release of particle-attached pathogens from bed sediment to a water column through a resuspension process) for the persistence and transport of pathogens in the estuaries (Smith et al. [1978]; Desmarais et al. [2002]). Previous studies have shown that pathogen growth and decay are influenced by environmental conditions. For instance, a study by Chandran and Hatha ([2005]) revealed that sunlight is a major factor that influences survival of pathogens like E. coli and S. typhimurium in the estuarine water.

Groundwater

Groundwater is heavily used all over the world as the primary source of domestic drinking water supplies, and contaminated groundwater certainly enhances risk to public health. Nationally, 40% of the U.S. domestic water supply originates from groundwater, and over 40 million people use groundwater as their drinking water via private wells (Alley et al. [1999]). Groundwater pathogen contamination has led to numerous disease outbreaks in the U.S.; for example, at least 46 outbreaks of disease occurred between 1992 and 1999, resulting in 2,739 cases of illness and several deaths (John and Rose [2005]). These are reported cases; due to underdiagnosis and underreporting, the actual morbidity is almost certainly higher.

Several studies have shown that microbial pathogens, such as Salmonella, E. coli, S. faecalis, and enteroviruses are relatively stable in groundwater (Bittion et al. 1983; Schijven and Hassanizadeh[2000]; Pang et al. [2004]) (Table 2). Controlling groundwater pathogen contamination has recently been emphasized in many countries, as pathogens can survive up to 400 days depending on the soil temperature (Nevecherya et al. [2005]; Filip and Demnerova [2009]). For example, identifying sources of groundwater pathogen contamination has received significant attention in France (Grisey et al. [2010]). Many studies reported that health risks caused by chlorine-resistant protozoans, such as Cryptosporidium spp. (Ferguson et al. [2003]; Kay et al. [2007]; Kay et al.[2008]), are considerable. One of the major concerns is that wetlands without lining might cause pathogen contamination of groundwater (Kay et al. [2007]). Similar concerns have been expressed in the United Kingdom by water regulators. The European Union (EU) has also emphasized protecting groundwater from pathogen contamination. Pathogen-contaminated groundwater can cause pollution in coastal environments. For example, a study of Buttermilk Bay has shown that groundwater is capable of transporting a large quantity of pathogens from surface to sub-surface water either by direct discharge or by discharge to rivers flowing into the bay (Moog[1987]; Weiskel et al. [1996]). The risk of contaminating groundwater particularly increases in areas where shallow aquifers exist. In these situations it is more likely that contaminated surface water or water from septic tanks can reach groundwater (Weiskel et al. [1996]). Precipitation events are likely to increase groundwater pathogen contamination because of contaminated ground water recharge.

Table 2: Pathogen contamination in freshwater environment (ground water, rivers and lakes and reservoirs)

Author(s) year	**Organisms**	**Results**	**Study remarks**
Groundwater			
Bitton et al. ([1983])	Salmonella, E. coli, S. faecalis, enteroviruses	S. faecalis decay rate was similar to viruses	Survival of pathogens in groundwater
Schijven and Hassanizadeh ([2000])	Viruses	Viruses attachment with soil was influenced by pH, and favorable sites	Soil passage impacts on virus removal at field-scale
Pang et al. ([2004])	E. coli and F-RNA phages	Pathogens were sorbed in aquifer material	Transport of E. coli and F-RNA phages
Nevecherya et al. ([2005])	Salmonella, viruses, E. coli, shigellos	Mathematical model was derived for temperature depends inactivation rate	Pathogenic bacteria and viruses survival in groundwater
Filip and Demnerova ([2009])	Bacillus megaterium and Staphylococcus	Pathogens survived 10 to 100 days	Pathogens survival in groundwater; FT-IR characterization
Grisey et al. ([2010])	Total coliforms, E. coli, Enterococci, Pseudomonas aeruginosa, Salmonella and Staphylococcus aureus	Bacterial density monitoring coupled with artificial trace experiments proved useful in locating pathogens sources	Pathogens survival in groundwater and landfill leachate

Rivers			
Chin ([2010])	Fecal coliform	Summer and rainfall raises pathogens	Urban areas impacts on stream pathogens
Smith et al. ([1973])	Salmonella, fecal coliforms, streptococci	Salmonella decline was close to fecal coliform	Usefulness of indicators organisms
Burton et al. ([1987])	Pseudomonas aeruginosa, Salmonella newport, E. coli	Clay in sediments improves E. coli survival	Survival of pathogens in fresh water sediments
Smith et al. ([1987])	E. coli, Fecal bacteria	U.S. rivers shows decline in fecal indicator	Water quality assessment from 1974 to 1981
Terzieva and McFeters ([1991])	E. coli, Campylobacter jejuni, Yersinia enterocolitica	Temperate zone surface water serve as a rersisitent verhicle in transimsision of bacteria between animals and humans	Survival and injury study of bacteria in agricultural surface water
Terzieva and McFeters ([1991])	Yersinia enterocolitica and E. coli	Experimental design and environmental play major role in pathogens survival	Survival in stream water, comparison between field and lab studies
Fraser et al. ([1998])	Fecal coliform	Model predicted pathogens	Modelling non-point source pollution
Lakes and reservoirs			
Beaver and Crisman ([1989])	Ciliates	Grazing habits of ciliates are discussed	Predators roles in fresh water
Rubentschik et al. ([1936])	Serratia marcescens	Adsorption of bacteria could be questionable	Adsorption of bacteria in salt lakes
Mac Kenzie et al. ([1994])	Cryptosporidium	C. oocysts study passes through the filtration system of water supply	Contaminated water from Milwaukee lake caused outbreak
Wcislo and Chrost ([2000])	E. coli	Predators controlled pathogen levels	Survival of pathogens in man-made reservoir
Kistemann et al. ([2002])	E. coli, coliform, fecal streptococcal, and Clostridium perfringens	Most of the pathogens increases during extreme runoff events	Microbial load in drinking water reservoir during rainfall events
Howe et al. ([2002])	Cryptosporidium oocysts	Animal feces was a major source of pathogens	Water supply's oocysts caused outbreak in northern England
Ishii et al. ([2006])	E. coli	E. coli survived longer in soil	Presence and growth of E. coli in Lake superior watershed

Pandey *et al.*

Pandey *et al.* *AMB Express* 2014 **4**:51, doi:10.1186/s13568-014-0051-x

Pathogen contamination (e.g., bacteria, protozoa, and viruses) poses a serious risk in water resources. The transport of pathogens from surface water to groundwater increases the vulnerability of groundwater (Jin and Flury [2002]). These authors reported that 70% of the water-borne microbial illness outbreaks in the United States have been associated with ground water. Pathogens such as viruses are much smaller than bacteria and protozoa, and many can potentially reach groundwater through porous soil matrices. Jin and Flury ([2002]) reviewed the fate and transport of viruses in porous media to understand mechanisms and modeling of virus sorption, and concluded that factors such as solution chemistry, virus properties, soil properties, temperature, and association with solid particle influences virus survival, transport, and sorption in porous media. Pang ([2009]) studied microbial removal rates in subsurface media, and reported that soil types considerably influence microbial removal rates. For instance, volcanic soils, pumice sand, fine sand, and highly weathered aquifer rocks showed high removal rates. The author found that microbial removal rates were inversely correlated with infiltration rates and transport velocity.

Considerable work recently has been done towards understanding pathogen transport in the vadose zone (Wang et al. [2014a]; [2014b]; Unc and Goss [2004]; Darnault et al. [2004]). Groundwater can be contaminated by seepage and percolation of contaminated water from the vadose zone (Darnault et al. [2004]). The macropores of agricultural land are also known to play a considerable role in polluting groundwater, particularly from fields where manure is applied (Jamieson et al. [2002]). Unc and Goss ([2004]) evaluated the influence of manure on the transport of bacteria from land receiving manure to water resources. These authors reported that manure application in the land influences pathogen transport in the vadose zone. The presence of straw and coarse organic matter influences the persistence of bacteria, and manure application changes the physical configuration of soil, the soil chemistry, and the properties of the microbial cells, which control the survival and persistence of bacteria in soils. Another recent study by Wang et al. ([2014]) assessed the transport of E. coli in soils with preferential flow. The authors reported that a decrease in macropore length resulted in a decreased apparent saturated hydraulic conductivity of the macropore and an increase in the mass transfer. Wang et al. ([2014a];[2014b]) concluded that macropore length has a considerable influence on preferential transport ofE. coli.

Reservoirs and Lakes

Previous studies have shown the presence of many pathogens in lakes and reservoirs (Table 2), and that these pathogens can pose risks to human health. In many countries surface reservoirs serve as the main source of drinking water, and these surface water bodies are often vulnerable to pathogen contamination (Kistemann et al. [2002]). In the developed world, although there is increased awareness of water treatment for pathogen contamination and water quality, outbreaks of water-borne disease via public water supplies continue to be reported (Gibson et al. [1998]; Howe et al. [2002]; Brookes et al. [2004]).

In the past, more than 403,000 residents of the greater Milwaukee, Wisconsin area experienced gastrointestinal illnesses due to infection with the parasite Cryptosporidium parvum following contamination of the city's water supply, which was associated with inadequate filtration of contaminated water from Lake Michigan (Mac Kenzie et al. [1994]; Cicirello et al. [1997]). In the 1990s, Cryptosporidiosis became the most common cause of outbreaks associated with public drinking water supplies in the United Kingdom (Howe et al. [2002]). In developing countries, diseases such as diarrhea and cholera are the leading cause of morbidity (Nelson et al. [2009]). Overall, diarrhea associated with drinking contaminated water is responsible for 2 to 2.5 million deaths annually (Fenwick [2006]). In lakes and reservoirs, increased pathogens are often associated with storm events, and the stream inflow is considered to be the major source of pathogens during storm events. Elevated flows in rivers most likely agitate bed sediment, which causes enhancement of pathogen levels of the water column (Jamieson et al. [2005a]; Jamieson et al. [2005b]; Pandey and Soupir [2013]; Bai and Lung [2005]). During the rainy season, the influx of contaminated water from rivers to lakes and reservoirs can substantially increase pathogen levels (Kistemann et al. [2002]). The quantity of pathogen influxes from tributaries of lakes and reservoirs during the rainy season is of particular importance in determining pathogen transport and distribution (Brookes et al. [2004]).

Rivers

Pathogen contamination is a major cause of stream impairments. The sources of impairment and health risks induced by water-borne pathogens are extensively reported (Table 2). In the U.S. pathogen contamination is the leading cause of stream water pollution. The EPA's National Water Quality Inventory Report suggests that about 53% of the assessed rivers are impaired, and a majority of them are contaminated by pathogens (U.S. EPA [2012a]). The cost to implement the total maximum daily load (TMDL) plans to improve stream water is estimated as $0.9 to $4.3 billion per year (U.S. EPA [2010b]).

Pathogen influxes into rivers from agricultural lands (Figure 4) are the main cause of stream impairments (Chin [2010]; U.S. EPA [2012a]). A weak understanding of pathogen transport from agricultural lands to rivers is considered to be a major challenge in implementing and deriving suitable land management practices capable of improving stream water quality. For instance, despite common knowledge that agricultural land's non-point source pollution is a leading cause of stream impairment, it is difficult to identify points of origin of pathogens and the pathways by which they enter streams. As an example, pathogens are likely to enter rivers from many potential sources, including lateral inputs from pastures and riparian zones, influx of pathogen-contaminated groundwater, direct deposit of fecal matter from livestock and wildlife, discharge of contaminated sanitary sewer flows, and wastewater treatment plant effluents. In rainy events, pathogens in rivers are influenced by fresh input from watersheds as well as sub-surface flow. In addition, the resuspension of legacy pathogens from bed sediments can considerably increase pathogen levels (Cho et al. [2010]; Droppo et al. [2009]; Jamieson et al. [2005b]; Kiefer et al. [2012]; Nagels et al. [2002]; Muirhead et al. [2004]; Kim et al. [2010]; Smith et al. [2008]).

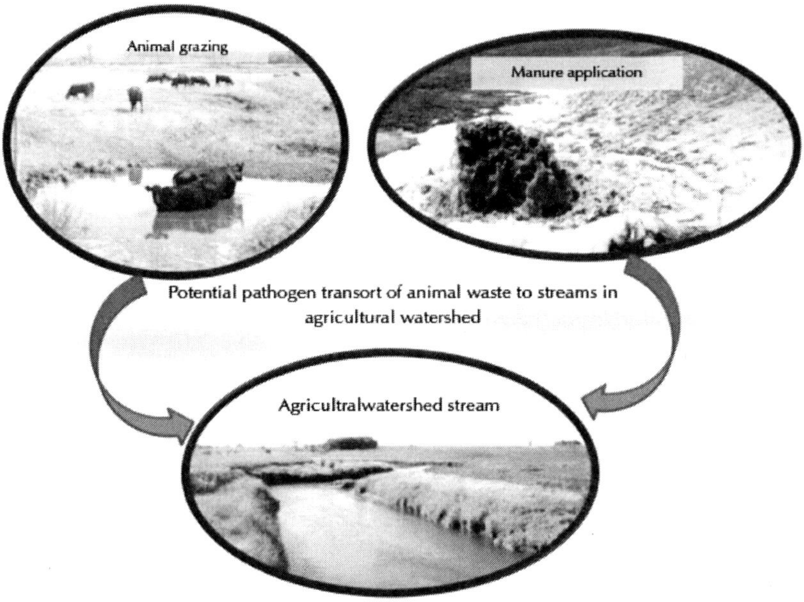

Figure 4: Simplified path of animal waste pathogen transport from agricultural land to rivers.

Controlling pathogen contamination from livestock/wildlife to streams is challenging (Terzieva and McFeters [1991]). For example, it is doubtful that pathogen contamination can be prevented by fencing off riparian buffers, and even if buffers are useful in controlling stream water pathogens, it is not certain what their width must be (Nagels et al. [2002]). There are review studies that elaborate on stream water pathogen contamination (Fraser et al. [1998]; Jamieson et al. [2004]; Pachepsky et al. [2006]).

Many studies have emphasized the use of mathematical models to understand pathogen transport from agricultural land to rivers (Kim et al. [2010]; Muirhead et al. [2004]; Jamieson et al. [2005a]; Jamieson et al. [2005b]). Previous studies (Gerba and Smith [2005]; Pandey et al. [2012b]; Pandey and Soupir [2013]; Pachepsky and Shelton [2011]; Martinez et al. [2014]) have emphasized the need to improve existing models for calculating the fate and transport of pathogens at the watershed scale. Currently, empirical as well as mechanistic models are being used to calculate microbial fate and transport (Muirhead and Monaghan [2012]). Numerous studies are available for exploiting watershed scale models such as WATFLOOD (Dorner et al. [2006]), the Soil and Water Assessment Tool (SWAT) (Neitsch et al. [2005]), the Spatially Explicit Deliver Model (SEDMOD) (Fraser [1999]), and KINEROS/STWIR (Guber et al. [2011]) for predicting pathogen transport. Though numerous watershed scale models are available, which can be exploited for calculating pathogen transport at watershed scale, considerable difficulties exist while using the models (Pandey et al. [2012b]; Pandey and Soupir [2013]). For instance, correctly identifying the model input parameter values is a daunting task. Recently, considerable emphasis has been given to understand the sensitivity of the input parameters to the model output (Martinez et al. [2014]; Parajuli et al. [2009]).

When implementing watershed scale models for predicting pathogen transport, difficulties related to the selection of model input parameters are common (Martinez et al. [2014]). A study by Parajuli et al. ([2009]) evaluated the sensitivity of fecal coliform bacteria loads modeled with SWAT, and the authors reported that many of the parameters (e.g., bacterial die-off rates, the temperature adjustment factor) were insensitive to the model output. Similarly, Coffey et al. ([2010]) reported that initial concentration of E. coli and the bacterial partition coefficient parameters of the SWAT model were overly sensitive in affecting the model's output. Another recent study by Martinez et al. ([2014]) evaluated the KINEROS/STWIF model input parameter sensitivities to the output. These authors reported that environmental controls such as soil saturation, rainfall duration, and rainfall intensity had the most sensitivity, while parameters such as soil and manure properties were the least sensitive in affecting model output. Many previous studies (Pandey and Soupir [2012a], [2012b]; Kim et al. [2010]; Martinez et al. [2014]; Parajuli et al. [2009]) reported that identification and selection of model input parameters are major challenges when implementing the model for predicting fate and transport of pathogens at the watershed scale.

Blooming of Cyanobacteria

While water-borne pathogens are a serious concern, excessive algal bloom (Figure 5) in water resources can potentially limit their uses for recreation activities as well as for drinking water. Cyanobacteria (blue-green algae) have unique roles in oxygenation of the atmosphere (Hofer[2013]); however, their excessive growth or dense algal bloom in water resources diminishes the quality and quantity of light in the water column ([U.S. EPA 2014b]). When blooms are excessive, the risk of toxin contamination (released by harmful algal bloom (HABs)) is likely to be elevated. The HAB includes many types of algal taxa such as dinoflagellates, diatoms, and cyanobacteria. Eutrophication caused by excessive algal bloom can cause fish kills and reduce the diversity of aquatic life ([U.S. EPA 2014b]). In hypoxic water, dissolved oxygen levels can be less than 2 – 3 ppm (U.S. EPA [2014c]). For example, in the hypoxic zone in the northern Gulf of Mexico, an area along the Louisiana-Texas coast, less than 2 ppm of dissolved oxygen concentration has been reported. This is believed to be caused by excess nutrients delivered from the Mississippi River, in combination with seasonal stratification of Gulf waters (U.S.G.S., [2014]). The largest U.S. hypoxic zone, which occurred in 2002 in the Gulf of Mexico, was about 13,518 square kilometers (U.S.G.S.[2012]).

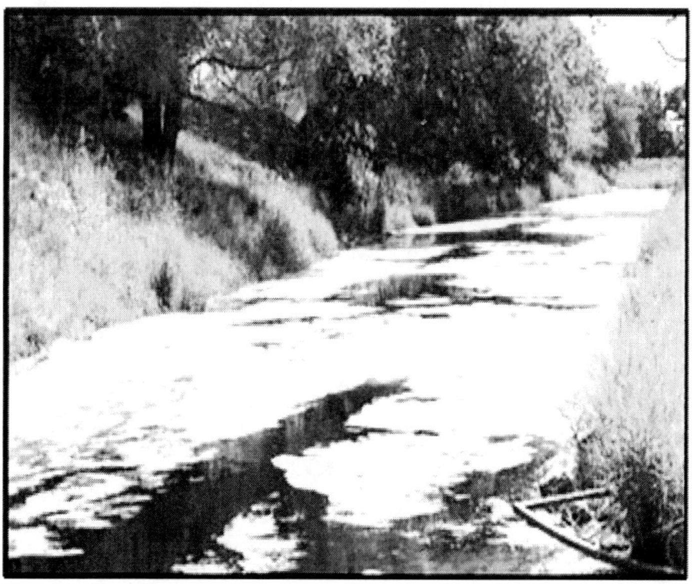

Figure 5: Algal bloom in Squaw Creek, Iowa, U.S.

Freshwater cyanobacterial blooms produce highly potent cyanotoxins and cyanobacterial HABs, which can affect the liver, nervous system, and skin (U.S. EPA [2014b]). Cyanobacterial blooms can be potentially detrimental to human and animal health, aquatic habitats, and aquaculture industries (Kaloudis et al. [2013]; Carmichael [2001];

Falconer [2005]; Codd et al. [1999]). Previous studies (Mackintosh et al. [1990]; Yoshizawa et al. [1990]) have shown that microcystins (i.e., cynotoxins) are hepatotoxic and act as tumor promoters through the inhibition of protein phosphatases, which play a key role in cellular regulation. Eutrophic water conditions combined with warm surface water temperatures (15 – 30°C) can potentially enhance cyanobacterial blooms in water (Oikonomou et al. [2012]; Vareli et al. [2009]). Currently more than 400 hypoxic zones exist in the world affecting 245,000 square kilometers (Diaz and Rosenberg [2008]). These dead zones in coastal waters have spread exponentially since the 1960s and have considerably impacted ecosystems. The increase in these dead zones is likely to be influenced by climate change. Various factors such as how climate change affects water-column stratification and how nutrient runoff affects organic matter production will determine further expansion of the dead zones (Diaz and Rosenberg [2008]). For instance, climate predictions of the Mississippi River basin indicate a 20% increase in river discharge, which will enhance nutrient loading and result in expansion of the oxygen depleted area (IPCC [2007]). Considering the importance of fresh water, estuarine, and marine environment to public health and aquatic life, identifying approaches capable of controlling excessive algal blooms is required before these dead zones spread globally.

Impact of Water Resources Development

Water resources development involves altering the natural flow path of rivers and lakes, as well as designing irrigation schemes and dams. These activities have been alleged to be responsible for causing new diseases and enhancing health risks (Fenwick [2006]; Steinmann et al. [2006]).

The influence of water resources development in spreading diseases, such as schistosomiasis, a parasitic disease which is ranked second only to malaria with regard to the number of people infected, has been reported extensively; one estimate says that about 103 million out of 779 million infected people live in close proximity to large reservoirs and irrigation schemes (Steinmann et al. [2006]).

Designing dams and irrigation schemes in tropical and subtropical climate zones has often resulted in disease outbreaks caused by water-borne pathogens. Consider, for example, the Sennar Dam on the Blue Nile River and Sudan's Gezira Scheme, the world's largest irrigation project. Because of the dam's commercial success, irrigation in the region has doubled from the 1940s and 1950s. After the 1950s, infections from malaria and schistosomiasis increased significantly, becoming the subject of the first integrated disease-control program, the Blue Nile Health Project, implemented from 1978 to 1990. The project failed to have any impact in controlling the prevalence of schistosomiasis (Eltoum et al. [1993]; Fenwick [2006]; Steinmann et al. [2006]). Another example is China's Three Gorges Dam, built across the Yangtze River and completed in 2009, which created a 50,700 km^2 reservoir and submerged more than 220 counties. Hotez et al. ([1997]) reported that the reservoir would produce environmental changes that could lead to the transmission of schistosomiasis in the area served by the dam. A recent study by Schrader et al. ([2013]) found major high risk areas for schistosomiasis occurrence in the large lakes and flood plain regions of the Yangtze River. Another study by Gray et al. ([2012]) reported that the Three Gorges Dam will likely to impact the transmission of schistosomiasis in China.

In the U.S., because of increasing concern for produce safety, pathogen-free irrigation water is attracting considerable attention (Martinez et al. [2014]). Painter et al. ([2013]) reported that produce accounted for nearly half of food-borne illnesses in the U.S. between 1998 and 2008. Growing concern about the safety of food and water will likely help in developing improved strategies while planning and designing large dams for irrigation purposes.

Challenges and Recommendations

Infectious diseases caused by pathogens are the third leading cause of death in the United States, and the leading cause in the world (Binder et al. [1999]). The past two decades have seen the emergence of many new pathogenic infectious diseases (Daszak et al. [2000]). Many of these are caused by anthropogenic changes, such as water resources development, climate warming, and interactions between humans and animals, both domestic and wild (Krause [1994]; Epstein [2001]; Woolhouse [2002]; Fenwick [2006]; Schriewer et al. [2010]).

Multidisciplinary knowledge about how ambient water bodies, wildlife, domestic animals, and human populations interact with and impact each other are crucial in dealing with future challenges. Generally, domestic animals, wildlife, and humans are considered to be major sources of water-borne pathogens; however, finding the specific culprit—the primary pathogen source—is challenging (Malakoff [2002]). A watershed, for example, can have many pathogen sources, such as agricultural land, riparian areas, agricultural feeding operations, livestock, wildlife, and humans.

Developing models that are reliable in predicting pathogen survival and transport at the watershed scale can be helpful in implementing/evaluating the strategies for mitigating ambient water body pathogen levels. Evaluating the impacts of various environmental factors on pathogen survival in water resources is crucial. Various publications (i.e., Dorner et al. [2006]; Kim et al. [2010]; Rehmann and Soupir [2009]; Droppo et al., [2011]; Cho et al. [2010]; Pandey et al. [2012b]; Pandey and Soupir [2013]) are available describing models capable of predicting pathogen contamination levels in ambient water bodies; however, further work is required to improve model predictions. The evaluation of predictions by existing models clearly demonstrates the need for improvement. Many pathogen transport models use only temperature-induced mortality and growth, and do not include interactions among other environmental factors (e.g., pH, nutrients, DO, solar radiation); future inclusion of these environmental factors will likely to improve the model predictions.

Typically most studies have relied on E. coli and other indicator bacteria to indicate pathogen levels in water. Although widely used in monitoring contamination levels, E. coli alone can lead to mercurial and misleading information (Gordon [2001]). Schriewer et al. ([2010]) suggested that with improved pathogen detection technology (i.e., PCR-based detection) an indicator organism, such as E. coli, can be sufficiently accurate in most cases. Overall, improving technology to identify causative agents more accurately, creating standard epidemiological data for diseased populations, and enhancing the knowledge of disease dynamics can improve the understanding of risks caused by interactions among various populations (Harvell et al. [1999]; Daszak et al.[2000]; Harvell et al. [2002]).

In the past, a number of studies on pathogen contamination have been conducted on a scale where the conditions of ambient water bodies were simulated in laboratories. These studies are helpful in understanding pathogen behavior only up to a point. For enhancing the understanding of pathogen interactions in the environment, more emphasis should be given to field-scale studies.

CONCLUSIONS

This review examines studies from various disciplines to understand pathogen contamination in ambient water bodies. The worldwide prevalence of pathogen contamination is a serious concern, and enhancing the understanding of major pathogen sources and their significant impacts on water resources is crucial. A considerable number of studies on pathogen contamination have been conducted on a laboratory-scale; more emphasis should be given to field-scale studies for enhancing the understanding of pathogen interactions in the environment. Developing new models, and improving existing modeling approaches commonly used for predicting water-borne pathogen levels will likely to help in assessing pathogen contamination at watershed-scale. Considering the limited ability of existing models to predict pathogen contamination, improvement and development of new models are needed so that pathogen levels can be predicted more accurately. Integrating knowledge from multiple fields (e.g., hydrology, microbiology, and ecology) would increase the understanding of pollution levels and potential causes of pollution, and can also help devise long-term strategies to improve water quality.

ACKNOWLEDGMENTS

The authors thank the Division of Agriculture and Natural Resources and Veterinary Medicine Extension, University of California, Davis, and National Science Foundation (award No. CBET-0967845) for supporting this work.

1. REFERENCES

2. Alley WM, Reilly TE, Franke OL (1999) Sustainability of Groundwater Resources. U.S. Geological Survey (U.S.GS), Denver, CO.
3. Arnone RD, Walling JP (2007) Waterborne pathogens in urban watersheds. J Water Health 5(1):149-162

4. Bai S, Lung WS (2005) Modeling sediment impact on the transport of fecal bacteria. Water Res 39:5232-5240
5. Baker-Austin C, McArthur J, Lindell A, Wright M, Tuckfield R, Gooch J, Warner L, Oliver J, Stepanauskas R (2009) Multi-site analysis reveals widespread antibiotic resistance in the marine pathogen: Vibrio vulnificus. Microb Ecol 57(1):151-159
6. Beaver JR, Crisman TL (1989) The role of ciliated protozoa in pelagic freshwater ecosystems. Microb Ecol 17(2):111-136
7. Binder S, Levitt AM, Sacks JJ, Hughes JM (1999) Emerging infectious diseases: public health issues for the 21st Century. Science 284(5418):1311-1313
8. Bitton G, Farrah SR, Ruskin RH, Butner J, Chou YJ (1983) Survival of pathogenic and indicator organisms. Groundwater 21(4):405-410
9. Bradford SA, Morales VL, Zhang W, Harvey RW, Packman AI, Mohanram A, Welty C (2013) Transport and fate of microbial pathogens in agricultural settings. Crit Rev Env Sci Tec 43:775-893
10. Brookes JD, Antenucci J, Hipsey M, Burch MD, Ashbolt NJ, Ferguson C (2004) Fate and transport of pathogens in lakes and reservoirs. Environ Int 30(5):741-759
11. Burton GA, Gunnison D, Lanza GR (1987) Survival of pathogenic bacteria in various freshwater sediments. Appl Environ Microbiol 53(4):633-638
12. Cabelli VJ (1983) Public health and water quality significance of viral diseases transmitted by drinking water and recreational water. Water Sci Technol 15(5):1-15
13. Carmichael WW (2001) Health effects of toxin-producing cyanobacteria: the CyanoHABs. Hum Ecol Risk Assess 7:1393-1407
14. (2011) Cholera in Haiti: One Year Later.
15. (2014) Salmonella.
16. Chandran A, Mohamed Hatha AAM (2005) Relative survival of Escherichia coli and Salmonella typhimurium in a tropical estuary. Water Res 39(7):1397-1403
17. Chin DA (2010) Linking pathogen sources to water quality in small urban streams. J Environ Eng 136(2):249-253

18. Cho KH, Pachepsky YA, Kim JH, Guber AK, Shelton DR, Rowland R (2010) Release of Escherichia coli from the bottom sediment in a first-order creek: Experiment and reach-specific modeling. J Hydrol 391(3–4):322-332
19. Cicirello HG, Kehl KS, Addiss DG, Chusid MJ, Glass RI, Davis JP, Havens PL (1997) Cryptosporidiosis in children during a massive waterborne outbreak in Milwaukee, Wisconsin: clinical, laboratory and epidemiologic findings. Epidemiol Infect 119(1):53-60
20. Codd G, Bell S, Kaya K, Ward C, Beattie K, Metcalf J (1999) Cyanobacterial toxins, exposure routes and human health. Eur J Phycol 34:405-415
21. Coffey R, Cummins EO, Flaherty V, Cormican M (2010) Pathogen sources estimation and scenario analysis using the Soil and Water Assessment Tool (SWAT). Hum Ecol Risk Assess 16(4):913-933
22. Colwell RR (1996) Global climate and infectious disease: The Cholera Paradigm. Science 274(5295):2025-2031
23. Craun GF, Fraun MF, Calderon RL, Beach MJ (2006) Waterborne outbreaks reported in the United States. J Water Health 4:19-30
24. Darnault CJD, Steenhuis TS, Garnier P, Kim YJ, Jenkins MB, Ghiorse WC, Baveye PC, Parlange JY (2004) Preferential flow and transport of Cryptosporidium parvum oocysts through the vadose zone: Experiments and modeling. Vadose Zone J 3(2):262-270
25. Daszak P, Cunningham AA, Hyatt AD (2000) Emerging infectious diseases of wildlife – threats to biodiversity and human health. Science 287:443-449
26. Desmarais TR, Solo-Gabriele HM, Palmer CJ (2002) Influence of soil on fecal indicator organisms in a tidally influenced subtropical environment. Appl Environ Microbiol 68(3):1165-1172
27. Diaz RJ, Rosenberg R (2008) Spreading dead zones and consequences for marine ecosystems. Science 321:926-929
28. Dickerson JW, Crozier JB, Hagedorn G, Hassall A (2007) Assessment of 16 s-23srDNA interagenic spacer regions in Eterococcus spp. for microbial source tracking. J Environ Qual 36:1661-1669.
29. Diffey BL (1991) Solar ultraviolet-radiation effects on biological-systems. Phys Med Biol 36(3):299-328

30. Dorner SM, Anderson WB, Slawson RM, Kouwen N, Huck PM (2006) Hydrologic modeling of pathogen fate and transport. Environ Sci Technol 40(15):4746-4753

31. Droppo IG, Liss SN, Williams D, Nelson T, Jaskot C, Trapp B (2009) Dynamic existence of waterborne pathogens within river sediment compartments: Implications for water quality regulatory affairs. Environ Sci Technol 43(6):1737-1743

32. Droppo IG, Krishnappan BG, Liss SN, Marvin C, Biberhofer (2011) Modeling sediment-microbial dynamics in the South Nation River, Ontario, Canada: Towards the prediction of aquatic and human health risk. Water Res 45:3797-3809

33. Dufour A (1984) Health Effects Criteria for Fresh Recreational Waters. Toxicology and Microbiology Division, U.S. Environmental Protection Agency Report EPA- 600-1-84-2004. Cincinnati, OH

34. Edge TA, Hill S, Seto P, Marsalek J (2010) Library-dependent and library independent microbial source tracking to identify spatial variation in faecal contamination sources along a Lake Ontario beach (Ontario, Canada). Water Sci Technol 62:719-727

35. Eltoum IA, Sulaiman SM, Elturabi H, Mahgoub E, Homeida MMA (1993) Infection with Schistosoma-Mansoni in 2 different endemic areas – a comparative population – based study in Elzidab and Gezira-Managil irrigation schemes, Sudan. J Trop Med Hyg 96(2):100-106

36. Epstein PR (2001) Climate change and emerging infectious diseases. Microbes Infect 3(9):747-754

37. Falconer IR (2005) Is there a human health hazard from microcystins in the drinking water supply? Acta Hydrochim Hydrobiol 33:64-71

38. Fayer R, Trout JM (2005) Zoonotic protists in the marine environment. In: Belkin S and Colwell RR (ed) Oceans and Health:. Pathogens in the Marine Environment, Springer, New York, U.S.

39. Fenwick A (2006) Waterborne Infectious Diseases-Could they be consigned to History? Science 313:1077-1081

40. Ferguson C, Husman AMD, Altavilla N, Deere D, Ashbolt N (2003) Fate and transport of surface water pathogens in watersheds. Crit Rev Environ Sci Technol 33(3):299-361

41. Filip Z, Demnerova K (2009) Survival in groundwater and FT-IR characterization of some pathogenic and indicator bacteria. In: Jones JAA, Vardanian TG, Hakopian C (ed). Threats to Global Water Security, Springer, Dordrecht, The Netherlands.
42. Fraser RH (1999) SEDMOD: A GIS-based delivery model for diffuse source pollutants. Yale University, PhD dissertation, School of Forestry and Environmental Studies.
43. Fraser RH, Barten PK, Pinney DAK (1998) Predicting stream pathogen loading from livestock using a geographical information system-based delivery model. J Environ Qual 27(4):935-945
44. Frias-Lopez J, Zerkle AL, Bonheyo GT, Fouke BW (2002) Partitioning of bacterial communities between seawater and healthy, black band diseased, and dead coral surfaces. Appl Environ Microbiol 68(5):2214-2228
45. Gerba CP, McLeod JS (1976) Effect of sediments on the survival of Escherichia coli in marine waters. Appl Environ Microbiol 32(1):114-120
46. Gerba CP, Smith J (2005) Sources of pathogenic microorganisms and their fate during land application of wastes. J Environ Qual 34:42-48
47. Gibson CJ, Haas CN, Rose JB (1998) Risk assessment of waterborne protozoa: current status and future trends. Parasitology 117:S205-S212
48. Gordon DM (2001) Geographical structure and host specificity in bacteria and the implications for tracing the source of coliform contamination. Microbiology 147(5):1079-1085
49. Goyal SM, Gerba CP, Melnick JL (1977) Occurrence and distribution of bacterial indicators and pathogens in canal communities along Texas Coast. Appl Environ Microbiol 34(2):139-149
50. Grave AK, Hagedorn C, Brooks A, Hagedorn RL, Martin E (2007) Microbial source tracking in a rural watershed dominated by cattle. Water Res 41:3729-3739
51. Gray DJ, Thrift AP, Williams GM, Zheng F, Li Y-S, Guo J, Chen H, Wang T, Xu XJ, Zhu R, Zhu H, Cao CL, Lin DD, Zhao ZY, Li RS, Davis GM, McManus DP (2012) Five-year longitudinal assessment of the downstream impact on schistosomiasis

transmission following closure of the Three Gorges Dam. PLoS Negl Trop Dis 6(4):e 1588 doi:10.1371/journal.pntd.0001588

52. Grisey E, Belle E, Dat J, Mudry J, Aleya L (2010) Survival of pathogenic and indicator organisms in groundwater and landfill leachate through coupling bacterial enumeration with tracer tests. Desalination 261(1–2):162-168

53. Guber AK, Pachepsky YA, Yakirevich AM, Shelton DR, Sadeghi AM, Goodrich DC, Unkrich CL (2011) Uncertainty in modelling of faecal coliform overland transport associated with manure application in Maryland. Hydrolical Process 25(15):2393-2404

54. Harvell CD, Kim K, Burkholder JM, Colwell RR, Epstein PR, Grimes DJ, Hofmann EE, Lipp EK, Osterhaus AD, Overstreet RM, Porter JW, Smith GW, Vasta GR (1999) Emerging marine diseases-climate links and anthropogenic factors. Science 285(5433):1505-1510

55. Harvell CD, Mitchell CE, Ward JR, Altizer S, Dobson AP, Ostfeld RS, Samuel MD (2002) Climate warming and disease risks for terrestrial and marine biota. Science 296:2158-2162

56. Hipsey MR, Antenucci JP, Brookes JD (2008) A generic, process-based model of microbial pollution in aquatic systems. Water Resour Res 44(7):

57. Hofer U (2013) Getting to the bottom of Cyanobacteria. Nat Rev Microbiol 11:818-819

58. Hotez PJ, Feng Z, Xu LQ, Chen MG, Xiao SH, Liu SX, Blair D, McManus DP, Davis GM (1997) Emerging and reemerging helminthiases and the public health of China. Emerg Infect Dis 3(3):303-310

59. Howe AD, Forster S, Morton S, Marshall R, Osborn KS, Wright P, Hunter PR (2002) Cryptosporidiumoocysts in a water supply associated with a cryptosporidiosis outbreak. Emerg Infect Dis 8(6):619-624

60. Ibekwe AM, Murinda SE, Graves AK (2011) Genetic diversity and antimicrobial resistance ofEscherichia coli from human and animal sources uncovers multiple resistances from human sources. PLoS One 6:e20819 doi:10.1371/journal.pone.0020819

61. (2007) IPCC Fourth Assessment Report, Summary for Policymakers.

62. Ishii S, Ksoll WB, Hicks RE, Sadowsky MJ (2006) Presence and growth of naturalized Escherichia coli in temperate soils from Lake Superior watersheds. Appl Environ Microbiol 72(1):612-621
63. Jamieson R, Gordon R, Sharples K, Stratton G, Madani A (2002) Movement and persistence of fecal bacteria in agricultural soils and subsurface drainage water: A review. Can Biosyst Eng 44:1.1-1.90
64. Jamieson R, Gordon R, Joy D, Lee H (2004) Assessing microbial pollution of rural surface waters: A review of current watershed scale modeling approaches. Agric Water Manag 70(1):1-17
65. Jamieson R, Joy DM, Lee H, Kostaschuk R, Gordon R (2005) Transport and deposition of sediment-associated Escherichia coli in natural streams. Water Res 39(12):2665-2675
66. Jamieson RC, Joy DM, Lee H, Kostaschuk R, Gordon RJ (2005) Resuspension of sediment-associated Escherichia coli in a natural stream. J Environ Qual 34(2):581-589
67. Jin Y, Flury M (2002) Fate and transport of viruses in porous media. Adv Agron 77:39-102
68. John DE, Rose JB (2005) Review of factors affecting microbial survival in groundwater. Environ Sci Tech 39(19):7345-7356
69. Jordan EO, Russell HL, Zeit FR (1904) The longevity of the typhoid bacillus in water. J Infect Dis 1(4):641-689
70. Kaloudis T, Zervou S, Tsimeli K, Triantis TM, Fotiou T, Hiskia A (2013) Determination of microcystins and nodularin (cyanobacterial toxins) in water by LC-MS/MS. Monitoring of Lake Marathonas, a water reservoir of Athens, Greece. J Hazard Mater 263:105-115
71. Kapuscinski RB, Mitchell R (1983) Sunlight-induced mortality of viruses and Escherichia coli in coastal seawater. Environ Sci Technol 17(1):1-6
72. Kay D, Edwards AC, Ferrier RC, Francis C, Kay C, Rushby L, Watkins J, McDonald AT, Wyer M, Crowther J, Wilkinson J (2007) Catchment microbial dynamics: the emergence of a research agenda. Prog Phys Geogr 31(1):59-76
73. Kay D, Crowther J, Stampleton CM, Wyer MD, Fewtrell L, Anthony S, Bradford M, Edwards A, Francis CA, Hopkins M, Kay C, McDonald AT, Watkins J, Wilkinson J (2008) Faecal indicator

organism concentrations and catchment export coefficients in the UK. Water Res 42:2649-2661

74. Ketchum BH, Ayers JC, Vaccaro RF (1952) Processes contributing to the decrease of coliform bacteria in a tidal estuary. Ecology 33(2):247-258
75. Kiefer LA, Shelton DR, Pachepsky Y, Blaustein R, Santin-Duran M (2012) Persistence of E. coli introduced into streabe dsedient with goose, deer and bovine animal waste. Lett Appl Microbiol 55(5):345-353
76. Kim JW, Pachepsky YA, Shelton DR, Coppock C (2010) Effect of streambed bacteria release on E. coli concentrations: Monitoring and modeling with the modified SWAT. Ecol Model 221(12):1592-1604
77. Kistemann T, Classen T, Koch C, Dangendorf F, Fischeder R, Gebel J, Vacata V, Exner M (2002) Microbial load of drinking water reservoir tributaries during extreme rainfall and runoff. Appl Environ Microbiol 68(5):2188-2197
78. Krause RM (1994) Dynamics of emergence. J Infect Dis 170(2):265-271
79. Liang Z, He Z, Zhou X, Powell C, Yang Y, He LM, Stoffella PJ (2013) Impact of mixed land-use practices on the microbial water quality in a subtropical coastal watershed. Sci Total Environ 449:426-433
80. Lipp EK, Rodriguez-Palacios C, Rose JB (2001) Occurrence and distribution of the human pathogen Vibrio vulnificus in a subtropical Gulf of Mexico estuary. Hydrobiologia 460(1):165-173
81. Ma LP, Li B, Zhang T (2014) Abundant rifampin resistance genes and significant correlations of antibiotic resistance genes and plasmids in various environments revealed by metagenomic analysis. Appl Microbiol Biotechnol 98:5195-5204 doi:10.1007/s00253-014-5511-3
82. Mac Kenzie WR, Hoxie NJ, Proctor ME, Gradus MS, Blair KA, Peterson DE, Kazmierczak JJ, Addiss DG, Fox KR, Rose JB, Davis JP (1994) A massive outbreak in Milwaukee of Cryptosporidiuminfection transmitted through the public water supply. N Engl J Med 331(3):161-167

83. MacKintosh C, Beattie KA, Klumpp S, Cohen P, Codd GA (1990) Cyanobacterial microcystin-LR is a potent and specific inhibitor of protein phosphatases 1 and 2A from both mammals and higher plants. FEBS Lett 264:187-192
84. Malakoff D (2002) Water quality: microbiologists on the trail of polluting bacteria. Science 295(5564):2352-2353
85. Martinez G, Pachepsky YA, Whelan G, Yakirevich AM, Guper A, Gish T (2014) Rainfall-induced fecal indicator organisms transport from manured fields: Model sensitivity analysis. Environ Int 63:121-129
86. Moog PL (1987) The hydrogeology and freshwater influx of Buttermilk Bay, Massachusetts, with regard to the circulation of coliforms and pollutants: a model study and development of methods for general application. Boston University, Boston, MA.
87. Muirhead RW, Monaghan RM (2012) A two reservoir model to predict Escherichia coli losses to water from pastures grazed by dairy cows. Environ Int 40:8-14
88. Muirhead RW, Davies-Colley RJ, Donnison AM, Nagels JW (2004) Faecal bacteria yields in artificial flood events: quantifying in-stream stores. Water Res 38(5):1215-1224
89. Nagels JW, Davies-Colley RJ, Donnison AM, Muirhead RW (2002) Faecal contamination over flood events in a pastoral agricultural stream in New Zealand. Water Sci Technol 45(12):45-52
90. Nasser AM, Zaruk N, Tenenbaum L, Netzan Y (2003) Comparative survival of Cryptosporidium, coxsackievirus A9 and Escherichia coli in stream, brackish-and sea waters. Water Sci Technol 47(3):91-96
91. Neitsch SL, Arnold JG, Kiniry JR, Williams JR, King KW (2005) Soil and water assessment tool: theoretical documentation, version 2005. Texas, U.S.A, Elsevier.
92. Nelson EJ, Harris JB, Glenn Morris J, Calderwood SB, Camilli A (2009) Cholera transmission: the host, pathogen and bacteriophage dynamic. Nat Rev Microbiol 7(10):693-702
93. Nevecherya IK, Shestakov VM, Mazaev VT, Shlepnina TG (2005) Survival rate of pathogenic bacteria and viruses in groundwater. Water Resources 32(2):209-214

94. Oikonomou A, Katsiapi M, Karayanni H, Moustaka-Gouni M, Kormas KA (2012) Plankton microorganisms coinciding with two consecutive mass fish kills in a newly reconstructed lake. Sci World J 2012:1-14 doi:10.1100/2012/504135
95. Okun DA (1996) From cholera to cancer to cryptosporidiosis. J Environ Eng 122(6):453-458
96. Pachepsky YA, Shelton DR (2011) Escherichia coli and fecal coliforms in freshwater and estuarine sediments. Crit Rev Env Sci Tec 41(12):1067-1110
97. Pachepsky YA, Sadeghi AM, Bradford SA, Shelton DR, Guber AK, Dao T (2006) Transport and fate of manure-borne pathogens: Modeling perspective. Agric Water Manag 86(1–2):81-92
98. Painter JA, Hoekstra RM, Ayers T, Tauxe RV, Braden CR, Angulo FJ, Griffin PM (2013) Attribution of foodborne illnesses, hospitalizations, and deaths to food commodities by using outbreak data, United States, 1998–2008. Emerg Infect Dis 19(3):407-415
99. Pandey PK, Soupir ML (2012a) Non-point Source Pollution. Berkshire Encyclopedia of Sustainability: Ecosystem Management and Sustainability. Berkshire Publishing Group, LLC, Great Barrington, MA, U.S.
100. Pandey PK, Soupir ML (2013) Assessing the impacts of E. coli laden streambed sediment on E. coliloads over a range of flows and sediment characteristics. J Am Water Resour Assoc 49(6):1261-1269
101. Pandey PK, Soupir ML, Rehmann CR (2012b) A model for predicting resuspension of Escherichia coli from streambed sediments. Water Res 46:115-126
102. Pang L (2009) Microbial removal rates in subsurface media estimated from published studies of field experiments and large intact soil cores. J Environ Qual 38:1531-1559 doi:10.2134/jeq2008.0379
103. Pang L, Close M, Goltz M, Sinton L, Davies H, Hall C, Stanton G (2004) Estimation of septic tank setback distances based on transport of E. coli and F-RNA phages. Environ Int 29(7):907-921
104. Parajuli PB, Douglas-Mankin KR, Barnes PL, Rossi CG (2009) Fecal bacteria source characterization and sensitivity analysis of SWAT 2005. Trans ASAE 52:1847-1858

105. Rao VC, Seidel KM, Goyal SM, Metcalf TG, Melnick JL (1984) Isolation of enteroviruses from water, suspended solids, and sediments from Galveston Bay: survival of poliovirus and rotavirus adsorbed to sediments. Appl Environ Microb 48(2):404-409
106. Rehmann CR, Soupir ML (2009) Importance of interactions between the water column and the sediment for microbial concentrations in streams. Water Res 43(18):4579-4589
107. Rhodes MW, Kator HI (1990) Effects of sunlight and autochthonous microbiota on Escherichia coli survival in an estuarine environment. Curr Microbiol 21(1):65-73
108. Rippey SR (1994) Infectious-diseases associated with molluscan shellfish consumption. Clin Microbiol Rev 7(4):419-425
109. Roberts MC, Soge OO, No D (2013) Comparison of multi-drug resistant environmental methicillin-resistant Staphylococcus aureus isolated from recreational beaches and high touch surfaces in built environment. Front Microbiol 4(74):1-8, doi:10.3389/fmicb.2013.00074
110. Rubentschik L, Roisin MB, Bieljansky FM (1936) Adsorption of bacteria in Salt Lakes. J Bacteriol 32(1):11-31
111. Rudolfs W, Falk LL, Ragotzkie RA (1950) Literature review on the occurrence and survival of enteric, pathogenic, and relative organisms in soil, water, sewage, and sludge, and on vegetation. Sewage Ind Wastes 22(10):1261-1281
112. Ruediger GF (1911) Studies on the self-purification of streams. Am J Public Health Assoc 1(6):411-415
113. Sayler GS, Nelson JD, Justice A, Colwell RR (1975) Distribution and significance of fecal indicator organisms in the Upper Chesapeake Bay. Appl Environ Microb 30(4):625-638
114. Schijven JF, Hassanizadeh SM (2000) Removal of viruses by soil passage: overview of modeling, processes, and parameters. Crit Rev Env Sci Tec 30(1):49-127
115. Schrader M, Hauffe T, Zhang Z, Davis GM, Jopp F, Remais JV, Wilke T (2013) Spatially explicit modeling of Schistosomiasis risk in eastern China based on a synthesis of epidemiological, environmental, and intermediate host genetic data. PLoS Negl Trop Dis 7(7):e2327

116. Schriewer A, Miller WA, Byrne BA, Miller MA, Oates S, Conrad PA, Hardin D, Yang HH, Chouicha N, Melli A, Jessup D, Dominik C, Wuertz S (2010) Presence of bacteroidales as a predictor of pathogens in surface waters of the Central California coast. Appl Environ Microbiol 76(17):5802-5814

117. Scott TW, Takken W, Knols BGJ, Boete C (2002) The ecology of genetically modified mosquitoes. Science 298(5591):117-119

118. Simons GW, Hilscher R, Ferguson HF, Gage SDM (1922) Report of the committee of bathing places. Am J Public Health 12(1):121-123

119. Sinton LW, Finlay RK, Lynch PA (1999) Sunlight inactivation of fecal bacteriophages and bacteria in sewage-polluted seawater. Appl Environ Microb 65(8):3605-3613

120. Smith RJ, Twedt RM, Flanigan LK (1973) Relationships of indicator and pathogenic bacteria in stream waters. Journal (Water Pollution Control Federation) 45(8):1736-1745

121. Smith EM, Gerba CP, Melnick JL (1978) Role of sediment in the persistence of enteroviruses in the estuarine environment. Appl Environ Microb 35(4):685-689

122. Smith RA, Alexander RB, Wolman MG (1987) Water-quality trends in the Nation's rivers. Science 235(4796):1607-1615

123. Smith J, Edwards J, Hilger H, Steck RTR (2008) Sediment can be a reservoir for coliform bacteria released into streams. J Gen Appl Microbiol 54:173-179

124. Snow J (1854) A Map of Cholera Deaths in London, 1840's. York University

125. Solo-Gabriele HM, Wolfert MA, Desmarais TR, Palmer CJ (2000) Sources of Escherichia coli in a coastal subtropical environment. Appl Environ Microb 66(1):230-237 [10.1890/13-1242.1]

126. Staley ZR, Rohr JR, Senkbeil JK, Harwood VJ (2014) Agrochemicals indirectly increase survival of E.coli O157:H7 and indicator bacteria by reducing ecosystem services. Ecol Appl, http://dx.doi.org/

127. Steinmann P, Keiser J, Bos R, Tanner M, Utzinger J (2006) Schistosomiasis and water resources development: systematic review, meta-analysis, and estimates of people at risk. Lancet Infect Dis 6(7):411-425

128. Terzieva SI, McFeters GA (1991) Survival and injury of E. coli, Campylobacter jejuni, and Yersinia Enterocolitica in stream water. Can J Microbiol 37(10):785-790 [http://water.epa.gov/scitech/datait/tools/waters/index.cfm]
129. U.S. Environmental Protection Agency (U.S. EPA) (1986) Ambient Water Quality Criteria for Bacteria. EPA 44015-84-002. Office of Regulations and Stand, Washington, DC, Accessed May 8 2014
130. U.S. Environmental Protection Agency (U.S. EPA) (2001) Protocol for Developing Pathogen TMDLs. National Summary of Impaired Waters and TMDL Information Washington, DC., Accessed May 8 2014
131. U.S. Environmental Protection Agency (U.S. EPA) (2010b) Protocol for Developing Pathogen TMDLs. National Summary of Impaired Waters and TMDL Information. Washington, DC, http://iaspub.epa.gov/waters10/ attains_nation_cy.control?p_report_type=T. Accessed May 8 2014
132. U.S. Environmental Protection Agency (U.S. EPA) (2012a) Impaired Waters and Total Maximum Daily Loads., Accessed May 8 2014
133. U.S. Environmental Protection Agency (U.S. EPA) (2012b) Drinking Water Contaminants. National Primary Drinking Water Regulations., http://water.epa. gov/drink/contaminants/#one. Accessed May 18 2014
134. U.S. Environmental Protection Agency (U.S. EPA) (2014a) Protocol for Developing Pathogen TMDLs. National Summary of Impaired Waters and TMDL Information. Washington, DC, http://iaspub.epa.gov/waters10/ attains_nation_cy.control?p_report_type=T. Accessed May 8 2014
135. U.S. Environmental Protection Agency (U.S. EPA) (2014b) Cyanobacterial Harmful Algal Blooms., http://www2.epa.gov/nutrient-policy-data/cyanobacterialharmful-algal-blooms-cyanohabs. Accessed May 8 2014
136. U.S. Environmental Protection Agency (U.S. EPA) (2014c) Hypoxia., http://water.epa.gov/type/watersheds/named/msbasin/hypoxia101.cfm. Accessed May 8 2014.
137. U.S. Geological Survey (U.S.G. S.) (2012) Dead Zone: the Source of the Gulf of Mexico's Hypoxia., http://www.usgs.gov/blogs/

features/usgs_top_story/deadzone-the-source-of-the-gulf-of-mexicos-hypoxia/. Accessed Apr 28 2014.

138. U.S. Geological Survey (U.S.G. S.) (2014) The Gulf of Mexico Hypoxic Zone.,
139. http://toxics.usgs.gov/hypoxia/hypoxic_zone.html. Accessed May 8 2014.
140. U.S. Geological Survey (U.S.G. S.) (2012) Dead Zone: the Source of the Gulf of Mexico's Hypoxia. http://toxics.usgs.gov/hypoxia/hypoxic_zone.html. Accessed May 8 2014
141. U.S. Geological Survey (U.S.G. S.) (2014) The Gulf of Mexico Hypoxic Zone. http://toxics.usgs.gov/hypoxia/hypoxic_zone.html. Accessed May 8 2014
142. Unc A, Goss MJ (2004) Transport of bacteria from manure and protection of water resources. Appl Soil Ecol 25:1-18
143. United Nation Children's Fund (UNICEF) (2014) World Water Day 2025: 4,000 children die each day from a lack of safe water. , http://www.unicef.org/wash/index_25637.html
144. Vareli K, Briasoulis E, Pilidis G, Sainis I (2009) Molecular confirmation of Planktothrix rubescens as the cause of intense, microcystin—synthesizing cyanobacterial bloom in Lake Ziros, Greece. Harmful Algae 8:447-453
145. Viau EJ, Goodwin KD, Yamahara KM, Layton BA, Sassoubre LM, Burns SL, Tong HI, Wong SHC, Lu Y, Boehm AB (2011) Bacterial pathogens in Hawaiian coastal streams — associations with fecal indicators, land cover, and water quality. Water Res 45:3279-3290
146. Wade TJ, Calderon RL, Sams E, Beach M, Brenner KP, Williams AH, Dufour AP (2006) Rapidly measured indicators of recreational water quality are predictive of swimming-associated gastrointestinal illness. Environ Health Perspect 114:24-28
147. Wang Y, Bradford SA, Simunek J (2014a) Estimation and upscaling of dual-permeability model parameters for the transport of Ecoli D21g in soils with preferential flow. J Contam Hydrol 159:57-66 [10.2136/vzj2013.07.0120]
148. Wang Y, Bradford SA, Simunek J (2014b) Physicochemical factors influencing the preferential transport of Escherichia coli in soils. Vadose Zone J 13(1) doi:10.2136/vzj2013.07.0120.

149. Wcislo R, Chrost RJ (2000) Survival of Escherichia coli in freshwater. Pol J Environ Stud 9(3):215-222

150. Weiskel PK, Howes BL, Heufelder GR (1996) Coliform contamination of a coastal embayment: Sources and transport pathways. Environ Sci Technol 30(6):1872-1881

151. White DL, Bushek D, Porter DE, Edwards D (1998) Geographic information systems (GIS) and kriging: analysis of the spatial and temporal distributions of the oyster pathogen Perkinsus marinusin a developed and an undeveloped estuary. J Shellfish Res 17(5):1473-1476

152. WHO (2011) Millennium Development Goals: progress towards the health-related Millennium Development Goals. http://www.who.int/mediacentre/factsheets/ fs290/en/index.html. Accessed 25 June 2012

153. Wilkes G, Brassard J, Edge TA, Gannon V, Jokinen CC, Jones TH, Lapen DR (2014) Coherence among different microbial source tracking markers in a small agricultural stream with or without livestock exclusion practices. Appl Environ Microbiol 79(20):6207-6219

154. Woolhouse MEJ (2002) Population biology of emerging and re-emerging pathogens. Trends Microbiol 10(10):s3-s7 [http://www.worldbank.org/en/topic/waterresourcesmanagement]

155. World Bank (2010) Water Resource Management. Washington, D. C, Accessed 26 Apr 2012

156. World Health Organization (WHO) (2010) Water Sanitation and Health. http:// www.who.int/water_sanitation_health/diseases/en/. Accessed 20 Apr 2012

157. World Health Organization (WHO) (2014) Water Quality and Health. Drinking water chlorination – A review of disinfection practices and issues, http:// www.waterandhealth.org/drinkingwater/wp.html. Accessed 28 Apr 2014

158. Yoshizawa S, Matsushima R, Watanabe MF, Harada K, Ichihara A, Carmichael WW, Fujiki H (1990) Inhibition of protein phosphatases by microcystis and nodularin associated with hepatotoxicity. J Cancer Res Clin Oncol 116:609 614

Citations

CHAPTER 1

Ponnerassery S. Sudheesh, Aliya Al-Ghabshi, Nashwa Al-Mazrooei, and Saoud Al-Habsi, "Comparative Pathogenomics of Bacteria Causing Infectious Diseases in Fish," International Journal of Evolutionary Biology, vol. 2012, Article ID 457264, 16 pages, 2012. doi:10.1155/2012/457264.

CHAPTER 2

Robin A. Bernhoft, "Mercury Toxicity and Treatment: A Review of the Literature," Journal of Environmental and Public Health, vol. 2012, Article ID 460508, 10 pages, 2012. doi:10.1155/2012/460508.

CHAPTER 3

Patricia Martínez Cruz, Ana L. Ibáñez, Oscar A. Monroy Hermosillo, and Hugo C. Ramírez Saad, "Use of Probiotics in Aquaculture," ISRN Microbiology, vol. 2012, Article ID 916845, 13 pages, 2012. doi:10.5402/2012/916845.

CHAPTER 4

Sharmin Ferdewsi Rakhi, Abdul Hakim Mohammad Mohsinul Reza, Mohammad Shafaet Hossen, and Zakir Hossain, Alterations in histopathological features and brain acetylcholinesterase activity in stinging catfish Heteropneustes fossilis exposed to polluted river water, doi: 10.1186/2008-6970-5-7.

CHAPTER 5

Leila Sievanen, How Do Small-Scale Fishers Adapt to Environmental Variability? Lessons from Baja California, Sur, Mexico, doi: 10.1186/s40152-014-0009-2.

CHAPTER 6

Mohammad Mahmudul Islam and Ratana Chuenpagdee, Negotiating Risk and Poverty in Mangrove Fishing Communities of the Bangladesh Sundarbans, doi: 10.1186/2212-9790-12-7.

CHAPTER 7

Amalia Mitsoura, Ifigenia Kagalou, Nikolaos Papaioannou, Panagiotis Berillis, Eleni Mente, and Theodoti Papadimitriou, The Presence of Microcystins in Fish Cyprinus Carpio Tissues: a Histopathological Study, doi:10.1186/2008-6970-5-8.

CHAPTER 8

Elizabeth Hoover, Cultural and Health Implications of Fish Advisories in a Native American Community, doi:10.1186/2192-1709-2-4.

CHAPTER 9

Pramod K Pandey,Philip H Kass, Michelle L Soupir, Sagor Biswas, and Vijay P Singh, Contamination of Water Resources by Pathogenic Bacteria, doi:10.1186/s13568-014-0051-x.

Index

W

Z